HOW NOT TO DIET

Also by Michael Greger, M.D., FACLM

How Not to Die
The How Not to Die Cookbook

HOW NOT TO DIET

THE GROUNDBREAKING SCIENCE
OF HEALTHY, PERMANENT WEIGHT LOSS

MICHAEL GREGER,
M.D., FACLM

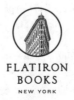

FLATIRON
BOOKS
NEW YORK

HOW NOT TO DIET. Copyright © 2019 by NutritionFacts.org Inc. All rights reserved. Printed in the United States of America. For information, address Flatiron Books, 120 Broadway, New York, NY 10271.

www.flatironbooks.com

Designed by Steven Seighman

Graphs and charts by Dustin Kirkpatrick

The Library of Congress Cataloging-in-Publication Data is available upon request.

ISBN 978-1-250-19922-5 (hardcover)
ISBN 978-1-250-19924-9 (ebook)

Our books may be purchased in bulk for promotional, educational, or business use. Please contact your local bookseller or the Macmillan Corporate and Premium Sales Department at 1-800-221-7945, extension 5442, or by email at MacmillanSpecialMarkets@macmillan.com.

First Edition: December 2019

10 9 8 7 6 5 4 3 2 1

To my mom,
the source of everything good in my life

Contents

HOW NOT
TO DIET

Preface

DOWN THE RABBIT HOLE

Surely, if there were a safe, simple, side effect–free solution to obesity, we would know about it by now, right?

I'm not so sure.

It takes an estimated average of seventeen years before evidence from scientific research is incorporated into day-to-day clinical practice.[1] One example that was particularly poignant for my family: heart disease. Decades ago, Dr. Dean Ornish and colleagues published evidence in one of the most prestigious medical journals in the world that our leading cause of death could be reversed with diet and lifestyle changes alone[2]—yet this monumental discovery was effectively ignored at the time.[3] Even now, hundreds of thousands of Americans continue to perish every year from what we learned nearly thirty years ago is an arrestable, reversible condition. In fact, I had seen such a reversal with my own eyes.

My dear grandmother was cured of her end-stage heart disease by one of Ornish's contemporaries, Nathan Pritikin, using similar methods. She was sixty-five when she was given her medical death sentence, but—thanks to a healthy diet—was able to live another thirty-one years to age ninety-six, to continue enjoying her six grandkids, including me.

If effectively the cure to the number-one killer of men and women could be ignored and get lost down some rabbit hole, what else might be buried in the medical literature? I've made it my life's mission to find out. That's why I went to medical school in the first place and why I started NutritionFacts.org.

So, like heart disease, might there already be a cure for obesity? That's what I intended to uncover.

Here's the problem: I hate diet books. Furthermore, I hate diet books that *purport* to hate diet books yet relish in all the same absurdities. This book is for those who want facts, not filler, fantasy, or fluff. If you want testimonials and before-and-after pictures, you've come to the wrong place. You don't need anecdotes when you have evidence. A Harvard sociologist of science calls those arguments by anecdotes in diet books "a deliberate attempt at credibility engineering."[4] When you don't have the science to back you up, all you have are "success" stories.

I'm not interested in offering dueling anecdotes, nor am I interested in dietary dogma, beliefs, or opinions. What I am interested in is the science. When it comes to making life-and-death decisions that concern something as important as your own health and that of your family, as far as I'm concerned, there's only one question: *What does the best available balance of evidence say right now?* That's what I've tried to encapsulate in this book.

Often, diet books deal in pseudoscientific twaddle swaddled in the trappings of science. But how is the untrained reader supposed to know the difference between the two and decide among the competing claims? It's no wonder people tend to flock to their respective gurus to have their minds made up for them. However, no one is born with this knowledge—and you have a right to demand to know where diet book authors got the information they're trying to sell you so you can check the credibility of the source and confirm its veracity. That's why I prefer presenting the science in video format on my website, where I can show the original data and link to downloads of all the primary sources. And here in this book, I've tried to cite each substantive statement of fact.

My goal was to create the oxymoron: an evidence-based diet book.

CAVEAT EATER

No other area of the national health probably is as abused by deception and misinformation as nutrition. Many travesties cheat the public of enormous sums of money, and of good health as well.

—WHITE HOUSE CONFERENCE ON FOOD, NUTRITION, AND HEALTH[5]

Frustrated by the current political climate of alternative facts and echo chambers? Welcome to my world. The entire diet industry is built upon a foundation of fake news. The nutrition field has been dealing with bald-faced lies since back in the pre-post-truth era, and diet books can be the worst offenders. "Often the loudest, most extreme voices drown out the well informed," wrote two noted nutrition professors on the subject of diet books. "There is also money to be made."[6]

Lots of money. Every month seems to bring us a trendy new diet or weight-loss fad, and they always sell because they always fail. The diet industry may rake in up to $50 billion a year, and the business model is based on repeat customers.[7] Racked with the guilt and self-hatred of failure, people often line right back up to be fooled again. I hope this book can help break that cycle by cutting through the BS.

Beyond the corrupting influence of commercial interests are the ideological biases. Too often in diet books, the rule is to obfuscate rather than illuminate, cherry-pick facts to push some pet theory, and ignore the rest to promote your own agenda. It's the opposite of science. In true scholarship, your conclusions follow from the evidence, not the other way around.

Unfortunately, even just sticking to the peer-reviewed scientific literature is not enough. An article in *The New England Journal of Medicine* on obesity myths concluded that "false and scientifically unsupported beliefs about obesity are pervasive" in medical journals as well.[8] In that case, the only way to get at the truth is to dive deep into the primary literature and read all the original studies yourself rather than taking some contemporary reviewer's word for it. But who's got time for that? There are more than half a million scientific papers on the subject of obesity, with a hundred new ones published every day. Even researchers in the field might only be able to keep track of what's going on in their narrow, subspecialized domains. But that's precisely what we do at NutritionFacts.org. We comb through tens of thousands of studies a year so you don't have to.

This is the kind of book I was made for. My research team and I were allowed to really flex our muscles, and the sorer those muscles got, the further we stretched ourselves, the more valuable we realized this contribution would be. Even "simple" questions on weight loss, like whether you should eat breakfast or skip it, or whether it's better to exercise before or after meals, turned into major, thousand-article research projects. If our nose-to-the-grindstone research team had trouble sifting through the stacks, a practicing physician would have no chance and the public would be totally lost.

Whether you're morbidly obese, just overweight like the average American, or at your ideal weight and wanting to keep it that way, our goal was to give you every possible tweak and technique we could find to build the optimal weight-control solution from the ground up.

I went into this project with the goal of creating a distillation of all the best science, but to my delight, I discovered all sorts of exciting new tools and tricks along the way. We did indeed uncover a treasure trove of buried data, like simple spices proven in randomized, double-blind, placebo-controlled studies to accelerate weight loss for pennies a day. With so little profit potential, it's no wonder those studies never saw the light of day.

And we were even able to traverse beyond the existing evidence base to propose a novel method to eliminate body fat. The proposed technique appears to have a strong theoretical basis but has never been put to the test because apparently no one has ever thought of it before. It can't be monetized either, but the only profiting I care about is your health. That's why I donate to charity 100 percent of the proceeds I get from my DVDs, speaking engagements, and books, including the one you're holding right now. I just want to do for everyone's family what Pritikin did for mine.

Introduction

SOMETIMES BIGGER IS BETTER

My literary agent told me that no one wants a fat diet book. They want it to be as slim as they envision their future selves. Sorry to disappoint, but I couldn't help it. I wanted to document every evidence-based tip, trick, tweak, and hack to give people every possible advantage—whether you're obese, overweight, or just wanting to maintain your ideal weight.

In *How Not to Diet,* I cover everything from cultivating a healthy microbiome in your gut to manipulating your metabolism through chronobiology, matching meal timing to your circadian rhythms. Every section could have been a book in its own right. We certainly attempted book-length research on each subject and then tried to distill down the most compelling, actionable takeaways from each of the most promising strategies. To that end, this is really more like forty books packed into one. For those of you now wielding a physical copy of the book and thinking, *This is the compact version?*, take comfort in the fact that you can use it to curl for a little extra resistance exercise.

It was important to me to include all the details so you can make as informed a decision about your health as possible, but you can always skip down to the summaries at the end of each section for my take-home suggestions. I wanted to be sure to clearly articulate how I arrived at each recommendation, because I don't want to be anyone's diet guru. I don't want you to take anything on faith but rather on evidence.

In the References section, I've included a website address and a QR code for the full list of the nearly five thousand citations referenced throughout this book. The advantage of presenting them online for you (beyond trimming five hundred pages and saving a few trees) is that it allowed me to hyperlink each and every citation to take you directly to the source, so you can download the PDFs and access the original research yourself.

Some of my conclusions are scientific slam dunks, but others are more uncertain, and I try to make the distinctions clear. That way, you can make up your own mind when trying to decide whether to incorporate any particular piece of my advice into your life. If you find yourself unconvinced by the data presented to support a particular recommendation, don't do it. The benefit of laying it all out is that you can decide for yourself. As famed scientist Carl Sagan (who also happened to be my next-door neighbor at Cornell!) put it: "Science by itself cannot advocate courses of human action, but it can certainly illuminate the possible consequences of alternative courses of action."[9]

WHAT ARE YOUR DIGITS?

Before we dive in, what does it really mean to be overweight? Obese? In simple terms, being overweight means you have too much body fat, whereas being obese means you have way too much body fat. In technical terms, obesity is operationally defined as a body mass index (BMI) of 30 or more, while being overweight means you have a BMI of 25 to 29.9. A BMI between 18.5 and 24.9 is considered "ideal weight."

Calculating your BMI is relatively easy: You can visit one of the scores of online BMI calculators, or you can grab a calculator and calculate it on your own. To do so, multiply your weight in pounds by 703. Then divide that twice by your height in inches. For example, if you weigh 200 pounds and are 71 inches tall (five foot eleven), that would be $(200 \times 703) \div 71 \div 71 = 27.9$, a BMI indicating that you would be, unfortunately, significantly overweight.

In the medical profession, we used to call a BMI under 25 "normal weight." Sadly, that's no longer normal. Being overweight became the norm by the late 1980s in the United States[10] and appears to have steadily worsened ever since.[11]

ISN'T A CALORIE A CALORIE?

Now that we see where the lines are drawn in the weight spectrum from optimal to obese, let's review some basic assumptions. The notion that a calorie from one source is just as fattening as a calorie from any other source is a trope broadcast by the food industry as a way to absolve itself of culpability. Coca-Cola even put out an ad emphasizing this "one simple commonsense fact."[12] As the chair of Harvard's nutrition department put it, this "central argument" from industry is that the "overconsumption of calories from carrots would be no different from overconsumption of calories from soda."[13] If a calorie is just a calorie, why does it matter what kinds of foods we eat?

Let's take the example of carrots versus Coca-Cola. While it's true that in a tightly controlled laboratory setting, 240 calories of carrots—ten carrots—would have the same effect on calorie balance as the 240 calories in a bottle of Coke,[14] this comparison falls flat on its face out in the real world. You could chug down those liquid calories in less than a minute, but eating 240 calories of carrots could take you more than two and a half hours of constant chewing. (It's been timed.[15]) Not only would your jaw get sore, but 240 calories of carrots is about five cups—you might not even be able to fit them all in your stomach. Like all whole plant foods, carrots have fiber, which adds bulk without adding net calories. What's more, you wouldn't even absorb all the carrot calories. As anyone who's eaten corn can tell you, some bits of vegetable matter can pass right through you, flushing out any calories they contain. A calorie may still be a calorie circling your toilet bowl, but it's not going to end up on your hips.

A more relatable comparison might be something like Cheerios versus Froot Loops. As Kellogg's is practically giddy to point out, its Froot Loops cereal has about the same number of calories as its rival's health-hallowed Cheerios. So why does Toucan Sam get singled out? (I was deposed as an expert witness in a case against sugary cereal manufacturers, so I heard these arguments firsthand.) Yes, the two cereals may have similar calories, but that doesn't take into account all the appetite-stimulating effects of concentrated sugar.[16] In an experiment in which children were alternately offered high- versus lower-sugar cereals, had they eaten more Cheerios than Froot Loops, they could have gotten more calories, but the opposite happened. On average, the kids poured and ate 77 percent more of the sugary cereal. So even with comparable calorie counts, sugary cereals may end up nearly doubling caloric intake.[17] In a lab, a calorie is a calorie, but in life, far from it.

Even if you eat and absorb the same number of calories, a calorie may *still* not be a calorie. As you'll learn, the same number of calories eaten at a different time of the day, in a different meal distribution, or after different amounts of sleep can translate into different amounts of body fat.

It's not only what we eat but how and when.

And the same number on the scale can mean different things on different diets or in different contexts. You could be losing weight but actually gaining body fat if your body sheds water and muscle mass. So it's not just about calories in versus calories out, eating less, and moving more. We'll see an illustration of this later, with a famous series of studies on prisoners in Vermont that showed that, depending on what the researchers fed them, it could take up to one hundred thousand more calories to create the same amount of weight gain. So you'll learn how they effectively made one hundred thousand calories disappear. But I'm getting ahead of myself.

A DETECTIVE STORY IN FOUR PARTS

In part I, the book starts with an outline of our growing problem with obesity—the causes, the consequences, and the solutions tried to date. It answers questions such as: *What led to the explosive increase in obesity starting in the late 1970s? Is being overweight really as bad for your health as "they" say? And what about the safety and efficacy of nonlifestyle approaches, such as stomach stapling, diet drugs, and weight-loss supplements?*

Then, in my attempt to build the optimal weight-loss strategy from scratch, I spend part II exploring all the key ingredients that might go into creating the ideal recipe for losing body fat. In part III, we see how all the diets out there stack up against this list of criteria, and we piece together the foremost formula for healthy, sustainable weight control. You also get the tools to be able to assess all the newer-than-new diets that haven't even come out yet.

After that come the boosters. In part IV, I unveil all the tricks and tweaks for fast-tracking weight loss that I've found through my years of scouring the medical literature. These are ways in which any diet can be modified to maximize the dissolution of body fat. I arrange the boosters in a simple daily checklist so you can pick and choose a portfolio of techniques that works best for you. I have to warn against skipping to this section and going for the quick fixes while continuing to eat the same crappy foods. Though there are indeed different ways to eat the same foods to achieve better results, the boosters are strictly meant to be adjuncts to a healthy diet.

In the final section, I lay to rest all the burning questions on burning fat: *What are the best ways to exercise to achieve maximum weight loss? How can you safely boost your metabolism? What is the optimum amount of sleep? What does the science say about ketogenic diets, intermittent fasting, and high-intensity interval training?* I also introduce you to specific foods that double as fat blockers and fat burners, and starch blockers and appetite suppressants. And did you know that the different timing, frequencies, and combinations of foods can also matter? There's even a food that can prevent the metabolic slowing that your body uses to frustrate your weight-loss attempts.

Skeptical? You should be! I was too.

I went into this thinking I would just end up railing against all the gimmicky snake oil out there and put out much of the same standard advice on trimming calories and hitting the gym. I imagined what would set this work apart would be its comprehensiveness and strict grounding in science. I figured this book would distinguish itself—but more as a book of reference than revolution. I certainly never thought I'd stumble across some novel weight-loss strategy. I just didn't realize how many new paths would be opened up by our newfound transformations in understanding of so many fields of human physiology. It's been thrilling to weave together all these cutting-edge threads to design a weight-loss protocol based on the best available evidence.

This has been a mammoth but joyful undertaking. People sometimes ask me why I don't go on vacations or even take a day off. I have to explain that I feel as though my entire life is a holiday. I feel so blessed to be able to dedicate my time to helping people while doing what I love: learning and sharing. I can't imagine doing anything else.

I. The Problem

THE CAUSES

The Weight of the World

Obesity isn't new, but the obesity *epidemic* is. We went from a few corpulent queens and kings, like Henry VIII and Louis VI (known as Louis le Gros, or "Louis the Fat"),[18] to a pandemic of obesity, now considered to be perhaps the direst and most poorly contained public health threat of our time.[19] Today, 71 percent of American adults are overweight and 40 percent of men and women appear to have so much body fat that they can be classified as obese, and there's no end in sight.[20] Earlier reports had suggested the rise in obesity was at least slowing down, but that doesn't actually appear to be the case.[21] Similarly, we had thought we were turning the corner on childhood obesity after thirty-five years of unrelenting bad news, but the bad news marches on.[22] Child and adolescent obesity rates have continued to rise, now into the fourth decade.[23]

Over the last century, obesity appears to have jumped tenfold, from as few as one in thirty people[24] to now one in three, but it wasn't a steady rise. Something seems to have happened around the late 1970s, and not just in the United States.[25] The obesity pandemic took off at about the same time in most high-income countries around the globe in the 1970s and 1980s. The fact that the rapid rise appeared almost concurrently across the industrialized world suggests a common cause.[26]

What might that trigger have been?

Any potential driver would have had to be global in nature and coincide with the upswing of the epidemic, so the change would have had to have started about forty years ago and been able to spread rapidly around the world.[27] So how do the various theories stack up? Some have blamed changes in our "built environment," for instance, pointing to shifts in city planning that have made our communities less conducive to walking, biking, and grocery shopping.[28] But that doesn't meet our criteria for a credible cause because there was no universal, simultaneous change in global neighborhoods within that time frame.[29]

If you do a survey of hundreds of policy-makers, most blame the obesity epidemic on "lack of personal motivation,"[30] but that makes little sense. Here in the United States, for example, obesity shot up across the entire population in the late 1970s. Are you telling me that every sector of the U.S. population experienced some sort of simultaneous decline in willpower?[31] Each age, sex, and ethnic group, with all their different attitudes and experiences, coincidentally lost their collective capacity for self-control at the same time?

More plausible than a global change in the nature of our characters would be some global change in the nature of our lives.[32]

Fast Food vs. Slow Motion

The food industry blames inactivity. "If all consumers exercised," said the CEO of PepsiCo, "obesity wouldn't exist."[33] Coca-Cola went a step further and spent $1.5 million to create the Global Energy Balance Network to downplay the role of diet in the obesity epidemic. Leaked internal documents show the company planned on using the front group to serve as a "weapon" to "change the conversation" about obesity in its "war" with the public health community.[34]

This tactic is so common among food and beverage companies it even has a name: *leanwashing*. You've likely heard of greenwashing, where companies deceptively pretend to be environmentally friendly. *Leanwashing* is the term used to describe companies that try to position themselves as helping to solve the obesity crisis when, instead, they're directly contributing to it.[35] For example, Nestlé, the largest food company in the world, has rebranded itself the "world's leading nutrition, health and wellness company."[36] Yes, that Nestlé, of Nestlé Nesquik fame, makers of Cookie Crisp cereal and more than one hundred different brands of candy, including Butterfinger, Kit Kat,

Goobers, Gobstoppers, Runts, and Nerds. Another of its slogans is "Good Food, Good Life." Its Raisinets may have some fruit, but the company seems to me more Willy Wonka than wellness. Let's just say that on its "What is Nestlé doing about obesity?" web page, the "Read about our Nestlé Healthy Kids programme" link gave me a Page Not Found error.[37]

The constant corporate drumbeat of overemphasis on physical inactivity appears to be working. In response to a Harris poll question ("Which of these do you think are the major reasons why obesity has increased?"), a large majority (83 percent) chose lack of exercise, while only 34 percent chose excessive calorie consumption.[38] But blaming couch-potato-ness has actually been identified as one of the most common misconceptions about obesity.[39] The scientific community has come to a fairly decisive conclusion[40] that the factors governing caloric intake far more powerfully affect overall calorie balance.[41]

There's even debate in the scientific literature as to whether changes in physical activity had "any role whatsoever" in the obesity epidemic.[42] The increase in caloric intake per person is more than enough to explain the U.S.[43] and global[44] epidemics of obesity. In fact, if anything, the level of physical activity over the last few decades has gone up slightly in both Europe and North America, rather than declined.[45] Ironically, this bump may be a result of the extra energy it takes to haul around our heavier bodies, making changes in energy expenditure a consequence of the obesity problem rather than the cause.

Formal exercise is only a small part of our total daily activity, though. Think how much more physical work people used to do on the job, on the farm, or even in the home.[46] It's not just the shift in collar color from blue to white. Increasing automation, computerization, mechanization, motorization, and urbanization have all contributed to increasingly more sedentary lifestyles over the last century—and therein lies the problem with the theory: The occupational shifts and advent of labor-saving devices have been gradual and largely predate the dramatic, recent rise in weight gain the world over.[47] Washing machines, vacuum cleaners, and the Model T were all invented before 1910. And indeed, when put to the test using state-of-the-art methods to measure energy in and energy out, it was caloric intake, not physical activity, that predicted weight gain over time.[48]

The common misconception that obesity is due mostly to lack of exercise may not just be a benign fallacy, as personal theories of causation appear to impact people's weight. Those who blame insufficient exercise are significantly more likely to be overweight themselves. Put them in a room with chocolate, for instance, and they can be covertly observed consuming more candy compared to those who put the onus of obesity on poor diet.[49] But you can't know if such attitudes are playing a role in their weight problem until you put it to the test. So researchers randomized people to read a fictitious article implicating inactivity in the rise of obesity and found they indeed went on to eat significantly more sweets than those who instead were given an article that indicted diet.[50] A similar study evidently found that those presented with research blaming genetics subsequently ate significantly more cookies. The paper was entitled "An Unintended Way in Which the Fat Gene Might Make You Fat."[51]

Do These Genes Make Me Look Fat?

To date, about one hundred genetic markers have been linked to obesity, but when you put all of them together, they account for less than 3 percent of the difference in body mass index between people.[52] The "fat gene" you may have heard about (called FTO, short for "FaT mass and Obesity associated") is the gene most strongly linked to obesity,[53] but it explains less than 1 percent of the difference between people (a mere 0.34 percent).[54]

FTO codes for a brain protein that appears to affect your appetite.[55] Are you one of the billion people on Earth who carry a full complement of FTO susceptibility genes?[56] It doesn't really matter, because this only appears to result in a difference in intake of a few hundred extra calories *a year,*[57] while what it took to lead to the obesity epidemic is more like a few hundred calories *a day.*[58] FTO is the gene so far known to have the most effect on excessive weight gain,[59] but the chances of accurately predicting obesity risk based on FTO status are only slightly better than flipping a coin.[60]

When it comes to obesity, the power of your genes is nothing compared to the power of your fork. Even the small influence the FTO gene does have appears to be weaker among those who are physically active[61] and may be abolished completely in those eating healthier diets. FTO only appears to affect those eating diets higher in saturated fat (predominantly found in dairy, meat, and junk food). Those eating more healthfully appear to be at no greater risk of weight gain even if they inherited the "fat gene" from both their parents.[62]

Physiologically, FTO gene status doesn't appear to affect your ability to lose weight.[63] Psychologically, knowing you're at increased genetic risk for obesity may motivate some people to eat and live more healthfully,[64] but it may cause others to fatalistically throw their hands up in the air and resign themselves to thinking it just runs in their families.[65] Obesity does tend to run in families, but so do lousy diets.

Comparing the weight of biological versus adopted children can help tease out the contributions of lifestyles versus genetics. Children growing up with two overweight biological parents were found to be 27 percent more likely to be overweight themselves, whereas adopted children placed in a home with two overweight parents were only 21 percent more likely to be overweight.[66] So genetics certainly play a role, but this suggests that it's more the children's environment than their DNA.

Diet Trumps Genes

One of the most dramatic examples of the power of diet over DNA comes from the Pima Indians of Arizona, who have among the highest rates of obesity[67] and diabetes[68] in the world. This has been ascribed to their relatively fuel-efficient genetic makeup.[69] Their propensity to store calories may have served them well in times of periodic scarcity when they were living off the land, but when the area became "settled," their source of water, the Gila River, was diverted upstream. Those who survived the ensuing famine[70] had to abandon their traditional diet to live off government food programs, and chronic disease rates skyrocketed.[71] Same genes, but a different diet, leading to a different result.

In fact, a natural experiment was set up. The Pima living across the border in Mexico come from the same genetic pool but were able to maintain more of their traditional lifestyle, centered around the food staples known as *the three sisters*: corn, beans, and squash.[72] Same genes, but about five times less diabetes and obesity.[73]

Genes may load the gun, but diet pulls the trigger.

Survival of the Fattest

It's been said: "Nothing in biology makes sense except in the light of evolution."[74] The known genetic contribution to obesity may be small, but in a certain sense, you could argue it's actually all in our genes. That's because the excess consumption of available calories may be hardwired into our DNA.

We were born to eat. Throughout most of human history and beyond, we existed in survival mode, in a context of unpredictable scarcity, so we've been programmed with a powerful drive to eat as much as we can, while we can, and just store the calories we don't need right away on our bodies for later. Food availability could never be taken for granted, so those who ate more in the moment and were best able to store more fat for the future might better survive subsequent shortages to pass along their genes. Generation after generation, millennia after millennia, those with lesser appetites may have died out, while those who gorged themselves could have selectively lived long enough to pass along a genetic predisposition to eat and store more calories. That may be how we evolved into such voracious, calorie-conserving machines. Now that we're no longer in such lean times, though, we're no longer so lean.

What I just described is the "thrifty gene" concept,[75] the proposal that obesity is the result of a mismatch between the modern environment and the environment in which we evolved.[76] It's as if we're now polar bears in a jungle; fur and fat may provide an edge up in the Arctic but would be decidedly disadvantageous in the Amazon.[77] Similarly, a propensity to pack on the pounds may have been a plus in prehistoric times but can turn into a liability when our scarcity-sculpted biology is plopped down into the land of plenty.

So the prime cause for the obesity epidemic is neither gluttony nor sloth. Obesity may simply be a normal response to an abnormal environment.[78]

Much of our physiology is finely tuned to stay within a narrow range of upper and lower limits. If we get too hot, we sweat; if we get too cold, we shiver. Our bodies have mechanisms to keep us in balance. In contrast, our bodies have had little reason to develop an upper limit to the accumulation of body fat.[79] In the beginning, there may have been evolutionary pressures to keep lithe and nimble in the face of predation, but thanks in part to weapons and fire, we haven't had to outrun as many saber-toothed tigers over the last two million years or so.[80] This may have left our genes with the one-sided selection pressures to binge on every morsel in sight and stockpile as many calories onto our bodies as possible.[81]

What was once adaptive is now a problem, or at least so says the thrifty gene hypothesis that originated more than a half century ago.[82] The theory has since been refined and updated, but the basic premise remains largely accepted by the scientific community,[83] and the implications are profound.

In 2013, the American Medical Association voted to classify obesity as a disease[84] against the advice of its own Council on Science and Public Health.[85] Not that it necessarily matters what we call it—a rose by any other name would cause just as much diabetes—but disease implies dysfunction. Bariatric drugs and surgery are not fixing some physiological malfunction. Our bodies are just doing what they were designed to do in the face of excess calories.[86] Rather than some sort of disorder, weight gain may be largely a normal response, by normal people, to an abnormal situation.[87] And with more than 70 percent of Americans now overweight,[88] it's *literally* normal.

Won't Work for Food

The traditional medical view on obesity, as summed up nearly a century ago: "All obese persons are alike in one fundamental respect—they literally overeat."[89] While this may be true in a technical sense, it is in reference to overeating calories, not food. Our primitive urge to overindulge is selective. People don't tend to lust for lettuce. We have a natural, inborn preference for sweet, starchy, fatty foods, because that's where the calories are concentrated.

Think about hunting and gathering efficiency. We used to have to work hard for our food. Prehistorically, it wouldn't have made sense to spend all day collecting types of food that, on average, don't provide at least a day's worth of calories. You would have been better off staying back at the cave. So we evolved to crave foods with the biggest caloric bang for their buck.[90]

If you were able to steadily forage a pound of food an hour and it had 250 calories per pound, it might take you ten hours just to break even on your calories for the day. But if you were gathering something with 500 calories a pound, you could be done foraging in five hours and spend the next five focusing on your wall paintings. So the greater the energy density, the more calories per pound, the more efficient the foraging. We developed an acute ability to discriminate foods based on calorie density and instinctively desire the densest.[91]

If you study the fruit and vegetable preferences of four- and five-year-old children, what they like correlates with calorie density. They prefer bananas over berries and carrots over cucumbers. Isn't that just a preference for sweetness? No, they also prefer potatoes over peaches and green beans over melon,[92] just like monkeys prefer avocados over bananas.[93] We appear to have an inborn drive to maximize calories per mouthful.

The researchers in the studies of children only tested whole fruits and vegetables, so all the foods naturally had fewer than five hundred calories per pound, with bananas topping the chart at about four hundred. Something funny happens when you start going much above that: We lose our ability to differentiate between which foods have the highest caloric density. Over a natural range of calorie densities, we have an uncanny aptitude to pick out the subtle distinctions. However, once you start heading toward chocolate, cheese, and bacon territory, which can reach thousands of calories per pound, our perceptions become relatively numb to the differences. No wonder, since these foods were unknown to our prehistoric brains. Aberrant behavior explained by an evolutionary mismatch,[94] like sea turtle hatchlings crawling in the wrong direction toward artificial light rather than the moon and never reaching the ocean, or dodo birds failing to evolve a fear response because they had no natural predators—and we all know how that turned out.

Full of CRAP

The food industry exploits our innate biological vulnerabilities by stripping down crops into almost pure calories—straight sugar, oil (which is pretty much pure fat), and white flour (which is mostly refined starch). First, they remove the fiber, because it effectively has zero calories. Run brown rice through a mill to make it white, and you lose about two-thirds of the fiber. Turn whole-wheat flour into white flour and lose 75 percent of the fiber. Or you can run crops through animals (to make meat, dairy, and eggs) and remove 100 percent of the fiber.[95] What you're left with is CRAP, an acronym conceived by one of my favorite dietitians, Jeff Novick, for *calorie-rich and processed* foods.[96]

Calories are condensed in the same way plants are turned into addictive drugs like opioids and cocaine: concentration, crystallization, distillation, and extraction.[97] They even appear to activate the same reward pathways in the brain.[98] Put people with "food addiction" in an MRI scanner and show them a picture of a chocolate milkshake, and the areas that light up in their brains are the same[99] as when cocaine addicts are shown a video of smoking crack[100] or when alcoholics are given a whiff of whiskey.[101]

Food addiction is a misnomer. People don't suffer out-of-control eating behaviors to food in general. We don't tend to compulsively crave cabbage. But milkshakes are packed with sugar and fat, two of the signals to our brains for calorie density. When people are asked to rate different foods in terms of cravings and loss of control, most incriminated was a load of CRAP—highly processed foods like donuts, along with cheese and meat.[102] Those foods least related to problematic eating behaviors? Fruits and vegetables. Calorie density may be the reason people don't get up in the middle of the night and binge on broccoli.

Animals don't tend to get fat eating the foods they were designed to eat. There is a confirmed report of free-living primates becoming obese, but that was a troop of baboons who evidently stumbled across some dumpsters at a tourist lodge. The "garbage-feeding animals" weighed 50 percent more than their wild-feeding counterparts.[103] Sadly, we, too, can suffer the same mismatched fate and become obese by eating garbage. For millions of years before we learned how to hunt, our biology evolved largely on leaves, roots, shoots, fruits, and nuts.[104] Ironically, even the creationists agree that we started out plant-based in Eden's garden.[105] Maybe it would help if we went back to the basics and cut the CRAP.

Toxic Food Environment

It is hard to eat healthfully against the headwind of such strong evolutionary forces. No matter our level of nutrition knowledge, in the face of pepperoni pizza, the ancestral heritage baked into our genes screams, *Eat it now!*[106] Anyone who doubts the power of basic biological drives should see how long they can go without blinking or breathing. Any conscious decision to hold your breath is soon overcome by the compulsion to breathe. In medicine, shortness of breath is sometimes even referred to as *air hunger*.

The battle of the bulge is a battle against biology, so obesity is not some moral failing. I can't stress enough that becoming overweight is a normal, natural response to the abnormal, unnatural ubiquity of calorie-dense, sugary, and fatty foods.

The sea of excess calories in which we are now floating (and in which many of us are now drowning) has been referred to as a "toxic food envi-ronment."[107] This helps direct focus away from the individual and toward societal forces at work, such as the fact that the average child may be blasted with ten thousand food commercials a year. Or maybe I should say *pseudo-food* commercials, as 95 percent of the ads were found to be for candy, liquid candy (soft drinks), breakfast candy (sugary cereals), and fast food.[108]

Wait a second. If weight gain is just a natural reaction to the easy avail-ability of mountains of cheap, tasty calories, then why isn't everyone fat? Well, in a certain sense, most everyone is. It's been estimated that more than 90 percent of American adults are "overfat," defined as having excess body fat sufficient to impair health.[109] This can occur even in normal-weight indi-viduals (often due to excess abdominal fat), but even if you just look at the numbers on the scale, being overweight has become the norm. If you look at the bell curve, more than 70 percent of us are overweight. A little less than a third are on one side at normal weight and more than a third are on the other side, so overweight they're obese.[110]

But if it really is the food, why doesn't *everyone* get fat? That's like asking, "If cigarettes really are to blame, why don't *all* smokers get lung cancer?" This is where genetic dispositions and other exposures can weigh in to tip the scales.[111] Different people are born with a different susceptibility to can-cer, but that doesn't mean smoking doesn't play a critical role in exploding whatever inherent risk we have—and the same goes for obesity and our toxic food environment. We can try to tip the scales with smoking cessation and a more healthful diet.

If you lock up two dozen folks in a research study and feed each the exact same number of excess calories, they all gain weight, but some gain more than others. In one study, overfeeding the same thousand calories a day, six days a week for one hundred days caused weight gains rang-ing from about nine pounds to twenty-nine pounds. Some people are just more genetically susceptible. The twenty-four people in the study were twelve sets of identical twins, and the variation in weight gain between each of them was about a third less than between the unrelated subjects.[112] A similar study with weight loss from exercise found a similar result.[113] So, yes, genetics play a role, but that just means some people have to work harder than others. Ideally, inheriting a predisposition for extra weight gain shouldn't give reason for resignation but rather motivation to put in the extra effort to unseal your fate.

Fattening Grandchildren from the Womb

Identical twins don't just share DNA; they shared a uterus too. Might that also help account for some of their metabolic similarities? Fetal overnutrition, evidenced by an abnormally large birth weight, seems to be a strong predictor of obesity in childhood and later in life.[114] Could it be that you are what your mom ate?

Who do you think most determines the birth weight of a test-tube baby—the donor mom who provided all the DNA, or the surrogate mom who provided the intrauterine environment? When it was put to the test, the womb won. Incredibly, a baby born to an obese surrogate mother with a skinny biological mom may harbor a greater risk of becoming obese than a baby from a big biological mom born to a slim surrogate. The researchers concluded that "the environment provided by the human mother is more important than her genetic contribution to birth weight."[115]

The most compelling data come from comparing obesity rates in siblings born to the same mother before and after she had bariatric (weight loss) surgery.[116] Compared to their brothers and sisters born after the surgery, those born when the mom weighed about one hundred pounds more had higher rates of inflammation and metabolic derangements, and, most critically, three times the risk of severe obesity (affecting 35 percent of those born before the weight loss, compared to 11 percent born after). The researchers concluded that "these data emphasize how critical it is to prevent obesity and treat it effectively to prevent further transmission to future generations."[117]

But wait. Mom had the same DNA before and after the surgery. She passed down the same genes. How could her weight during pregnancy affect the weight destiny of her children any differently? We finally figured out the mechanism by which this can happen: epigenetics.

Epigenetics, which literally means *above genetics,* layers an extra level of information on top of the DNA sequence that can both be affected by our surroundings and potentially passed on to our children.[118] This is thought to account for the "developmental programming"[119] (also known as *metabolic imprinting*[120]) that can occur in the womb depending on the weight of the mother, or even the grandmother. Since all the eggs in an

(continued)

infant daughter's ovaries are already preformed before birth,[121] a mother's weight status during pregnancy could potentially affect the obesity risk of her grandchildren too.[122] Either way, you can imagine how this could result in a vicious intergenerational cycle where obesity begets obesity.

Is there anything we can do about it? Well, prevention may be the key. Given the epigenetic influence of maternal weight during pregnancy, a symposium of experts on pediatrics concluded that "planning of pregnancy, including prior optimization of maternal weight and metabolic condition, offers a safe means to initiate the prevention rather than treatment of pediatric obesity."[123] Easier said than done, but overweight moms-to-be may take comfort in the fact that even the moms in the study who had given birth to kids with three times lower risk of obesity were still, on average, obese themselves,[124] suggesting that significant weight loss can help even if you're not able to get down to a normal weight.

What Happened in the 1970s?

The rise in the number of calories provided by the U.S. food supply since the 1970s is more than sufficient to explain the entire obesity epidemic.[125] Similar spikes in calorie surplus were noted in developed countries around the world in parallel with,[126] and presumed primarily responsible for,[127] the expanding waistlines of their populations. By the year 2000, after taking exports into account, the United States was producing 3,900 calories a day for every man, woman, and child, nearly twice as much as many people need.[128]

The number of calories in the food supply actually declined over the first half of the twentieth century, only starting its upward climb to unprecedented heights in the 1970s.[129] The drop in the first half of the century was attributed to the reduction in hard manual labor. The population had decreased energy needs, so they ate decreased energy diets. They didn't need all the extra calories. But then, the so-called energy balance flipping point occurred. (*Energy balance* is the concept of calories in versus calories out.) Why did the "move less, stay lean" phase that had existed throughout most of the century turn into the "eat more, gain weight" phase that plagues us to this day?[130] What changed to bring about this flipping point?

What happened in the 1970s was a revolution in the food industry. In the 1960s, most food was prepared and cooked in the home. The average housewife spent hours a day cooking and cleaning up after meals (the husband averaged nine minutes).[131] But then a profound transformation took place. Technological advances in food preservation and packaging enabled manufacturers to mass prepare and distribute food for ready consumption. The metamorphosis has been compared to what had happened a century before in the Industrial Revolution with the mass production and supply of manufactured goods. This time, though, it was the mass production and supply of food. Using new preservatives, artificial flavors, and techniques such as deep freezing and vacuum packing, food companies could take advantage of economies of scale[132] to mass-produce ready-made, durable, palatable edibles that offer an enormous commercial advantage over fresh and perishable foods.[133] And the packaged food sector is now a multi*trillion*-dollar industry.[134]

Think ye of the Twinkie. With enough time and effort, any ambitious cook could create cream-filled cakes in their own kitchen, but today they are available at every turn for less than a dollar.[135] If every time we wanted a Twinkie we had to bake it ourselves, we'd probably eat far fewer of them.[136]

Consider the humble potato. We've long been a nation of potato eaters, but they were largely baked or boiled. Anyone who has made fries from scratch knows what a pain it is, with all the peeling, cutting, and splattering. But with sophisticated machinations of mechanization, french fry production became centralized so fries could be shipped at -40°F to any fast-food deep-fat fryer or supermarket frozen food section in the country to become America's favorite vegetable. Nearly all the increase in potato consumption in recent decades has been in the forms of french fries and potato chips.[137]

Cigarette production offers a compelling parallel. Before the automated rolling machine was invented, cigarettes had to be rolled by hand. It took fifty workers to produce the same number of cigarettes a machine could make in a single minute. After automation, cigarette prices plunged and production leaped into the billions.[138] Cigarette smoking went from being relatively uncommon to almost everywhere. In the twentieth century, the average per capita cigarette consumption rose from 54 cigarettes a year to 4,345 by the time of the 1964 Surgeon General's report.[139] The average American went from smoking about 1 cigarette a week to 70. That's a half pack a day.

Tobacco itself was just as addictive before and after mass marketing. What changed was the much greater opportunity for cheap, easy access. French fries have always been tasty, but they went from being rare even in restaurants to omnipresent around every corner. You can probably even find them next to the gas station where you can get your Twinkies and cigarettes.

The first Twinkie dates back to 1930, though, and Ore-Ida started selling frozen french fries in the 1950s.[140] So there has to be more to the story than just technological innovation.

Aiding and Abetting

The rise in calorie surplus sufficient to explain the obesity epidemic was less a change in food *quantity* than in food *quality,* with an explosion in cheap, high-calorie, low-quality convenience foods. The federal government very much played a role in making this happen. U.S. taxpayers unwittingly give billions in subsidies to prop up the likes of the sugar industry, the corn industry and its high-fructose syrup, and the soybean industry, which processes about half of its crop into vegetable oil and the other half into cheap animal feed to help make Dollar Menu meat.[141] When was the last time you sat down to some sorghum? Exactly. Why then do taxpayers give nearly a quarter billion dollars a year to the sorghum industry?[142] It's almost all fed to livestock.[143] We've created a pricing structure that favors the production of sugars, oils, and animal products.[144]

The first farm bill started out as an emergency measure during the Great Depression of the 1930s to protect small farmers, but subsequent ones were weaponized by Big Ag into cash cows with pork barrel politics.[145] Agricultural policies in the United States and Europe have been deliberately designed to lower the costs of basic cash crops like sugar and staples like meat, wheat, dairy, and eggs.[146] There is a lot of money at stake—and in steak. From 1970 to 1994, for example, global beef prices dropped by more than 60 percent.[147] If it weren't for taxpayers sweetening the pot with billions of dollars a year,[148] high-fructose corn syrup would cost the soda industry about 10 percent more.[149]

Subsidies are one of the reasons chicken is so cheap. After one of the farm bills, corn and soy were subsidized below the cost of production for cheap animal fodder, effectively handing the poultry and pork industries around $10 billion each.[150] That's not chicken feed. Or rather, it is!

This is changing what we eat. Thanks in part to subsidies, meats, sweets, eggs, oils, dairy, and soda were all getting relatively cheaper as the obesity epidemic took off (compared to the overall consumer food price index), whereas the relative cost of fresh fruits and vegetables *doubled*.[151] This may help explain why, during about the same period, the percentage of Americans getting five servings of fruits and vegetables a day dropped from 42 percent to 26 percent.[152] Why not subsidize produce instead? Because that's not where the money is.

Whole foods, or minimally processed foods such as canned beans or tomato paste, are what's referred to in the food business as *commodities*. They have such slim profit margins that they're sometimes even sold at or below cost as "loss leaders" to attract customers in the hopes they'll also buy the "value-added" products,[153] the most profitable of which (for producers and vendors alike) are the ultraprocessed, fatty, sugary, and salty concoctions of artificially flavored, artificially colored, and artificially cheap ingredients, thanks to taxpayer subsidies.

Different foods reap different returns. Measured in profit per square foot of supermarket selling space, confectionaries like candy bars consistently rank among the most lucrative. Fried snacks like potato chips and corn chips are also highly profitable. PepsiCo's subsidiary Frito-Lay brags that while its products represent only about 1 percent of total supermarket sales, they may account for more than 10 percent of the operating profits for supermarkets and 40 percent of profit growth.[154]

It's no surprise then that the entire system is geared toward garbage. The rise in the calorie supply wasn't just *more* food but more of a different *kind* of food. More than half of all calories consumed by most adults in the United States these days were found to originate from these subsidized foods, and we appear to be worse off for it. Those eating the most have significantly higher levels of chronic disease risk factors, including elevated cholesterol, inflammation, and body weight.[155]

There's a dumb dichotomy about the drivers of the obesity epidemic: Is it the sugar or the fat? Both are highly subsidized, and both took off during the unfolding epidemic. Along with a significant rise in refined grain products, the rise in obesity was accompanied by about a 20 percent increase in per capita pounds of added sugars and a 36 percent increase in added fats[156] (mostly in the form of oil,[157] presumably from fried fast food and processed junk).[158] Both added sugars and added fats now represent major sources of calories in the American diet.[159]

Quarter Pounder

In the 1970s, the U.S. government went from just subsidizing some of the worst foods to actually paying companies to make more of them. During that decade, the farm bills reversed long-standing policies aimed at limiting production to protect prices and instead started giving payouts in proportion to output.[160] Extra calories began pouring into the food supply.

Then, in 1981, the CEO of General Electric gave a speech that effectively launched the "shareholder-value movement," reorienting the primary goal of corporations toward maximizing short-term returns for investors.[161] This placed extraordinary pressures on food companies from Wall Street to post increasing profit growth every quarter to boost their share prices. There was already a glut of calories on the market, and now they had to sell even more.

This puts food and beverage CEOs into a near impossible bind. It's not like they're rubbing their sticky hands together at the thought of luring more Hansels and Gretels to their doom in their houses of candy. Food giants cannot necessarily do the right thing if they wanted; they are beholden to investors. If they stopped marketing to kids or tried to sell healthier food or attempted anything that could jeopardize their quarterly profit growth, Wall Street could demand a change in management.[162] Healthy eating is bad for business. It's not some grand conspiracy—it's not even anyone's fault. It's just how the system works.

Marketing Excesses

Given the constant demands for corporate growth and rapid returns in an already oversaturated marketplace, the food industry needed to get people to eat more. Like the tobacco industry before it, the food industry turned to the ad men—and in a big way.[163] Tens of millions of dollars are now spent annually advertising a single brand of candy bar.[164] McDonald's alone spends billions a year.[165] Thus far, the food industry has spent more money on advertising than any other sector of the economy.[166]

Reagan-era deregulation removed the limits placed on marketing food products on television to children.[167] In addition to the ten thousand food ads children may see on TV a year,[168] there is marketing content online, in print, at school, on their phones, at the movies, and everywhere in between.[169] Nearly all of it is for products detrimental to their health.[170]

Besides its massive early exposure[171] and ubiquity, food marketing has become highly sophisticated. With the help of child psychologists, companies learn how best to influence children to manipulate their parents. Packaging is designed to most effectively attract a child's attention and then placed at their eye level in the store.[172] You know those mirrored bubbles in the ceilings of supermarkets? They're not just for shoplifters. Closed-circuit cameras and GPS-like devices on shopping carts are used to strategize how best to guide shoppers toward the most profitable products.[173] Behavioral psychology is widely applied to increase impulse buying, and even eye-movement tracking technologies are utilized.[174]

The unprecedented rise in the power, scope, and sophistication of food marketing starting around 1980 aligns well with the blastoff slope of the obesity epidemic. Since then, some of the techniques, such as product placement, in-school advertising, and event sponsorships, skyrocketed from essentially nothing to multibillion-dollar industries. This led at least one noted economist to conclude that "the most compelling single interpretation of the admittedly incomplete data we have is that the large increase in obesity is due to marketing."[175] Innovations in manufacturing and political maneuvering led to a food supply bursting at the seams with nearly four thousand calories a day for each one of us, but the critical piece may have been the advancements in marketing manipulations used to try to peddle that surplus into our mouths.[176]

Wining and Dining

The opening words of the National Academy of Medicine's report on the threat posed by food ads: "Marketing works."[177] Yes, there's a large number of well-conducted randomized studies I could share with you to show how advertising exposure and other marketing methods can change your eating behavior and get you to eat more,[178] but what do you need to know beyond the fact that the industry spends tens of billions of dollars on it?[179] To get people to drink its brown sugar water, do you think Coca-Cola would spend a penny more than it thought it had to? It's like when my medical colleagues accept invitations to "drug lunches" from pharmaceutical representatives and take offense that I would suggest it might affect their prescribing practices. Do they really think drug companies are in the business of giving away free money for nothing? They wouldn't do it if it didn't work. There is no free lunch.

Just to give you a sense of marketing's insidious nature, let me share an interesting piece of research published in *Nature,* the world's leading[180] scientific journal. The article titled "In-Store Music Affects Product Choice" documented an experiment in which either French accordion or German Bierkeller music was played on alternate days in the wine section of a grocery store.[181] On the days the French music played in the background, people were three times more likely to buy French wine, and on German music day, shoppers were about three times more likely to buy German wine. Despite the dramatic effect—not just a few percent difference but a complete three-fold reversal—when approached afterward, the vast majority of shoppers denied the music had influenced their choices.[182]

Like a Kid in a Candy Store

In addition to the $10 billion or so spent on advertising each year, the food industry spends around another $20 billion on other forms of marketing, such as trade shows, incentives, consumer promotions, and supermarket "slotting fees,"[183] which are the purchasing of shelf space from grocery stores by food and beverage companies to prominently display their most profitable products. The practice is evidently known as *cliffing,* because companies are forced to bid against each other for eye-level shelf placement, with the loser being pushed "over the cliff."[184] With slotting fees up to $20,000 per item, per retailer, and per city,[185] you can imagine what kinds of products get the special treatment. Hint: It ain't broccoli.

To get a sense as to what types of products merit prime-shelf real estate, look no further than the checkout aisle. "Merchandising the power categories on every lane is critical," reads a trade publication on the "best practices for superior checkout merchandising." And what are the "power categories"? Candy bars and beverages. Evidently, even a 1 percent power category boost in sales could earn a store an extra $15,250 a year.[186] It's not that supermarkets don't care about their customers' health. It's more that publicly traded companies (like most of the leading grocery store chains) are impelled to increase profits above other considerations.[187]

Driven by Distraction

We all like to think we make important life decisions, such as what to eat, consciously and rationally. If that were the case, though, we wouldn't be in the midst of an obesity epidemic.[188] As I explore in the Habit Formation section, most of our day-to-day behavior does not appear to be dictated by careful, considered deliberations. Rather, we tend to make more automatic, impulsive decisions triggered by unconscious cues or habitual patterns, especially when we're tired, stressed, or preoccupied. The unconscious parts of our brains are thought to guide human behaviors as much as 95 percent of the time,[189] and this is the arena where marketing manipulations do most of their dirty work.

The parts of our brains that govern conscious awareness may only be able to process about fifty bits of information per second, which is roughly equivalent to a short tweet. Our entire cognitive capacity, on the other hand, is estimated to process in excess of ten million bits per second. Because we're only able to purposefully process a limited amount of information at a time, our decisions can become even more impulsive if we're distracted or otherwise unable to concentrate.[190] An elegant illustration of this "cognitive overload" effect was provided by an experiment involving fruit salad and chocolate cake.

Before calls could be made at a touch of a button or the sound of our voice, the seven-digit span of a phone number was based in part on the longest sequence most people can recall on the fly. We only seem able to hold about seven chunks of information (plus or minus two) in our immediate, short-term memory.[191] So this was the setup: Randomize people to memorize either a seven-digit number or a two-digit number to be recalled in another room down the hall. As they walk from one room to the other, offer each of them the choice of a fruit salad or a piece of chocolate cake. Memorizing a two-digit number is easy and presumably takes few cognitive resources. Under the two-digit condition, most chose the fruit salad. Faced with the same decision, most of those trying to keep seven digits in their heads just went for the cake.[192]

This can play out in the real world by potentiating the effect of advertising. Have people watch a TV show with commercials for unhealthy snacks, and, no surprise, they eat more unhealthy snacks compared to those exposed to nonfood ads. Or maybe that is a surprise. We all like to feel as if we're in control and not so easily manipulated. The kicker is we may be even more susceptible the less we're paying attention. Randomize people to the same two- or seven-digit memorization task while watching a TV show, and the snack-attack effect was magnified among those who were more preoccupied.[193] How many of us have the TV playing in the background or multitask during commercial breaks? This research suggests that doing so may make us even more impressionable to the subversion of our better judgment.

There's an irony in all of this. Calls for restrictions on marketing are often resisted by invoking the banner of freedom. What does that even mean in this context, when research shows how easily our free choices can be influenced without our conscious awareness?[194] A senior policy researcher at the RAND Corporation even went as far as to suggest that given the dire health consequences of our unhealthy eating habits, insidious marketing manipulations "should be considered in the same light as the invisible carcinogens and toxins in the air and water that can poison us without our awareness."[195]

Passive Overconsumption

Food and beverage companies frame body weight as a matter of personal choice. But even when we're not distracted, the power of the "eat more" food environment may sometimes overcome our conscious controls over eating.[196] One look around the room at a dietitians' convention can tell you that even nutrition professionals are vulnerable to the aggressively marketed ubiquity of tasty, cheap, convenient calories. This suggests there are aspects of our eating behaviors that defy personal insight by flying below the radar of conscious awareness.[197] Appetite physiologists call the result of these subconscious actions *passive overconsumption*.[198]

Remember that brain scan study where the thought of a milkshake lit up the same reward pathways in the brain as when cocaine addicts saw videos of smoking crack or alcoholics got a whiff of whiskey? That was triggered with just a *picture* of a milkshake. Intellectually, we know it's only an image, but our lizard brains just see survival. Dopamine gets released, cravings get activated, and we're motivated to eat. It's simply a reflexive response over which we have seemingly little control, which is why marketers ensure there are pictures everywhere of milkshakes and the like.[199]

Maintaining a balance between calories in and calories out feels like a series of voluntary acts under conscious control, but it may be more akin to bodily functions, such as blinking, breathing, coughing, swallowing, or sleeping. You can try to will yourself power over any of these, but, by and large, they just happen automatically, driven by ancient scripts.[200]

Portions Out of Proportions

During any given two-day period, it seems half of U.S. children consume fast food.[201] Though attempts have been made to tie fast-food consumption with burgeoning obesity,[202] it may just be a marker for a lousier diet in general.[203] Value-meal bundling and supersizing portions are not unique to the fast-food industry. Portion sizes have increased throughout the restaurant sector.

Compared to McDonald's original sizes in 1955, its burger, fries, and soda offerings have increased 250–500 percent.[204] But huge food is everywhere—half-pound muffins,[205] steak house steaks weighing a pound and a half,[206] and pasta bowls capable of harboring two pounds of Alfredo.[207] Have you seen some of the giant chocolate bars these days? At the movie theater, a "medium" popcorn today may hold sixteen cups of greased kernels and top off at a thousand calories.[208]

What role has expanding sizes played in expanding our sizes? To be a plausible driver of the obesity crisis, candidate factors would not only match the epidemic curve but also be shown demonstrably to cause weight gain. The increases in portion size do seem to parallel obesity trends, but the experimental data are limited.[209] Manipulating portion sizes at a meal or over the course of a day can reliably affect intake,[210] perhaps due to the tendency for people to take larger and faster bites when provided with bigger portions.[211] The longest big-portion-size study I could find only lasted eleven days. In that time, however, a 50 percent increase in portion sizes increased intake by more than four hundred calories a day. Critically, this effect was sustained throughout the duration of the study and did not appear to decline over time, suggesting that bigger servings may indeed lead to bigger curvings.[212]

Of course, it matters *what* you're overeating. Some foods, like many vegetables, have such a low calorie density that you would tire from

(continued)

chewing before you could overdo it. You'd have to eat a wheelbarrow full of cabbage before you'd ever need to begin worrying about overindulging. The portion-size effect has even been used to encourage healthier habits by dishing out extra veggies.[213] So "simply telling people to eat less of everything may not be the most effective message," wrote one of the principal investigators in the obesity field.[214] Thus, this is not a call to buy baby carrots and cherry tomatoes. Size may matter, but substance is more salient.

Every Day We Run the Gauntlet

Not only are food ads ubiquitous, but so, too, is the food being advertised. The types of establishments selling food products expanded dramatically in the 1970s and 1980s,[215] and now that jolt of dopamine and the artificially stimulated feelings of hunger are around every turn.[216] Candy and snacks can be found at the checkout counters of gas stations, drugstores, bookstores, and places that used to just sell clothes, hardware, building supplies, or home furnishings. The largest food retailer in the United States is Walmart.[217]

It has become socially acceptable to eat anywhere—in your car, on the street, at your desk, or even on a crowded bus. We've become a snacking society.[218] Vending machines are pervasive. Daily eating episodes seem to have gone up by about a quarter from the late 1970s, from about four occasions a day to five, which potentially accounts for twice the calorie increase attributed to increasing meal sizes.[219] Snacks and beverages alone could account for the bulk of the calorie surplus implicated in the epidemic.[220]

And think of the children. Here we are trying to do the best for our kids, role modeling healthy habits and feeding them healthy foods, but then they venture out into a veritable tornado of junk foods and manipulative messages. As a commentary in *The New England Journal of Medicine* asked, why should our efforts to protect our "children from life-threatening illness be undermined by massive marketing campaigns from the manufacturers of junk food?"[221] Pediatricians are now encouraged to have the "French Fry Discussion" with parents at the twelve-month "well-child visit" and no longer wait until kids are two years old.[222] And even that may be too late. Two-thirds of infants are fed junk food before their first birthday.[223]

Dr. David L. Katz may have said it best in *Harvard Health Policy Review*:

> *Those who contend that parental or personal responsibility should carry the*
> *day despite these environmental temptations might consider the implications*
> *of generalizing the principle. Perhaps children should be encouraged, but not*
> *required, to attend school and tempted each morning by alternatives, such as*
> *buses to the circus, zoo, or beach.*[224]

Is Big Food Making Us Big Too?

The plague of tobacco-related deaths wasn't just due to the mass manufacture and marketing of cheap cigarettes. Tobacco companies actively sought to make their products even more craveable by spraying the sheets of tobacco with nicotine and additives like ammonia to provide a bigger nicotine kick.[225] The food industry employs taste engineers to accomplish a similar goal: maximize the irresistibility of their products.

Taste is the leading factor in food choice.[226] Salt, sugar, and fat are used as the three points of the compass to create "superstimulating" "hyperpalatability" to tempt people into impulsive buys and compulsive consumption.[227] Foods are designed intentionally to hook into our evolutionary triggers and breach whatever biological barriers help keep consumption within reasonable limits.[228]

Big Food is big business. The processed food industry alone brings in more than $2 trillion a year.[229] That affords it the economic might to manipulate more than just taste profiles; it influences public policy and scientific inquiry as well. The food, alcohol, and tobacco industries have all used similar unsavory tactics: blocking health regulations, co-opting professional organizations, creating front groups, and distorting the science.[230] The common playbook shouldn't be surprising given the many common corporate threads—at one time, for example, cigarette giant Philip Morris owned both Kraft and Miller Brewing.[231]

In 2009, the food industry spent more than $50 million to hire 350 lobbyists to influence legislation, most of whom were "revolvers," former federal employees in the revolving door between industry and its regulators. They could push corporate interests from the inside and then turn around and be rewarded with cushy lobbying jobs after their "public service."[232]

In the following year, the food industry acquired a new weapon, a stick to go along with all those carrots. On January 21, 2010, the Supreme Court's 5—4 *Citizens United* ruling permitted corporations to spend unlimited amounts of money on campaign ads to trash anyone who dared stand against them.[233] No wonder our elected officials have so thoroughly shrunk from the fight,[234] leaving us largely with a government of Big Food, by Big Food, and for Big Food.[235]

Globally, a similar dynamic exists. Weak tea calls from the public health community for voluntary standards are met not only with vicious fights against meaningful change[236] but also massive transnational trade and foreign investment deals that cement protection of food industry profits into the laws of the lands.[237]

The corrupting commercial influence even extends to medical associations. Reminiscent of the "Just what the doctor ordered" cigarette ads of yesteryear,[238] the American Academy of Family Physicians has accepted millions from the Coca-Cola Company, in part to explicitly "develop consumer education content on beverages and sweeteners."[239] When the American Academy of Pediatrics was called out for its proud new corporate relationship with Coke and the company's "invaluable commitment to children's health,"[240] an executive vice president of the academy tried to quell protest by explaining that this alliance was not without precedent: The American Academy of Pediatrics had had relationships with Pepsi and McDonald's for some time.[241]

On the front line, fake grassroots "AstroTurf" groups are used to mask the corporate message. In the footsteps of Get Government Off Our Back, memorably acronymed GGOOB and created by R. J. Reynolds to fight tobacco regulation, the front group Americans Against Food Taxes may just as well be called Food Industry Against Food Taxes.[242] The power of front-group formation was enough to bind two bitter corporate rivals, the Sugar Association and the Corn Refiners Association, and have them link arms with the American Beverage Association and the National Confectioners Association to partner together as Americans for Food and Beverage Choice.[243]

Another tried-and-true tobacco industry tactic:[244] Research front groups like Coca-Cola's Global Energy Balance Network can be used to subvert the scientific process by shaping[245] or suppressing[246] science that deviates from the corporate agenda. The trans fat story is one of many examples. Food manufacturers have not only long denied that trans fat was associated with disease,[247] they actively worked to limit inquiry[248] and discredit research findings.[249]

One estimate places the global death toll from foods high in trans fat, saturated fat, salt, and sugar at fourteen million lost lives. Every year.[250] The inability of countries around the world to turn the tide on obesity "is not a failure of individual will-power," said the director-general of the World Health Organization.[251] "It is a failure of political will to take on the powerful food and soda industries."[252] She ended her keynote address entitled "Obesity and Diabetes: The Slow-Motion Disaster" before the National Academy of Medicine with these words: "The interests of the public must be prioritized over those of corporations."[253]

We Have to Stop Eating Like This

When it comes to uncovering the root causes of the obesity epidemic, there appears to be a sort of manufactured confusion. Major studies assert the causes are "extremely complex" and "fiendishly hard to untangle."[254] Having just reviewed the literature, it doesn't seem like much of a mystery to me.

It's the food.

Attempts at obfuscation—rolling out hosts of implausible explanations like sedentary lifestyles or lack of self-discipline—serve the needs of the manufacturers and marketers more than the public's health and the interest of truth.[255] When asked about the role of restaurants in the obesity epidemic, the president of the National Restaurant Association replied, "Just because we have electricity doesn't mean you have to electrocute yourself."[256] Yes, but much of the food industry is effectively attaching electrodes to shock and awe the reward centers in our brains to undermine our self-control.

Advances in processing and packaging, combined with government policies and handouts that fostered cheap commodities for the "food industrial complex,"[257] led to a glut of ready-to-eat, ready-to-heat, or ready-to-drink products. To help assuage impatient investors, marketing became ever-more pervasive and persuasive. All these factors conspired to create unfettered access to copious, convenient, low-cost, high-calorie foods often willfully engineered with chemical additives to be hyperstimulatingly sweet or savory, yet only weakly satiating.

As we each sink deeper into a quicksand of calories, more and more mental energy is required to swim upstream against the constant bombardment of advertising and 24–7 panopticon of arm's-length tempting treats.[258] There's so much food flooding the market now that much of it ends up in the trash. Food waste has progressively increased by about 50 percent since the 1970s.[259] Perhaps better in the landfill, though, than filling up our stomachs. And too many of these cheap, fattening foods prioritize shelf life over human life.

But dead people don't eat. Don't food companies have a vested interest in keeping their consumers healthy? A question such as this reveals a fundamental misunderstanding of the system. A public company's primary responsibility is to reap returns for investors. Consider the fact that the tobacco industry produces products that *kill* one in two of its most loyal customers.[260] It's not about customer satisfaction but shareholder satisfaction. The customer always comes second.

Just as weight gain may be a perfectly natural reaction to a fattening food environment, governments and businesses are just responding normally to the political and economic realities of our system.[261] Can you think of a single major industry that would benefit from people eating less junk? "Certainly not the agriculture, food product, grocery, restaurant, diet, or drug industries," emeritus professor Marion Nestle wrote in a *Science* editorial when she was chair of nutrition at New York University. "All flourish when people eat more, and all employ armies of lobbyists to discourage governments from doing anything" about it.[262]

If part of the problem is cheap, tasty convenience, is the solution hard-to-find food that's unappealing and expensive? Or might there be a way to get the best of all worlds—easy, healthy, delicious, satisfying meals that help you lose weight?

I wrote this book to find out.

THE CONSEQUENCES

As Queasy as ABC

The largest study in history on the health effects of being overweight analyzed data from more than fifty million people in nearly two hundred countries and found that too much excess body weight accounts for the premature deaths of about four million people every year. Most of these deaths are from heart disease, but the researchers found "convincing" or "probable" evidence linking obesity to twenty different disorders[263]—a veritable alphabet soup of potential health concerns.

A Is for *Arthritis*

In the ABCs of health consequences, *A* is for *arthritis*. Obesity can worsen rheumatoid arthritis[264] and increase the risk of another inflammatory joint disease,[265] gout, known as *the disease of kings* thanks to their overly rich diets. The most common joint disease in the world, though, is osteoarthritis,[266] and obesity may be its main modifiable risk factor.[267]

Osteoarthritis develops when the cushioning cartilage lining of joints breaks down faster than the body can build it back up.[268] The knees are the most commonly affected, leading to the assumption that the disease's relationship to obesity was simply the excess wear and tear from added load on the joints. Non-weight-bearing joints, like the hands and wrists, can also be affected, however, which suggests the link isn't purely mechanical. Obesity-related *dyslipidemia* may be playing a role,[269] with elevations in the amount of fat, cholesterol, and triglycerides in the blood aggravating inflammation in the joints.[270]

Losing just around a pound a year over a span of a decade may decrease the odds of developing osteoarthritis by more than 50 percent.[271] Weight reduction may even obviate the need for knee replacement surgery. Within just eight weeks, obese osteoarthritis sufferers who had been randomized to lose weight improved their knee function as much as those going through surgery. Researchers concluded that losing around twenty pounds of fat "might be regarded as an alternative to knee replacement."[272]

But isn't it easier to just get your knee replaced than lose twenty pounds? Rarely discussed is the fact that nearly one in two hundred knee replacement patients dies within ninety days of surgery. Given the extreme popularity of the operation—about seven hundred thousand are performed each year in the United States—an orthopedics journal editor suggested that "people considering this operation are inadequately attuned to the possibility that it may kill them."[273] A surgeon responded by questioning whether patients should be told about what is arguably the "single most-salient fact":[274]

To me, the real question is whether this knowledge will help the patient. Will it add to the anxiety of the already-anxious patient, perhaps to the point of denying that patient a helpful operation? Or will this knowledge motivate a less-handicapped patient to stick to a diet and physical activity regime? Ultimately, then, the question boils down to the surgeon's judgment.[275]

Even among the vast majority who survive the surgery, approximately one in five knee replacement patients describes being unsatisfied with the outcome.[276] Weight loss, on the other hand, may offer a nonsurgical alternative that instead treats the *cause* and offers only beneficial side effects.

B Is for *Back Pain* and *Blood Pressure*

Being overweight is also a risk factor for low back pain,[277] sciatica,[278] lumbar disc degeneration,[279] and herniation.[280] As with arthritis, this may be due to the combination of the hefty joint load plus the inflammation and cholesterol associated with being heavier.[281] Autopsy studies show that the lumbar arteries that feed the spine can get clogged with atherosclerosis and starve the discs in the lower back of oxygen and nutrients.[282]

B is also for *blood pressure*. Excess visceral fat can physically compress our kidneys,[283] and the increased pressure can effectively squeeze sodium back into our bloodstreams, increasing our blood pressures. Together, the combination of obesity and hypertension can have "disastrous health implications."[284] Ready for some good news? Even just a few pounds of weight loss can help take off the pressure. Losing weight has been described as a "vital strategy for controlling hypertension."[285] In fact, losing around nine pounds was shown to lower blood pressures[286] about as much as cutting salt intake[287] approximately in half.[288]

C Is for *Cancer*

As many as three-quarters of people surveyed were evidently unaware of the link between obesity and cancer[289] when in fact, based on a comprehensive review of a thousand studies, excess body fat raises the risk of most cancers, including esophageal, stomach, colorectal, liver, gallbladder, pancreatic, breast, uterine, ovarian, kidney, brain, thyroid, and bone marrow (multiple myeloma) cancers.[290] Why? It could be due to the chronic inflammation that comes with obesity[291] or the high insulin levels due to insulin resistance.[292] (Besides controlling blood sugars, insulin is a potent growth factor that can promote tumor growth.[293]) In women, it could also be the excess estrogen.[294]

After the ovaries shut down at menopause, fat takes over as the principal site of estrogen production. This is why obese women have up to nearly twice the estrogen levels circulating in their bloodstreams,[295] which is associated with increased risk of developing—and dying from—breast cancer.[296] A twenty-pound weight loss can reduce estrogen levels within the breast by 24 percent.[297] The data on prostate cancer aren't as strong,[298] though obesity is associated with increased risk of invasive penile cancer.[299]

One reason we're confident the link between obesity and cancer is cause and effect, and not just an indirect consequence of eating poorly, is because when people lose weight—even just through bariatric surgery—their overall risk of cancer goes down. Those experiencing a sustained loss of about forty pounds after surgery went on to develop around one-third fewer cancers over the subsequent decade or so, compared with a nonsurgical control group of matched individuals who continued to slowly gain weight over time.[300] The exception is colorectal cancer.[301]

Colorectal cancer appears to be the only malignancy for which the risk goes *up* after obesity surgery. After bariatric surgery, the rate of rectal cancer death may triple.[302] The rearrangement of anatomy involved in one of the most common surgeries—gastric bypass—is thought to increase bile acid exposure along the intestinal lining. This causes sustained pro-inflammatory changes even years after the procedure, which are thought to be responsible for the increased cancer risk.[303] In contrast, losing weight by dietary means has the potential to decrease obesity-related cancer risk across the board.

D Is for *Diabetes*

As laid out in a consensus statement from the International Diabetes Federation, obesity is considered the single most important risk factor for the development of type 2 diabetes,[304] which is now the leading cause of kidney failure, lower-limb amputations, and adult-onset blindness.[305] Ironically, many of the leading drugs used to treat diabetes, including insulin itself, actually cause further weight gain, creating a vicious cycle.[306] So, again, using lifestyle medicine to treat the underlying cause is not only the safest, simplest, and cheapest route but also can be the most effective.

E Is for *Encephalopathy*

Encephalopathy means *brain disease,* and there are consistent data linking obesity in middle age to higher risk of dementia later in life.[307] Overweight individuals have about one-third higher risk, and those who are obese in midlife seem to have about 90 percent greater risk of becoming demented.[308] The risk isn't just limited to future dysfunction, though. People with excess body weight don't appear to think as clearly at any age.

Obese individuals show broad impairments in what are called *executive functions of the brain,* such as working memory, decision-making, planning, cognitive flexibility, and verbal fluency.[309] These play a critical role in everyday life. People may think about their obesity and the resulting stigma they experience as much as five times every hour,[310] but the cognitive deficits do not appear to arise just from being distracted by these thoughts. There are actually structural brain differences between normal-weight and overweight individuals.

A review entitled "Does the Brain Shrink as the Waist Expands?" noted gray matter atrophy across all ages among those carrying excess body fat.[311] This reduced brain volume correlates with the lower executive function.[312] Compromised integrity of the rest of the brain, the white matter, has also been shown, which suggests accelerated brain aging even in young adults and children with obesity.[313] This implies that there's something about the obesity itself that is affecting brain function, rather than a later clinical consequence of corresponding conditions such as high blood pressure.[314] Purported mechanisms for such executive dysfunction include inflammation and oxidative stress, both related to obesity.[315]

Does weight loss improve cognitive function? Based on a meta-analysis of twenty studies, mental performance across a variety of domains can be significantly improved with even modest weight loss, though no studies have yet been done to determine if this then translates into a normalization of Alzheimer's disease risk.[316]

F Is for *Fertility*

F is for *fertility,* or rather *failed fertility.* Overweight couples struggling to have children "should be educated on the detrimental effects of fatness," one meta-analysis concluded, as weight loss is associated with an improvement in pregnancy rates among infertile women.[317] Men may also suffer impaired fertility. The heavier a man is, the greater his risk of having a low sperm count or being completely sterile.[318] This in part may be because of the effects of excess body fat on testosterone levels.

Fat isn't the primary site of estrogen production only in postmenopausal women but in men as well. There's an enzyme in body fat that actually converts testosterone into estrogen.[319] Even going from obese to just overweight could potentially raise testosterone levels in the blood of men by 13 percent.[320]

A more dramatic cause of infertility in obese men is called *hidden penis.* Also referred to in the medical literature as *buried penis, concealed penis,* or *inconspicuous penis,* it occurs when excess fat in the pubic area subsumes the male member. It's also called *trapped penis* because the moist enfolding skin can result in a chronic inflammatory dermatitis leading to scarring and requiring surgical intervention.[321] So *F* may also stand for *Free Willy.*

G Is for *Gallstones* and *GERD*

What is the number-one digestive reason people are hospitalized? Gallbladder attack. Every year, more than a million Americans are diagnosed with gallstones, and about seven hundred thousand have to get their gallbladders surgically removed.[322] It's a relatively safe procedure.[323] Immediate complication rates tend to be under 5 percent, and the mortality rate is only about one in a thousand.[324] However, 10 percent of patients may develop "post-cholecystectomy syndrome" with persistent gastrointestinal symptoms weeks or months after their gallbladders are removed.[325]

What are gallstones made of? In 80 to 90 percent of cases, gallstones are mostly just crystallized cholesterol, forming like rock candy in the gallbladder.[326] This was used to explain why some small, earlier studies found that nonvegetarians had a higher incidence of gallstones given their higher cholesterol levels,[327] but the results from larger, more recent studies are more equivocal.[328,329] The biggest purported cause-and-effect risk factor[330] may be obesity,[331] which increases risk as much as sevenfold.[332]

Ironically, rapid weight loss may also be a trigger of gallbladder attacks. A half pound a day has been deemed the "upper limit for medically safe weight loss" based on gallstone formation. Ultrasound studies found that above that limit, the incidence of new stones can go from less than one in two hundred a week up to one in thirty.[333] To help prevent a gallstone attack, you can increase your fiber intake. Not only is dietary fiber intake associated with less gallbladder disease,[334] but those placed on high-fiber foods during a weight-loss regimen suffered significantly less gallbladder sludging than those losing the same weight without the extra fiber.[335]

Fiber-rich food consumption can also decrease the risk of acid reflux (Gastroesophageal Reflux Disease, or GERD). The excess abdominal pressure due to obesity may push up acid into the throat, causing heartburn and inflammation.[336] The increased pressure on the abdominal organs associated with obesity may also explain why overweight women suffer from more vaginal prolapse,[337] where organs such as the rectum push out into the vaginal cavity.

H Is for *Heart Disease*

Of the four million deaths attributed to excess body weight every year around the world, nearly 70 percent are due to cardiovascular disease.[338] Is it just because those people had been eating poorly? Genetic studies suggest that people effectively randomized from conception to be heavier—just based on their genes—do indeed have higher rates of heart disease and stroke regardless of what they eat.[339] So, if we lose weight, does our risk drop?

The SOS trial, which stands for *Swedish Obese Subjects,* was the first long-term controlled trial to compare the outcomes of thousands of bariatric surgery patients to matched control subjects who started out at the same weight but went the nonsurgical route. The control group maintained their weights, whereas the surgical group maintained about a 20 percent weight loss over the next ten to twenty years. Over that time, the surgical weight-loss group not only developed 80 percent less diabetes but suffered significantly fewer heart attacks and strokes, so, not surprisingly, they significantly reduced their total mortality overall.[340]

I Is for *Immunity*

The SOS trial also found that those who lost weight got less cancer.[341] This may be because antitumor immunity appears to be affected by weight. Natural killer cells are our immune systems' first line of defense against cancer cells (as well as many viral infections), and their function is severely impaired by obesity. When obese individuals were randomized to a weight-loss program, there was a significant reactivation of natural killer cell function within just three months.[342] However, the program involved an exercise component, so it's hard to tease out the impact of the weight loss itself since physical activity alone can boost natural killer cell activity.[343]

On the other end of the spectrum, obesity is suspected to be a causal risk factor for the development of multiple sclerosis, an autoimmune disease.[344] This suggests obesity is associated with the worst of both worlds when it comes to immune function: underactivity when it comes to protecting against cancer and infection, but overactivity when it comes to certain inflammatory autoimmune conditions.[345]

J Is for *Jaundice*

Thanks to the obesity epidemic, nonalcoholic fatty liver disease (NAFLD) is now the most common liver disorder in the industrialized world.[346] Fat doesn't just end up in our bellies and thighs but inside some of our internal organs. More than 80 percent of individuals with abdominal obesity may have fatty infiltration into their livers,[347] and in those with severe obesity, the prevalence can exceed 90 percent.[348] This can lead to inflammation, scarring, jaundice, and, ultimately, cirrhosis and liver cancer.[349] Currently, the advanced form of NAFLD, nonalcoholic fatty hepatitis, is the leading cause of liver transplants in American women, and men are expected to catch up by 2020.[350]

K Is for *Kidneys*

Obesity is also one of the strongest risk factors for chronic kidney disease. Our kidneys compensate for the metabolic demands of excess weight by red-lining into what's called *hyperfiltration* to deal with the extra workload. The resulting increased pressure within the kidneys can damage the sensitive organs and increase the risk of kidney failure over the long term.[351]

. . . and *L, M, N, O, P* Through *Z*

If we wanted to keep singing the alphabet of obesity-related health concerns, *L* could be for *diminished lung function,*[352] *M* for a cluster of risk factors known as *metabolic syndrome,*[353] and so on. There's even an *X*—for *xiphodynia,* pain at the tip of the bottom of the breastbone from being bent outward by an expanding abdomen.[354]

Counting the Costs

Given the myriad health conditions associated with excess weight, medical spending attributable to obesity is nearly $2,000 per person per year,[355] with obese workers with multiple complications costing companies up to $10,000 more in health-care coverage compared to lean counterparts.[356] Beyond just brazen discrimination, this actually may account for some of the wage gap obese employees experience as companies try to make up for these costs.[357] Between health-care costs and diminished productivity in terms of lost workdays, the total per capita lifetime costs of long-term obesity have been estimated to exceed $200,000.[358]

Some estimates peg the current national cost of obesity at about $150 billion,[359] with another $50 billion per year added by 2030 as our increasingly heavy baby boomers continue to age.[360] The Milken Institute appraised the cost of obesity as a *trillion*-dollar drag on the economy,[361] more than twice what we spend on national defense.[362] Others diametrically disagree, based on the morbid fact that obese individuals may not live as long. Just as the medical costs of tobacco-related diseases may be more than offset by the shortened survival of smokers, the lifetime health-care costs of obese individuals may turn out to be lower because they are expected to die so much sooner.[363] So the true cost may be calculated in lives rather than dollars.

Larger Than Life

Martin Luther King Jr. warned that "human progress is neither automatic nor inevitable,"[364] and the same may be true of the human life span.[365] In 1850, life expectancy in the United States was less than forty years,[366] but it has steadily increased over the last two centuries,[367] gaining about two years per decade—until recently, that is. Longevity gains have faltered or even reversed, and the greatest victims will be our children. Thanks to the obesity epidemic, we may now be raising the first American generation to live shorter lives than their parents.[368]

The downward trend in longevity is expected to accelerate as the current, younger generation—who started out heavier from a younger age than ever before—matures into adulthood. If the obesity epidemic continues unchecked, current trends signal a potential "looming social and economic catastrophe."[369] In the coming decades, some predict we may lose two to five years—or more—of life expectancy in the United States. To put that into perspective, a miracle cure for *all* forms of cancer would only add three and a half years to the average American life span.[370] In other words, reversing the obesity epidemic might save more lives than curing cancer.

The Obesity Paradox

The evidence that being overweight increases our risk for debilitating diseases like diabetes is considered indisputable, but, surprisingly, there is controversy surrounding body weight and overall mortality.[371] In 2013, scientists from the Centers for Disease Control and Prevention (CDC) published a meta-analysis in *The Journal of the American Medical Association* suggesting that being overweight was actually advantageous. Yes, grade 2 or grade 3 obesity, which is like being the average American's height, five foot six,[372] and weighing about 215 pounds or more, was associated with living a shorter life, but grade 1 obesity (about 185–215 pounds at the same height) was not. And, being overweight (155–185 pounds at average height) appeared to be protective compared to those who were normal weight (115–155 pounds at five foot six). The overweight individuals, with a BMI of 25–30, appeared to live the longest.[373]

Headline writers were giddy: "Being Overweight Can Extend Life," "Dreading Your Diet? Don't Worry . . . Plump People Live LONGER,"[374] and "Extra Pounds Mean Lower Chance of Death."[375] Not surprisingly, the study ignited a firestorm of controversy in the public health community and was called "ludicrous,"[376] "flawed," and "misleading."[377] The chair of nutrition at Harvard lost his cool, calling it "really a pile of rubbish,"[378] fearing the food industry might exploit the study in the same way the petroleum industry misuses a manufactured controversy over climate change.[379]

Public health advocates can't just dismiss data they find inconvenient, though. Science is science. But how could being overweight increase the risk of life-threatening diseases, yet, at the same time, make you live longer? This became known as the *obesity paradox*.[380] The solution to the puzzle appears to lie with two major sources of bias, the first being confounding by smoking.[381]

As I'll explore in the Amping AMPK section, the nicotine in tobacco can lead to weight loss. So if you're skinnier because you smoke, then it's no wonder you'd live a shorter life with a slimmer waist. The failure to control for the effect of smoking in studies purporting to show an "obesity paradox" leads to the dangers of obesity being "grossly underestimated."[382]

The second major source of bias is reverse causality. Instead of lower weight leading to life-threatening diseases, isn't it more likely that life-threatening diseases lead to lower weight? Conditions such as hidden tumors, chronic heart or lung disease, alcoholism, and depression can all cause unintentional weight loss months or even years before a diagnosis is made.[383] As we've discussed, it's become normal to be overweight in this country.[384] People who are "abnormally" thin—that is, at an ideal weight—could actually be taking care of themselves, but they also may be heavy smokers, elderly and frail, or seriously ill with weight loss from their disease.[385]

Deadweight

To put the obesity paradox issue to the test once and for all, the Global BMI Mortality Collaboration was formed, reviewing data from more than ten million people from hundreds of studies in dozens of countries—the largest evaluation of BMI and mortality in history.[386] To help eliminate bias, the researchers omitted smokers and those with known chronic disease. They then excluded the first five years of follow-up to try to remove from the analysis those with undiagnosed conditions who had lost weight due to an impending death. The results were clear: Being overweight or any grade of obesity was associated with a significantly greater risk of dying prematurely.[387] In fact, adjusting for those biases leads to "eliminating the obesity paradox altogether."[388] In other words, the so-called obesity paradox appears to be just a myth.[389]

Indeed, when intentional weight loss is actually put to the test, people live longer. Bariatric surgery studies like the SOS trial show weight loss reduces long-term mortality,[390] and randomizing people to lose weight through lifestyle changes shows the same.[391] Losing a dozen pounds through diet and exercise was found to be associated with a 15 percent drop in overall mortality risk. Exercise alone may extend life span even without weight loss,[392] but there also appears to be a similar longevity benefit of weight loss through dietary means alone.[393]

The Optimal BMI for Optimal Longevity

The largest studies in the United States[394] and around the world[395] found that having a normal body mass index, a BMI of 20–25, is associated with the longest life span. Putting together all the best available studies with the longest follow-up, that can be narrowed down even further to a BMI of 20–22.[396] You can use this unisex chart to see what your optimal weight might be based on your height:

Height	Ideal Weight	Height	Ideal Weight	Height	Ideal Weight	Height	Ideal Weight
4'9"	92–102	5'2"	109–120	5'7"	128–140	6'	147–162
4'10"	96–105	5'3"	113–124	5'8"	132–145	6'1"	152–167
4'11"	99–109	5'4"	117–128	5'9"	135–149	6'2"	156–171
5'	102–113	5'5"	120–132	5'10"	139–153	6'3"	160–176
5'1"	106–116	5'6"	124–136	5'11"	143–158	6'4"	164–181

So even within a "normal" BMI, the risk of developing chronic diseases, such as type 2 diabetes, heart disease, and several types of cancer, starts to rise toward the upper end, starting as low as a BMI of 21. BMIs of 18.5 and 24.5 are both considered within the normal range, but a BMI of 24.5 may be associated with twice the heart disease risk compared to 18.5.[397] The ideal

BMI appears to be between 20 and 22, confirmed in a study of an "unusually slim cohort" from the Oxford Vegetarian Study.[398]

Just as there are gradations of risk within a normal BMI range, there is a spectrum within obesity. Grade 3 obesity, characterized as having a BMI greater than 40, can be associated with the loss of a decade of life or more. At a BMI greater than 45, such as a five-foot-six person at 280 pounds, life expectancy may shrink to that of a cigarette smoker.[399]

Health at Every Size™?

There are "obesity skeptics" who argue that the health consequences of obesity are unclear or even greatly exaggerated. They are a motley bunch of unlikely bedfellows, ranging from feminists, queer theorists, and new ageists to "far right wing, pro-gun, pro-America websites where the idea [is] that obesity alarmists are nanny-state communists who simply want to stop us from having fun."[400]

There are also many "fat activists" who try to downplay the risks of obesity. The director of medical advocacy for the Council on Size and Weight Discrimination routinely takes part in obesity conferences and government panels on obesity. She is quoted as saying, "I'm not actually particularly that interested in [health]" and "God, I hate science."[401] Unlike activists who, for example, organized to raise consciousness to stamp out the AIDS epidemic, the size-acceptance movement appears to have the opposite goal, rallying for *less* public awareness and treatment of the problem.[402] (They do have good slogans, though: "We're here, we're spheres, get used to it!"[403]) I'm all for fighting size stigma and discrimination, but the adverse health consequences of obesity are an established scientific fact. In a study of more than six hundred centenarians, those one hundred years old and older, fewer than 2 percent of the women and not a single one of the men were obese.[404]

Can't you be fat but fit? There appears to be a rare subgroup of obese individuals who don't suffer the typical metabolic costs of obesity, such as high blood pressure and high cholesterol.[405] This raised the possibility that there may be such a thing as "benign obesity."[406] It may just be a matter of time before the risk factors develop.[407] But even if they don't develop, followed long enough, even "metabolically healthy" obese individuals are at increased risk of diabetes,[408] fatty liver disease,[409] cardiovascular events such as heart attacks, and/or premature death.[410] Bottom line? There is strong evidence that "healthy obesity" is a myth.[411]

Hating Their Guts

The size-acceptance movement is definitely right about one thing, though: the extraordinary scourge of weight stigma. Described as the last "acceptable" form of bias,[412] weight stigma is the rampant discrimination and stereotyping of overweight individuals. Fifty overweight women were asked to keep a diary of all the times they felt they were stigmatized for their weights. Over just one week, more than a thousand instances were recorded.[413] An overweight woman may expect to be harassed (such as called names or insulted), encounter physical barriers (like being unable to fit into public seats), or be discriminated against (such as receiving perceived poorer service at restaurants or stores) on average about three times a day. Obese men report three times less discrimination than women of the same size,[414] so it may be only a daily occurrence for them.

This weight stigma starts surprisingly early. Children as young as three years old label overweight peers as "mean," "stupid," "lazy," and "ugly."[415] One of the most poignant illustrations comes from a famous study published in 1961. Children in summer camps and schools across a swath of different social, cultural, and ethnic backgrounds in California, Montana, and New York were asked to rank the following images as to whom they liked best:

1. a child in crutches with one leg in a brace
2. a child in a wheelchair
3. a child with one hand missing
4. a facially disfigured child
5. an obese child

In every population of kids they tested, there was "remarkable uniformity."[416] The obese child always came in dead last.

But that was ages ago. What happened when the original study was repeated? Researchers published the forty-year follow-up in 2003, and guess what they found? The title of the study gives it away: "Getting Worse: The Stigmatization of Obese Children." The obese child was liked even less.[417] This parallels trends throughout society with a 70 percent jump in perceived weight discrimination recorded in national surveys since the mid-1990s.[418]

Attitudes among educators may not be helping. More than a quarter of teachers and other school staff surveyed felt that becoming obese is "one of the worst things that could happen to a person."[419] Even parents can be biased, providing less support for college for their overweight daughters compared to thinner siblings.[420] As two prominent obesity researchers commented, "It is strong prejudice indeed when parents discriminate against their own children."[421]

What about doctors? One representative national survey found that more than half of physicians viewed obese patients as "awkward, unattractive, ugly, and noncompliant."[422] About a quarter of nurses agreed or strongly agreed with the statement "Caring for an obese patient usually repulses me."[423] This antagonism can have serious health consequences for those who may need care the most. For example, obese women are at higher risk for developing cervical,[424] endometrial, and ovarian cancers,[425] yet they are less likely to be screened. Morbidly obese patients only have about half the odds of getting their recommended pelvic exams.[426] Though some of this may be avoidance on the part of the patient, some doctors just turn away obese patients. *The Sun Sentinel* polled OB-GYN practices in Florida and found that as many as one in seven refused to see heavier women, for example, setting weight cut-offs for new patients starting at two hundred pounds.[427]

Even doctors who welcome obese patients have been found to give them short shrift. Physicians randomized to receive a medical chart of a migraine patient who either presented as average weight or obese said they would give the obese patient about 28 percent less of their time[428]—and it's less quality time too. Recorded doctor visits found physicians tend to build less emotional rapport with overweight patients.[429]

At least the doctors appear able to hide their disdain. In a study entitled "Obese Patients Overestimate Physicians' Attitudes of Respect," despite the negative attitudes doctors harbored toward their obese patients, the same patients expressed their satisfaction with their providers. The researchers concluded, "While physicians may be successfully playing the part, the lack of true respect suggests . . . the authenticity of the patient–physician relationship should be questioned."[430]

For Shame

Weight stigma may perpetuate a cycle of stress leading to obesity, leading to even more stress. I discuss this concept further in the Stress Hormone Relief section. Across thousands of individuals followed for four years, those reporting discriminatory experiences had more than twice the odds of becoming obese. As well, those who started out obese had more than three times the odds of staying that way compared to people who started out at the same weight but didn't experience discrimination.[431] This could be from stress-induced eating on one side of the calorie-balance equation or stigma-induced exercise avoidance on the other.

Obese individuals with more frequent experiences with weight stigma report greater avoidance of exercising in public, feeling judged and embarrassed.[432] These "too fat to exercise"[433] fears may be well grounded. Strong anti-fat biases have been documented in both fitness professionals and regular gym-goers,[434] which may present an unwelcoming environment in fitness centers and health clubs.[435]

Whichever side of the calorie equation gets tipped, those who experience weight stigma can end up suffering health consequences independent of any added weight. Those reporting more frequent fat prejudice exhibit higher levels of depression,[436] inflammation,[437] and oxidative stress,[438] as well as shorter life spans. Two studies following a total of nearly twenty thousand people both found about a 50 percent increase in mortality risk among those reporting greater daily discrimination.[439] Despite these hazards, some scholars advocate for even *more* fat shaming.

The president emeritus of the prestigious Hastings Center infamously advocated for "a kind of stigmatization lite," using social pressures to compel people to lose weight without resorting to outright discrimination. After all, he argued, what else has the potential to counter the persuasive force of the billions spent in advertising every year by the food and beverage industry? It worked against tobacco. He recalls his own battle with addiction: "The force of being shamed and beat upon socially was as persuasive for me to stop smoking as the threats to my health." The public health campaign to stigmatize cigarettes turned what had been considered "simply a bad habit into reprehensible behavior."[440]

When such campaigns have been tried, they have been met with fierce resistance. Georgia's Strong4Life campaign featured billboards of morose-looking obese children with such captions as "Warning: Chubby kids may not outlive their parents" and "It's hard to be a little girl when you're not."[441] The campaign sponsors defended the ads as an attempt to break through the denial in a state with some of the highest recorded childhood obesity rates[442]—but it's only defensible if it works.

So does it? Being labeled "too fat" in childhood was associated with a higher risk of becoming obese compared to children who weighed the same but were never told that.[443] Does this mean we should just ignore the elephant in the room? Many doctors apparently think so.

Just as veterinarians have been found to be reluctant to tell people their pets are obese,[444] many pediatricians are similarly quiet when it comes to discussing weight concerns with parents. Less than a quarter of parents of overweight children report having been told that about their children's weight status by their pediatricians.[445] One might think it would be obvious, but a Gallup survey found that parents appear to be "notoriously poor judges of their children's weight." Similarly, despite skyrocketing obesity, the percentage of adults who describe themselves as overweight has remained essentially unchanged over the past few decades. All this, Gallup concluded, helps "paint a picture of mass delusion in the United States about its rising weight."[446]

I think patients have the right to be informed. Those told by their doctors that they are overweight have nearly four times the odds of attempting weight loss[447] and about twice the odds of succeeding.[448] Just as physicians who smoke are less likely to challenge their patients who smoke, overweight physicians are less likely to bring up the subject of weight loss[449] or even document obesity in patient charts.[450] Ironically, overweight patients trust diet advice more from overweight doctors than those who are normal weight.[451]

As obesity rates have gone up, the rate of weight counseling advice from primary care physicians has inexplicably gone down.[452] Even when they do manage to counsel patients, doctors appear to have little to offer in terms of specifics. Fewer than half who were surveyed said they provide specific guidance to their patients.[453] Just telling patients *Watch what you eat*, is unlikely to be particularly helpful, but many primary care physicians may not even go that far. Physical inactivity was rated by physicians as significantly more important than any other cause of obesity, which is far from accurate, as I discuss on page 355. Most physicians said they would spend more time working with patients on weight management if only their time were "reimbursed appropriately."[454] Maybe we could even offer doctors a bonus to refrain from blaming the victim.[455] As one pair of commentators wrote in response to the pro-stigmatization camp, "If shaming reduced obesity, there would be no fat people."[456]

Blind, Deaf, Dumb, or Fat

I want to end this stigma section with the jaw-dropping findings of a study I think best illustrates how hard it is to live inside a fat body. If this doesn't foster sympathy among my medical colleagues, I don't know what will. Researchers talked with men and women who had lost and kept off more than 100 pounds to tap into their unique insights, having personally experienced what it was like to be morbidly obese and then, on average, 126 pounds lighter. Forty-seven such individuals were interviewed.

They were asked to think back to when they were heavier and make a choice: "If someone offered you a couple of million dollars if you stayed morbidly obese forever, would you have chosen the money? Or would you have chosen to be normal weight no matter what?"

- **Option 1:** "I would have chosen no money and being normal weight. It would have taken me one second to decide."
- **Option 2:** "I probably would have chosen being normal weight. But the possibility of having that much money would make me think about the choice."
- **Option 3:** "I wanted to be normal weight, but I really could use the money. If I would be a multimillionaire I think I could live with being morbidly obese."

One of the forty-seven people had to think about it, but the other forty-six jumped at Option 1. Not a single person chose Option 3. They all said they would give up being a multimillionaire to be normal weight.[457]

If that shocked you, buckle your seat belt. They were then asked about being obese compared to other disabilities. Normally when you ask people to choose between living with their own disability or switching to a different one, there is a strong proclivity to stay with their own.[458] For example, even though most people would rather be deaf than blind, blind people prefer to remain blind by a large margin rather than having sight without sound. They already know how to cope with their own disability, so there's safety in familiarity. The exact opposite happened when the formerly obese were asked.

Each of the forty-seven men and women said they'd rather be deaf for the rest of their lives than obese. Every single one said they'd rather be unable to read, be diabetic, have very bad acne, or have heart disease than be obese. And then the true jaw-dropper: More than 90 percent said they'd rather have a leg amputated, and, similarly, about nine out of ten said they'd rather be *blind* their whole lives than obese. Obesity appears to be the only handicap where nearly everyone wants to switch disabilities no matter what the cost. To quote one study subject, "When you're blind, people want to help you. No one wants to help when you're fat."[459]

How Much Weight Does It Take?

We seem to have become inured to the mortal threat of obesity. If you go back in the medical literature a half century or so, when obesity wasn't run of the mill, the descriptions are much grimmer: "Obesity is always tragic, and its hazards are terrifying."[460] But it doesn't have to be frank obesity. Of the four million deaths every year attributed to excess body fat, nearly 40 percent of the victims are just overweight, not obese.[461] According to two famous Harvard studies, as little as eleven pounds of weight gain from early adulthood through middle age increases the risk of major chronic disease.[462]

The flip side is that even modest weight *loss* can have major health benefits.

The good news is the riskiest fat is the easiest to lose. Our bodies appear to preferentially shed the villainous visceral fat first.[463] Although it may take losing as much as 20 percent of your weight to realize significant improvements in quality of life for most individuals with severe obesity,[464] disease risk drops almost immediately. At 3 percent weight loss (only six pounds for someone weighing two hundred), your blood sugar control and triglycerides start to get better.[465] At 5 percent weight loss, blood pressure and cholesterol improve. Furthermore, a 5 percent weight loss—just ten pounds for someone starting at two hundred—may cut the risk of developing diabetes in half.[466]

What About Weight Cycling?

There was a book originally published in the 1980s and then repeatedly republished ever since entitled *Dieting Makes You Fat*. Since most people who lose weight go on to regain it, the concern is there may be adverse health effects to so-called yo-yo dieting.[467] This idea emerged from animal studies[468] that showed, for example, detrimental effects of starving and refeeding obese rats.[469] This captured the media's attention, leading to a pervasive common belief about the "dangers" of weight cycling, discouraging people from even trying.[470]

Even the animal data are inconclusive, though. For example, weight cycling mice makes them live *longer*.[471] Most importantly, other than perhaps a greater risk of gallstones,[472,473] a review of the human data concluded that "evidence for an adverse effect of weight cycling appears sparse, if it exists at all."[474] In fact, as I write this, the current issue of *Obesity,* the official journal of the leading scientific society dedicated to the field, published a commentary entitled "Yo-Yo Dieting Is Better Than None."[475]

The Skinny on Fat

Let's take a closer look at the best way to measure and define excess body fat.

BODY MASS INDEX VS. BODY FAT PERCENTAGE

Most of the population studies that have explored the relationship between obesity and disease have relied on BMI,[476] body mass index. (Calculate your own on page 6.) BMI takes height into account but doesn't take the *composition* of the weight into account. Bodybuilders are heavy for their heights but can be extremely lean. The gold-standard measure of obesity is percentage of body fat,[477] but accurate calculations for this can be complicated and expensive.[478] All that's needed to measure BMI is a scale and a tape measure, but it may underestimate the true prevalence of obesity.

The World Health Organization[479] and the American College of Endocrinology[480] define obesity as a body fat percentage over 25 percent in men or 35 percent in women. At a BMI of 25, which is considered just barely overweight, body fat percentages in a representative U.S. sample of adults varied between 14 and 35 percent in men and 26 and 43 percent in women.[481] So you could be normal weight, but actually obese.[482] Using the BMI cutoff for obesity, only about one in five Americans were obese back in the 1990s, but based on their body fat, the true proportion back then was closer to 50 percent.[483] Even by the '90s, half of America was not just overweight but obese.

By using only BMI, doctors may misclassify more than half of obese individuals as being just overweight or even normal weight and miss an opportunity to intervene.[484] The important thing, however, is not the label but the health consequences. Ironically, BMI appears to be an even better predictor of cardiovascular disease death than body fat percentage.[485] This suggests that excess weight from any source—fat or lean—may not be healthy in the long run.[486] The life spans of professional bodybuilders do seem to be cut short. They have about a third higher mortality rate than the general population, with an average age of death around forty-eight years,[487] but this may be due in part to the toxic effects of anabolic steroids on the heart.[488]

WEIGHT VS. WAIST

Preeminent nutritional physiologist Ancel Keys (after whom K rations were named[489]) suggested the mirror method: "If you really want to know whether you are obese, just undress and look at yourself in the mirror. Don't worry about our fancy laboratory measurements; you'll know!"[490] All fat is not the same, though. There is the pinchable, superficial flab you may see jiggling about your body, and then there's the riskier, visceral fat that coils around and infiltrates your internal organs, bulging out your belly.[491] Measuring BMI is simple, cheap, and effective, but it doesn't take into account the distribution of fat on the body—whereas waist circumference can provide a measure of the deep underlying abdominal fat.

Both BMI and waist circumference can be used to predict the risk of death due to excess body fat,[492] but even at the same BMI, there appears to be nearly a straight-line increase in mortality risk with widening waistlines.[493] Someone with "normal-weight central obesity"—meaning someone not even considered to be overweight according to BMI, but who carries fat around the middle[494]—may have up to twice the risk of dying compared to someone who's overweight or obese according to their weight and height. This is why the World Health Organization,[495] National

(continued)

Institutes of Health,[496] and American Heart Association[497] recommend measuring both BMI and waist circumference. This may be especially important for older women, who lose approximately 13 pounds of bone and muscle as they age from twenty-five to sixty-five, while quadrupling their visceral fat stores. (Men's visceral fat stores tend only to double.)[498] So even if a woman doesn't gain any weight according to the bathroom scale, she may be gaining fat.

What's the healthy waistline cutoff?[499] Increased risk of metabolic complications starts at an abdominal circumference of 31.5 inches in women and 37 inches in most men, but closer to 35.5 inches for Chinese, Japanese, and South Asian men.[500] The benchmark for substantially increased risk starts at about 34.5 inches for women and 40 inches for men.[501] Once you get greater than an abdominal circumference of about 43 inches in men, mortality rates shoot up about 50 percent compared to men with 8-inch-smaller stomachs, and women suffer 80 percent greater mortality risk at 37.5-inch waists compared to 27.5 inches.[502] The reading of a measuring tape may translate into years off one's life span.

Surprisingly, there is no universal protocol for assessing waist circumference. Some guidelines recommend measuring at the level of the last rib, others at the top of the hip bones, and others still suggest halfway between those landmarks, or at the belly button, or at the narrowest point.[503] While the belly button may be the most intuitive and easiest to measure (and the preferred location for a one-time visceral fat assessment),[504] the halfway point between the top of the hip bones and bottom of the rib cage appears to be the most effective at tracking changes in visceral fat over time.[505]

KEEP YOUR WAIST LESS THAN HALF YOUR HEIGHT

Unlike waist circumference, body mass index has the advantage of taking height into account. Waist-to-height ratio may offer the best of both worlds, and the cutoff value is the simplest to remember: Keep your waist less than half your height.[506] The goal for adults and children six years or older is to get a waist-to-height ratio under 0.5.[507]

Waist-to-height ratio may be a better predictor of both body fat percentage and visceral fat mass than BMI or waist circumference alone.[508] In terms of screening for cardiometabolic risk (for example, heart disease and diabetes), waist-to-height ratio appears superior to BMI in adults[509] and seems to work as well as BMI for assessing body fat in children.[510] So the ideal may be a combination of BMI and a measure of abdominal obesity, such as waist-to-height ratio.[511]

THE SOLUTIONS

Bringing a Butter Knife to a Gunfight

Now that you have a sense of the causes and consequences of obesity, let's look at the panoply of solutions that have been undertaken to combat excess body fat—and whether or not they actually address the root cause. The treatment of obesity has long been stained by the snake-oil swindlings of profiteers, hustlers, and quacks. Even the modern field of bariatric medicine (derived from the Greek word *baros,* meaning *weight*) is pervaded by an "insidious image of sleaze."[512] Beguiled by advertising for fairy-tale magic bullets of rapid, effortless weight loss, people blame themselves for failing to manifest the miracle or imagine themselves to be metabolically broken. On the other end of the spectrum are overly pessimistic practitioners of the opinion that "people who are fat are born fat, and nothing much can be done about it."[513] The truth lies somewhere in between.

The difficulty of curing obesity has been compared to learning a foreign language; it's an achievement virtually anyone can attain with a sufficient investment of energies, but it always takes considerable time and effort.[514] Research suggests that most obese individuals don't stay in treatment. Of those who do, most don't adhere to it sufficiently to lose the excess weight. But, even among those who try to stick with it, most will regain much of the weight.[515] To me, this speaks to the difficulty, rather than the futility. It may take smokers an average of thirty quit attempts to finally kick the habit.[516] Like quitting smoking, it helps to think of losing excess weight as just something that has to be done. As the chair of the Association for the Study of

Obesity put it, it doesn't take willpower to do essential tasks like getting up at night to feed a baby—it's just something that has to be done.[517]

Our collective response to the obesity epidemic doesn't seem to match the rhetoric or reality.[518] If obesity is such a "national crisis" "reaching alarming proportions,"[519] dubbed by the post-9/11 Surgeon General as "every bit as devastating as terrorism," why has our reaction been so tepid?[520] For example, governments meekly suggest the food industry take "voluntary initiatives to restrict the marketing of less healthy food options to children."[521] Have we just given up and ceded control to Big Business?

Our timid response to the obesity epidemic is encapsulated by a national initiative promulgated by the Joint Task Force of the American Society for Nutrition, Institute of Food Technologists, and International Food Information Council: the "small-changes approach."[522] Since small changes are "more feasible,"[523] suggestions include "using mustard rather than mayonnaise" and "eating 1 rather than 2 doughnuts in the morning."[524] Seems a bit like bringing a butter knife to a gunfight. Proponents of the small-changes approach lament that unlike other addictions, such as alcohol, cocaine, gambling, or tobacco, we can't counsel our obese patients to give up the addictive element completely, as "no one can give up eating."[525] But just because we have to breathe doesn't mean it has to be through the end of a cigarette. Similarly, just because we have to eat doesn't mean we have to eat junk.

Bariatric Surgery

Liposuction Sucks

The first surgical attempt at body fat sculpting was in 1921. A dancer wanted to "improve" the shape of her ankles. The surgeon apparently scraped away too much tissue and tied the stitches too tight, resulting in necrosis, amputation, and the first recorded malpractice suit in the history of plastic surgery.[526] Modern liposuction is much safer, killing only about one in five thousand patients.[527]

Liposuction currently reigns as the most popular cosmetic surgery in the world, and its effects are indeed only cosmetic.[528] A study published in *The New England Journal of Medicine* assessed fifteen obese women before and after having about twenty pounds of fat sucked out of their bodies, resulting in nearly a 20 percent drop in their total body fat.[529] Normally, if you lose even just 5–10 percent of your body weight in fat, you get significant improvements in blood pressure, blood sugars, inflammation, cholesterol, and triglycerides,[530] but none of those benefits materialized after the massive liposuction.[531]

This suggests subcutaneous fat, the fat under our skin, is not the problem. The metabolic insults of obesity arise from the *visceral* fat surrounding or even infiltrating our inner organs, like the fat marbling our muscles and livers. The way you lose that fat, the dangerous fat, is to take in fewer calories than you burn.

Under the Knife

What about bringing a scalpel to the gunfight instead? The use of bariatric surgery has exploded from about forty thousand procedures per year, as noted in the first international survey in 1998,[532] to hundreds of thousands now performed each year in the United States alone.[533] The first technique developed, the intestinal bypass, involved carving out about twenty feet of intestines.[534,535] More than thirty thousand intestinal bypass operations were performed[536] before the "catastrophic,"[537] "disastrous outcomes" were recognized.[538] This included protein deficiency–induced liver disease[539] progressing to "fatal hepatic necrosis."[540] Its inauspicious start is remembered as "one of the dark blots in the history of surgery."[541]

Today, death rates after bariatric surgery are considered "very low," occurring on average in perhaps one in three hundred[542] to one in five hundred patients.[543] The most common procedure is stomach stapling, also known as a *sleeve gastrectomy,* in which most of the stomach is permanently removed,[544] leaving only a narrow sleeve or tube of stomach so as to restrict how much food people can eat at any one time.[545] It's ironic that many patients choose bariatric surgery, convinced that "diets don't work" for them, when, in reality, that's all the surgery may be—an enforced diet.[546] Bariatric surgery can be thought of as a form of internal jaw wiring.

Gastric bypass is the second most common bariatric surgery.[547] It combines restriction—stapling the stomach into a pouch smaller than the size of a golf ball—with malabsorption, by rearranging our anatomy to bypass the first part of our small intestines.[548] It appears to be more effective than just cutting out most of the stomach—resulting in a loss of 63 percent of excess weight compared to 53 percent with a gastric sleeve[549]—but gastric bypass carries a greater risk of serious complications.[550] Many are surprised to learn that new surgical procedures don't require premarket testing or approval by the Food and Drug Administration (FDA)[551] and are largely exempt from rigorous regulatory scrutiny,[552] potentially making new surgeries even riskier than new medications.

It's Complicated

The third most common bariatric procedure is a revision to fix a previous bariatric procedure.[553] Up to 25 percent of bariatric patients have to go back into the operating room to rectify problems caused by their first bariatric surgery or for additional procedures. Reoperations are riskier, carrying up to ten times the mortality rate,[554] and offer no guarantee of success.[555] Complications include leaks,[556] fistulas, ulcers, strictures, erosions, obstructions, and severe acid reflux.[557]

The extent of risk may depend on the skill of the surgeon. In a study published in *The New England Journal of Medicine,* bariatric surgeons voluntarily submitted videos of themselves performing surgery to a panel of their peers for evaluation. Technical proficiency varied widely and was related to the rates of complications, hospital readmissions, reoperations, and death. Patients operated on by the less competent surgeons suffered nearly three times the complications and five times the risk of death.[558]

As with athletes and musicians, some surgeons may simply be more talented than others, but practice may help make perfect.[559] Gastric bypass is such a complicated procedure that its learning curve may require hundreds of cases for a surgeon to master it. Risk of complications plateaus after about five hundred cases, with the lowest risk found among surgeons who've performed more than six hundred bypasses.[560] So if you do choose to undergo the procedure, I'd recommend asking your surgeon how many they've done and also choosing an accredited Bariatric Center of Excellence, since surgical mortality appears to be two to three times lower at those institutions than at nonaccredited ones.[561]

Even if the surgery goes perfectly, lifelong nutritional replacement and monitoring are required to avoid vitamin and mineral deficits[562]—the consequences of which include more than just a little anemia, osteoporosis, or hair loss.[563] Bariatric surgeries have resulted in full-blown cases of potentially life-threatening deficiencies, such as beriberi, pellagra, kwashiorkor, and nerve damage[564] that can manifest as vision loss years or even decades after surgery (in the case of copper deficiency).[565] Tragically, in cases of severe deficiency of a B vitamin called thiamine, nearly one in three patients progressed to permanent brain damage before they were even diagnosed.[566]

The malabsorption of nutrients is on purpose for procedures like gastric bypass. By cutting out segments of the intestine, we can successfully impair the absorption of calories—but at the expense of impairing the absorption of necessary nutrition. Even people who simply undergo restrictive procedures like stomach stapling can be at risk for life-threatening nutrient deficiencies because of persistent vomiting.[567] Indeed, vomiting is reported by up to 60 percent of patients after bariatric surgery due to "inappropriate" eating behaviors—that is, by trying to eat normally.[568]

"Dumping syndrome" can work the same way. A large percentage of gastric bypass patients can suffer from abdominal cramps, diarrhea, nausea, bloating, fatigue, or palpitations after eating calorie-rich foods as they bypass the stomach and dump straight into the intestines. As surgeons describe it, this is a feature, not a bug: "Dumping syndrome is an expected and desired part of the behavior modification caused by gastric bypass surgery; it can deter patients from consuming energy-dense food."[569]

Bariatric Surgery: Metabolic or Hyperbolic?

The surgical community objects to the characterization of bariatric surgery as internal jaw wiring, the cutting up of healthy organs just to discipline people's behavior. The field has gone as far as to rename it "metabolic surgery," suggesting the anatomical rearrangements cause changes in digestive hormones that offer unique physiological benefits.[570] As evidence, the surgical community points to the remarkable remission rates for type 2 diabetes.

After bariatric surgery, about 55 percent of obese diabetics and 75 percent of "super-obese" diabetics go into remission, meaning they have normal blood sugars off all diabetes medications.[571] The normalization in blood sugars can happen within just days after the surgery.[572] Fifteen years after surgery, 30 percent may remain diabetes-free (compared to a 7 percent cure rate in a nonsurgical control group).[573] But are we sure it was the surgery that did this? Could their improvement in blood sugars just be from the extreme caloric restriction that typically precedes and also follows surgery, rather than some surgical sort of metabolic magic? Researchers decided to put it to the test.

At a bariatric surgery clinic at the University of Texas, patients with type 2 diabetes scheduled for a gastric bypass volunteered to first undergo an identical period of caloric restriction. They were placed in the hospital and, for ten days, were put on the same diet they would be on immediately before and after the surgery, averaging fewer than five hundred calories a day to mimic the surgical situation. The researchers then waited a few months so the subjects would gain back the weight before putting them through the actual surgery, matched day for day to the diets they had been on before. Same patients, same diets—just with or without the actual surgery. If there were some sort of metabolic benefit to the anatomical rearrangement, they would have done better with the actual surgery, but in some ways, they actually did worse. The caloric restriction alone resulted in similar improvements in blood sugar, pancreatic function, and insulin sensitivity, but several measures of diabetic control improved significantly more *without* the surgery.[574] So, if anything, the surgery seemed to put them at a metabolic disadvantage.

The bottom line is that type 2 diabetes is reversible with weight loss if you catch it early enough. With the loss of 15 percent of body weight, nearly 90 percent of those who've had type 2 diabetes for fewer than four years can achieve remission, whereas it may only be reversible in 50 percent of those who've lived with the disease for longer than eight years.[575] That's losing weight with diet alone, though. The remission numbers for diabetics losing more than twice as much weight with bariatric surgery may only be around 62 percent and 26 percent, respectively.[576] So losing weight with your fork can be more than twice as effective as the surgeons' knives.

Losing weight without resorting to surgery may offer other benefits as well. In the Anti-Inflammatory section, I'll discuss the slimming hormone leptin. Losing weight with diet alone can improve leptin sensitivity,[577] but losing weight from gastric bypass apparently does not.[578] Diabetics losing weight with diet alone can also improve markers of systemic inflammation, such as tumor necrosis factor, whereas levels significantly worsened when about the same amount of weight was lost from a gastric bypass.[579]

The Blind Leading the Blind

What about diabetic complications? Two of the reasons we don't want diabetes are that we don't want to go blind and we don't want to go on dialysis.

Reversing diabetes with bariatric surgery can improve kidney function[580] but, surprisingly, may not prevent the appearance[581] or progression of diabetic vision loss.[582] Perhaps this is because bariatric surgery affects diet quantity but not necessarily diet quality. This reminds me of a famous study published in *The New England Journal of Medicine* that randomized thousands of diabetics to an intensive lifestyle program that focused on weight loss. Ten years in, the study was stopped prematurely because the diabetics weren't living any longer or having any fewer heart attacks.[583] This may be because they remained on the same heart-clogging diet, but just with smaller portions.

There is a diet that has been shown to reverse diabetic eye disease: Dr. Kempner's rice and fruit diet. More than a half century ago, Walter Kempner at Duke University showed that his plant-based diet, ultralow in sodium, fat, cholesterol, and animal protein, could not only reverse advanced heart and kidney failure[584] but diabetic retinopathy as well, with some patients going from not even being able to read headlines to having normal vision.[585]

How do we treat severe diabetic retinopathy these days? With intravitreal drugs (meaning injections straight into your eyeball). If those don't work, there's always panretinal laser photocoagulation, in which laser burns are etched over nearly the entire back of your eye[586] in the hope that the little pieces left behind may get more of the blood flow.[587] When I see this, along with Kempner's work, I can't help but feel like history has been reversed. It would be one thing if, a half century ago, the best we had was a barbaric burn-out-your-eye-socket surgery but, thankfully, we've since learned that we can reverse the vision loss through dietary means alone. But instead of learning, medicine seems to have forgotten.

Kempner also proved massive obesity could be corrected "without drastic intervention," showing people could lose hundreds of pounds through lifestyle changes alone, without resorting to hospitalization, drugs, or surgery.[588] His diet was itself pretty drastic (certainly not to be undertaken without medical supervision),[589] but at least it didn't entail getting one's internal organs cut open and stapled. "Even if surgery proves sustainably effective," wrote the founding director of the Yale-Griffin Prevention Research Center, "the need to rely on the rearrangement of natural gastrointestinal anatomy as an alternative to better use of feet and forks [exercise and diet] seems a societal travesty."[590]

Through Thick and Thin

How sustainable is weight loss with bariatric surgery? Over the first year or two after the procedure, most gastric bypass patients do end up regaining some of the weight they had lost,[591] but five years later, three-quarters maintain at least a 20 percent weight loss.[592] The typical trajectory for someone who starts out obese at 285 pounds, for example, would be to drop to an overweight 178 pounds two years after bariatric surgery but then regain back up to an obese 207 pounds.[593] This has been chalked up to "grazing" behavior, where compulsive eaters may shift from bingeing, which becomes more difficult post-surgery, to constantly eating smaller amounts throughout the day.[594] Eight years out, about half of gastric bypass patients continue to describe episodes of disordered eating.[595] As one pediatric obesity specialist described, "I have seen many patients who put chocolate bars into a blender with some cream, just to pass technically installed obstacles" such as a gastric band.[596]

Bariatric surgery advertisements are filled with happily-ever-after fairy-tale narratives of cherry-picked outcomes, offering, as one ad analysis put it, "the full Cinderella-romance happy ending."[597] This may contribute to the finding that patients often overestimate the amount of weight they're going to lose and underestimate the difficulty of the recovery process.[598] Surgery forces profound changes in eating habits, requiring slow, small, thoroughly chewed bites. The stomach goes from the volume of two softballs down to about the size of half a tennis ball in stomach stapling and about half a Ping-Pong ball in the case of gastric bypass or banding.[599]

As you can imagine, weight regain after surgery can have devastating psychological effects, as patients may feel they failed their last resort.[600] This could help explain why bariatric surgery patients are at a higher risk of depression[601] and suicide.[602] Severe obesity alone may increase risk of suicidal depression,[603] but even at the same weight, those going through surgery appear to be at higher risk.[604] At the same BMI, age, and gender, bariatric surgery recipients have about four times the odds of suicide.[605] Most convincingly, before-and-after "mirror-image analysis" shows the risk of serious self-harm increases post-surgery in the same individuals.[606]

Nearly one in fifty bariatric surgery patients ends up being hospitalized for self-harm or attempted suicide.[607] Furthermore, this only includes confirmed self-harm episodes, excluding masked attempts[608] such as overdoses of "undetermined intention."[609] Bariatric surgery patients also have an elevated risk of "accidental death,"[610] though some of this may be due to changes in alcohol metabolism. When gastric bypass patients have two shots of vodka, for example, because of their altered anatomy, their blood alcohol levels shoot up past the legal driving limit within minutes.[611] It's unclear, however, whether this plays a role in the 25 percent increase in prevalence of alcohol problems noted during the second postoperative year.[612]

Even those who successfully lose the excess weight and keep it off appear to have a hard time coping. Ten years out, though health-related quality of life improves, general mental health tends to significantly deteriorate compared to presurgery levels—even among the biggest losers.[613] Ironically, there's a common notion that bariatric surgery is for "cheaters"[614] who take the "easy way" out by choosing the "low-effort" method of weight loss.[615] Shedding the pounds may not shed the stigma of even prior obesity. Studies suggest that, in the eyes of others, knowing someone was fat in the past leads them to always be treated more like a fat person. And there's a strong anti-surgery bias on top of that, such that those who choose the scalpel to lose weight are rated most negatively (for example, thought of as least physically attractive).[616] One can imagine how remaining a target of prejudice even after joining the "in-group" could potentially undercut psychological well-being.

Weighing the Options

In the Middle Ages, starving peasants dreamed of gastronomic utopias where food rained down from the sky. The English called it the Kingdom of Cockaigne. Little could medieval fabulists predict that many of their descendants would not only take permanent residence there but also cut out parts of their stomachs and intestines to combat the abundance.[617]

A body gaining weight when excess calories are available for consumption is behaving as it should.[618] Efforts to curtail such weight gain with drugs or surgery are not efforts to correct an anomaly in human physiology but rather to deconstruct and reconstruct its normal operations at the core. Critics have pointed out this irony of surgically altering healthy organs to make them dysfunctional ("malabsorptive") on purpose,[619] especially when it comes to operating on children. Bariatric surgery for kids and teens is becoming widespread[620] and is being performed in children as young as five years old.[621]

Surgeons defend the practice by arguing that growing up fat can leave emotional scars and "lifelong social retardation."[622]

Promoters of preventive medicine argue that bariatric surgery is the proverbial "ambulance at the bottom of the cliff."[623] In response, a proponent of pediatric bariatric surgery said, "It is often pointed out that we should focus on prevention. Of course, I agree. However, if someone is drowning, I don't tell them, 'You should learn how to swim'; no, I rescue them."[624]

A strong case can be made that the benefits of bariatric surgery far outweigh the risks if the alternative is remaining morbidly obese, which is estimated to shave off up to thirteen years of one's life.[625] Although there are no data from randomized trials yet to back it up, compared to obese individuals who hadn't been operated on, those getting bariatric surgery would be expected to live significantly longer on average.[626] It's no wonder surgeons consistently frame the elective surgery as a life-or-death necessity,[627] but this is a false dichotomy. The benefits only outweigh the risks if there are no other alternatives.

Like Lead Balloons

With much fanfare, the 1980s brought us intragastric balloons that could be implanted into the stomach and inflated with air or water to fill up much of the space.[628] Sadly, surgical devices are often brought to market before there is adequate evidence of safety and effectiveness,[629] and the balloons were no exception.

The "Gastric Bubble" had its bubble burst when a study at the Mayo Clinic found that eight out of ten balloons spontaneously deflated (which is potentially dangerous, as they could pass into the intestines and cause an obstruction[630]), but not before causing gastric erosions—that is, damage to the stomach lining—in half the patients.[631] The kicker is that, in terms of inducing weight loss, the device didn't even work.[632] It was eventually pulled from the market, but now balloons are back.

After a thirty-three-year hiatus, the FDA started approving a new slew of intragastric balloons in 2015,[633] resulting in more than five thousand placements.[634] By then, the Sunshine Act had been passed in order to shine a disinfecting light on industry enticements by forcing drug companies and the surgical and medical device industry to disclose any payments they were making to physicians.[635] Most people now know about the overly cozy financial relationships doctors can have with Big Pharma, but fewer realize that surgeons can also get payments from the companies manufacturing the devices they use.[636] The hundred top recipients of industry payments received an unbelievable $12 million from device companies in a single year. Yet when these doctors published papers, only a minority disclosed the blatant conflict of interest.[637]

The benefit of balloons over most types of bariatric surgery is that they're reversible, but that doesn't mean they're benign. The FDA has released a series of advisories about their risks, which includes cases of patient fatalities due to a stomach rupture.[638] How could someone suffer a gastric perforation from a smooth, rounded object? By causing the patient to puke so much they rip open their stomach and die.[639] Nausea and vomiting are unsurprising and very common side effects, affecting the majority of those who have balloons placed.[640] Persistent vomiting likely also explains cases of life-threatening nutrient deficiencies after balloon implantation.[641]

Some complications, such as bowel obstruction, are due to the balloon deflating,[642] but others, oddly enough, are due to the balloons suddenly overinflating,[643] causing pain, vomiting, and abdominal distention.[644] This was first noticed in breast implants, as documented in reports such as "The Phenomenon of the Spontaneously Autoinflating Breast Implant."[645] Out of nowhere, the implants just started growing, increasing breast volume by an average of more than 50 percent.[646] "It remains," one review noted, "an underreported and poorly understood phenomenon."[647] (Interestingly, breast implants were actually used as some of the first failed experimental intragastric balloons.[648])

As with any medical decision, though, it's all about risks versus benefits. Industry-funded trials display notable weight loss, but it's hard to tease out the effect of the balloon alone from the accompanying supervised diet and lifestyle changes prescribed along with the devices in the studies.[649] In drug trials, you can randomize subjects to sugar pills, but how do you eliminate the placebo effect of undergoing a procedure? You perform sham surgery.

In 2002, a courageous study was published in *The New England Journal of Medicine*. Knee arthroscopy, the most common orthopedic surgery, was put to the test. Billions of dollars are spent sticking scopes into knee joints and cutting away damaged tissue in osteoarthritis and knee injuries, but does the surgery actually work? Knee pain sufferers were randomized to get either the real surgery or a sham surgery in which surgeons sliced into people's knees and pretended to perform the procedure, complete with splashing saline, but never actually did anything within the joint.

The trial caused an uproar. How could anyone randomize people to get cut open for fake surgery? Professional medical associations questioned the ethics of the surgeons and the sanity of the patients who agreed to be part of the trial.[650] But guess what happened? Yes, the surgical patients got better, but so did the placebo patients. The surgeries had no actual effect.[651,652] Currently, heart stents[653] and rotator cuff shoulder surgery are facing the same crisis of confidence.[654]

When intragastric balloons were put to the test, sham controlled trials show both older[655] and newer[656] devices sometimes fail to offer any weight-loss benefit. Even when they do work,[657] the weight loss may be temporary because balloons are only allowed to stay in for six months, at which point the deflation risk gets too great. Why can't we keep putting in new ones? That's been tried, and it failed to improve long-term weight outcomes.[658] A sham controlled trial showed that any effects of the balloon on appetite and satiety may vanish with time,[659] perhaps as our bodies get used to the new normal.

What sham-surgery trials have shown us is that some of our most popular surgeries are themselves shams. Doctors like to pride themselves on being men and women of science. We rightly rail against the anti-vaccination movement, for example. Many of us in medicine have been troubled by the political trend of people choosing their own "facts." When I read that some of these still-popular surgeries are not only useless[660] but may actually make things worse—for example, increasing the risk of progression to a total knee replacement[661]—I can't help but think we doctors are not immune to our own versions of "fake news" and "alternative facts."[662]

Diet Drugs

One Pill Makes You Smaller

We worship medical magic bullets in this country. Yet, despite the full menu of FDA-approved medications for weight loss these days, they've only been prescribed for about one in fifty obese patients.[663] What gives? One of the reasons anti-obesity drugs are so highly stigmatized[664] is that, historically, they've been anything but magical; the bullets have been blanks, or worse.[665]

To date, most weight-loss drugs, despite their initial approval, have been pulled from the market for unforeseen side effects that turned them into a public threat.[666] As I explore in the Fat Burners section, it all started with DNP, a pesticide with a promise to safely melt away fat[667]—but instead melted away people's eyesight.[668] (The DNP disaster, in fact, helped lead to the passage of the Federal Food, Drug, and Cosmetic Act in 1938.[669]) Thanks to online accessibility, DNP has made a comeback with predictably lethal results.[670]

Then came the amphetamines. Currently, more than half a million Americans are addicted to amphetamines like crystal meth,[671] but the original amphetamine epidemic was generated by doctors and drug companies.[672] By the 1960s, pharmaceutical companies were churning out about eighty thousand kilos a year, which is nearly enough for a weekly dose for every man, woman, and child in the United States. Literally billions of doses were taken each year, and weight-loss clinics were raking in huge profits. A dispensing diet doctor could buy one hundred thousand amphetamine tablets for less than $100 and turn around and sell them to patients for $12,000.[673]

At a 1970 Senate hearing, Senator Thomas Dodd, father of Dodd-Frank senator Chris Dodd, suggested America's speed freak problem was no "accidental development." He said the pharmaceutical industry's "multihundred million dollar advertising budgets, frequently the most costly ingredient in the price of a pill, have, pill by pill, led, coaxed and seduced post–World War II generations into the 'freakedout' drug culture."[674] I'll leave drawing the Big Pharma parallels to the current opioid crisis as an exercise for the reader.

Aminorex was a widely prescribed appetite suppressant before it was pulled for causing lung damage.[675] Eighteen million Americans were on fen-phen before it was pulled[676] for causing severe damage to heart valves.[677] Meridia was pulled for heart attacks and strokes,[678] Acomplia for psychiatric side effects including suicide,[679] and the list goes on.[680]

The fen-phen debacle resulted in some of the largest litigation payouts in the industry's history, but it's all baked into the formula.[681] A new weight-loss drug may injure and kill so many that "expected litigation cost" could exceed $80 million, but Big Pharma consultants estimated in the journal *PharmacoEconomics* that, if successful, the drug could bring in excess of $100 million.[682] You do the math.

Think Outside the Black Box

Current options for weight-loss medications include Qsymia, a combination of phentermine, the *phen* in fen-phen, and topiramate, a drug that can cause seizures if you abruptly stop taking it.[683] Qsymia was explicitly rejected multiple times for safety reasons in Europe but remains for sale in the United States. Belviq (lorcacerin) is in a similar boat, allowed here but not in Europe out of concerns about it possibly causing cancers, psychiatric disorders, and heart valve problems.[684] It's sold in the United States for about $200 a month, a bargain compared to the latest addition: Saxenda (liraglutide).

A drug requiring daily injections, Saxenda is listed at $1,281.96 for a thirty-day supply.[685] It carries a black box warning—FDA's strictest caution about potentially life-threatening hazards—for thyroid cancer risk.[686] Paid consultants and employees of the company that makes it argue the greater number of breast tumors found among drug recipients may be due to "enhanced ascertainment," meaning easier breast cancer detection due to the drug's effectiveness.[687] Contrave (bupropion/naltrexone) is another option if you choose to ignore its own black box warning about a potential increase in suicidal thoughts.[688]

Alli (orlistat) is the final choice. That's the drug that blocks fat absorption and causes side effects such as "flatus with discharge."[689] The drug evidently "forces the patient to use diapers and to know the location of all the bathrooms in the neighborhood in an attempt to limit the consequences of urgent leakage of oily fecal matter."[690] A Freedom of Information Act exposé found that although company-sponsored studies claimed "all adverse events were recorded,"[691] one trial apparently conveniently failed to mention 1,318 of them.[692]

What's a little bowel leakage compared to the ravages of obesity, though?[693] As always, risks versus benefits, right? But in an analysis of more than one hundred clinical trials of anti-obesity medications lasting up to forty-seven weeks, drug-induced weight loss never exceeded nine pounds.[694] Since you're not treating the underlying cause—a fattening diet—the weight tends to come right back when people stop taking these drugs,[695] so you'd have to take them every day for the rest of your life. How well are people able to stay on them? Using pharmacy data from a million people, most Alli users stopped after the first purchase, and most Meridia users didn't even make it three months. Taking weight-loss meds is so disagreeable that 98 percent of people stopped taking them within the first year.[696]

Studies show many doctors tend to overestimate the amount of weight loss caused by these drugs.[697] One reason may be that some clinical practice guidelines, like those of the Endocrine Society, go out of their way to advocate pharmacotherapy for obesity.[698] Are they seriously recommending drugging 40 percent of Americans—more than one hundred million people?[699] At this point, you will not be surprised to learn that the principal author of the guidelines had a "significant financial interest or leadership position" in six separate pharmaceutical companies that all, coincidentally, work on obesity drugs.[700] In contrast, independent expert panels, like the Canadian Task Force on Preventive Health Care, explicitly recommend against weight-loss drugs given their poor track records of safety and efficacy.[701]

Weight-Loss Supplements

Bad Manufacturing Practices

According to a national survey, a third of adults who've made serious efforts at weight loss have tried using dietary supplements,[702] for which Americans spend literally billions of dollars every year.[703] Most people surveyed mistakenly thought that over-the-counter appetite suppressants, herbal products, and weight-loss supplements had to be approved for safety by a government agency like the FDA before being sold to the public—or at least include some kind of warning on the label about potential side effects. Nearly half even thought they had to demonstrate some sort of effectiveness.[704] None of that is true.

The FDA estimates that dietary supplements in general cause fifty thousand adverse events annually,[705] most commonly liver and kidney damage.[706] Meanwhile, prescription drugs don't just adversely affect but actually kill more than one hundred thousand Americans every year.[707] But at least with prescription meds, you notionally have the opportunity to parse out the risks versus the benefits, thanks to testing and monitoring requirements typically involving thousands of individuals.[708] When the manufacturer of the ephedrine-containing dietary supplement Metabolife 356 had it tested in a study that ended up with just twenty-four people, only minor side effects were found (like dry mouth, headache, and insomnia).[709] However, once unleashed on the populace, nearly fifteen thousand adverse effects were reported before it was pulled from the market, including heart attacks, strokes, seizures, and deaths.[710]

Given the lack of government oversight, there's no guarantee that what's on the label is even inside the bottle. FDA inspectors have found that 70 percent of supplement manufacturers violated so-called Good Manufacturing Practices, which are considered the *minimum* quality standards,[711] such as basic sanitation and ingredient identification. Not 7 percent, but 70 percent.

DNA testing of herbal supplements across North America found that most could not be authenticated. In 68 percent of the supplements tested, the main labeled ingredient was missing completely and substituted with something else. For example, a "St. John's Wort" supplement contained nothing but senna,[712] a laxative that can cause anal blistering.[713] Only two out of twelve supplement companies had products that were accurately labeled.[714]

The problem isn't limited just to fly-by-night phonies in some dark corner of the internet. The New York State Attorney General commissioned DNA testing of seventy-eight bottles of commercial herbal supplements sold by Walgreens, Walmart, Target, and GNC. Four out of five bottles didn't contain any of the herbs listed on their labels. Instead, capsules were often stuffed with little more than cheap fillers like powdered rice "and houseplants."[715]

Getting More Than You Paid For

Weight-loss supplements are also infamous for being adulterated with drugs.[716] Of 160 "100% natural" weight-loss supplements sampled, more than half were tainted with drugs, ranging from antidepressants to erectile dysfunction meds.[717] Diuretic drugs are frequent contaminants, which makes sense.[718] In the Intermittent Fasting section, I talk about rapid water loss as the billion-dollar gimmick that has sold low-carb diets for more than a century.

Researchers in Denver tested every weight-loss supplement they could find within a ten-mile radius and alarmingly found a third were adulterated with *banned* ingredients, and 90 percent contained "discouraged-use" components.[719] The most common illegal adulterant of weight-loss supplements is sibutramine, the Meridia drug that was yanked off the market back in 2010 for heart attack and stroke risk,[720] and is now blamed for cases of slimming supplement–induced psychosis.[721] An analysis of weight-loss supplements bought off the internet and advertised with claims such as "purely natural," "harmless," or "traditional herbal" found that a third contained a high dose of sibutramine and the rest contained caffeine. Wouldn't we be able to tell if caffeine were added to a supplement? Perhaps not if the supplement also contained temazepam, a controlled-substance benzodiazepine downer sedative found in half of the caffeine-tainted supplements.[722]

Doesn't the FDA demand recalls of adulterated supplements? Yes, but the pills just pop up again on store shelves. Twenty-seven supplements purchased at least six months after recalls were retested, and two-thirds still contained banned substances. At the follow-up testing, seventeen supplements out of twenty-seven had the same pharmaceutical adulterant found originally, and six contained one or more *additional* banned ingredients.[723] And unfortunately, the manufacturers aren't sufficiently penalized for noncompliance. As a founding fellow of the Institute for Science in Medicine put it, "Fines for violations are small compared to the profits."[724]

Slim Pickings

One of the ways supplement makers can skirt the law is by labeling them "not intended for human consumption," for example, labeling the fatal fat-burner DNP as an industrial or research chemical.[725] That's how designer street drugs can be sold openly at gas stations and convenience stores as "bath salts."[726] Another way is to claim that synthetic stimulants added to slimming supplements are actually natural food constituents, like listing the designer drug dimethylamylamine as "geranium oil extract." The FDA banned dimethylamylamine in 2012 after it was determined DMAA was "not found in geraniums." (Who eats geraniums anyway?[727]) Despite being tentatively tied to cases of sudden death[728] and hemorrhagic stroke,[729] DMAA has continued to be found in weight-loss supplements with innocuous names like Simply Skinny Pollen made by Bee Fit with Trish.[730]

There is little doubt that certain banned supplements like ephedra could help people lose weight.[731] "There's only one problem," wrote a founding member of the American Board of Integrative Medicine. "This supplement may kill you."[732]

Are there any safe and effective dietary supplements for weight loss? When nine popular slimming supplements were put to the test in a randomized placebo-controlled trial, not a single one could beat out placebo sugar pills.[733] A systematic review of diet pills came to a similar conclusion: None appears to generate appreciable impacts on body weight without undue risks.[734] One such systematic review of "nutraceutical" supplements out of the Weight Management Center at Johns Hopkins University ended with this:

> In closing, it is fitting to highlight that perhaps the most general and safest alternative/herbal approach to weight control is to substitute low–energy density foods for high–energy density and processed foods, thereby reducing total energy intake. By taking advantage of the low–energy density and health-promoting effects of plant-based foods, one may be able to achieve weight loss, or at least assist weight maintenance without cutting down on the volume of food consumed or compromising its nutrient value.[735]

Licensed to Swill

Even if harmless, there's a way weight-loss supplements could actually make you gain weight, thanks to a fascinating glitch of human psychology called *self-licensing*.[736] This is when we unwittingly justify doing something that pulls us away from our goals, right after we've done something that moves us toward them. We reward ourselves with an indulgence that sets us back.

When smokers were told they were given "vitamin C" supplements, they subsequently smoked more cigarettes than if they had been given what were identified as "placebo" pills—even though both groups had been given identical sugar pills. The "vitamin C" group smoked nearly twice as much, perhaps thinking at some subconscious level that since they had just done something good for their health by taking a "supplement," they could afford to "live a little," when, in effect, it may have indeed occasioned them to live a little . . . less.[737]

You can see how self-licensing can translate into other lifestyle arenas. Other studies have shown that those given placebo pills they believed to be dietary supplements not only expressed less desire to subsequently engage in exercise but followed through by walking about a third less. Compared to those who were told the pills were placebos, misled participants were also more likely to choose a buffet over a "healthful, organic meal."[738] Would they eat more too? A seminal study entitled "The Liberating Effect of Weight Loss Supplements on Dietary Control" put it to the test.

Participants were randomized to take a known placebo or a purported weight-loss supplement that was actually just the same placebo, and they were later covertly observed at a buffet. Not only did the "supplement" subjects eat more foods, they chose less-healthy items.[739] They also ate about 30 percent more candy in a bogus "taste test" and ordered more sugary drinks.[740] "Hence," the investigators concluded, "people who rely on dietary supplements for health protection may pay a hidden price: the curse of licensed self-indulgence."[741]

Policy Approaches

System Failure

The public health community appears to have all but given up on ending the obesity epidemic. The latest World Health Organization goals include a 2025 obesity target of just trying to shoot for a zero increase in further prevalence.[742] Even such a modest-sounding low bar may represent one of the greatest challenges facing global health. Though there have been isolated pockets of patchy progress, no country has yet reversed the epidemic.

The promotion of the overconsumption of high-calorie, low-nutrient foods and beverages has been identified as the major driver of the obesity pandemic.[743] Now that we have rid much of the world of pestilence and famine, some public health proponents have gone as far as to suggest that the "new vectors of disease" are taking the form of "trans-national food corporations that market salt, fat, sugar, and calories in unprecedented quantities."[744] Blame has been laid at the feet of lobbying efforts of the food industry,[745] which is considered the world's biggest industry.[746] The processed food makers alone may bring in trillions.[747] "Put simply," concluded a senior director at the George Institute for Global Health, "the enormous commercial success enjoyed by the food industry is now causing what promises to be one of the greatest public health disasters of our time."[748]

But remember—corporations just do what they're set up to do. Their goal is not to make people fat but to make people money.[749] The food industry manipulates ingredients like salt, sugar, and fat and throws in caffeine and flavor-enhancing chemicals for reasons no more nefarious than maximizing profits. Markets often incentivize companies to cater to, and take advantage of, human weaknesses.[750] The food and beverage CEOs simply have a fiduciary responsibility to maximize quarterly profits for their shareholders.

But why not sell apples instead of Apple Jacks or oranges instead of Orange Crush? To quote from Slick Willie Sutton's apocryphal answer to why he robbed banks: "That's where the money is." The reason some of the unhealthiest foods are marketed is one of simple economics: Real food goes bad.[751] Fruits and vegetables are perishable. What shareholders want is a snack cake that lasts for weeks on the shelf.

On top of that, real food doesn't have brand names. Why would a broccoli grower put an ad on TV when you'd just as likely buy their competitor's broccoli? The system is simply not set up to reward the sale of health-promoting food.

And finally, real food costs money to grow. Shareholders don't want dirt—they want dirt-cheap commodities such as corn syrup, preferably discounted by taxpayer subsidies, that they can then mix with carbonated water and sell for a few bucks a bottle. Burgers on the Dollar Menu are there thanks in part to hundreds of billions of dollars of federal subsidies for cheap animal feed.[752] Those who resist calls for "heavy-handed" government regulation may not realize those heavy hands are already pressing down the scale on the side of Big Business.

Using the Anti-Tobacco Playbook

What we learned from the tobacco experience, wrote two preeminent public health scholars, is how powerfully profits can motivate "even at the cost of millions of lives and unspeakable suffering." Here they quote a U.S. district judge ruling on a tobacco case:

All too often in the choice between the physical health of consumers and the financial well-being of business, concealment is chosen over disclosure, sales over safety, and money over morality. Who are these persons who knowingly and secretly decide to put the buying public at risk solely for the purpose of making profits, and who believe that illness and death of consumers is an apparent cost of their own prosperity?[753]

Tobacco is one of our great public health victories. The share of adults who smoke declined from 42 percent in 1965[754] down to just 15 percent today.[755] That's about five out of twelve down to fewer than two out of twelve. Thanks to the decline, cigarettes now only kill about a half million Americans a year, whereas our diets kill many thousands more. Currently, the leading cause of death in America is the American diet.[756]

Might we be able to use the same strategies that were so successful in the battle against Big Tobacco? It may be no coincidence that three of the most cost-effective policy interventions against obesity seem to be taken straight from the tobacco wars: (1) taxes on unhealthy products, (2) front-of-pack labeling, and (3) a restriction on advertising to children.[757]

Death and Taxes

Excise taxes on cigarettes have been cited as the single most effective weapon in slashing smoking rates.[758] A twenty-five-cents-per-pack tax to help deal with some of the societal costs of smoking was tied to as much as a 9 percent decrease in smoking rates.[759] The World Health Organization has estimated that a 70 percent global increase in the price of cigarettes could prevent up to a quarter of all tobacco-related deaths worldwide.[760]

Extending taxes on alcohol and tobacco to foodstuffs was proposed by none other than Adam Smith in his 1776 *Wealth of Nations*: "Sugar, rum, and tobacco, are commodities which are nowhere necessaries of life, which are become objects of almost universal consumption, and which are, therefore, extremely proper subjects of taxation."[761] People have the right to smoke, drink, and eat fattening foods, the logic goes, but perhaps they should help defray some of the publicly funded medical costs that result from their unhealthy habits.[762]

A penny-per-ounce tax on sugar-sweetened beverages could bring in more than a billion dollars a year in states like Texas and California.[763] A 10 percent tax on fattening foods on a national level could yield half a trillion dollars over ten years.[764] Even if such a tax were combined with a subsidy that lowered the cost of fruits and vegetables by 10 percent, it would be expected to net hundreds of billions of dollars. But would it change anyone's eating habits? Just a small price differential of about 10 percent between unleaded and leaded gas was able to shift the entire auto industry away from lead.[765] What we want to know now is whether such a price difference could also shift Americans to apples from apple pie.

A systematic review of the available evidence suggests that dietary financial incentives and disincentives do work. The cheaper we make fruits and vegetables, the more people said they'd buy, and the more we tax unhealthy foods, the lower their consumption drops.[766] Based on this kind of modeling, a tax on saturated fat (found mostly in fatty meat, dairy, and junk) could potentially save thousands of lives a year.[767]

But wouldn't such a tax disproportionately affect the poor? Yes, in that we would expect the impoverished to *benefit* the most. It's like cigarette taxes.[768] The classic tobacco industry argument is that cigarette taxes are "unfair" and "regressive," burdening the poor the most, to which the public health community responded: "Cancer is unfair." Indeed, cancer disproportionately burdens the poor,[769] so these types of taxes would be expected to affect the greatest health gains for the least well-off.

The fact that the tobacco industry fought tooth and nail against cigarette taxes—doing everything from inventing industry front groups to overtly buying off politicians[770]—suggests that taxes can indeed be a powerful tool to shift people's habits, but much of the evidence on changing food behaviors has not been based on real-life data. When people are put through high-tech, 3-D supermarket simulators, researchers have shown that a 25 percent discount on fruits and vegetables appears to boost produce purchasing by the same amount—up to nearly two pounds a week.[771] Virtual vegetables, however, don't actually do you any good. Does this work in the real world with real food?

South Africa's largest private health insurer started offering up to 25 percent cash back on healthy food purchases to hundreds of thousands of households, up to the U.S. equivalent of $799 per month.[772] Why would the insurer give money away? Because it apparently increases consumption of fruits, vegetables, and whole grains, while at the same time decreasing consumption of foods high in added sugar, salt, and fat, including processed meats and fast food—which then would be expected to translate into reduced disease rates, saving the insurer money.[773]

Why not just pay people to lose weight directly? A systematic review found that eleven out of twelve studies on financial incentives for weight loss described positive results.[774] The one that failed to find a benefit of direct monetary inducements had only offered $2.80 a day.[775] With kids, you can get away with just giving them a nickel or a sticker to get them to choose dried fruit over a cookie as an afterschool snack, but as soon as the enticements ended, so did the change in behavior.[776]

Even if the incentives have to be made permanent, they might still pay for themselves. In the United States, every $1 spent taxing processed foods or milk might net an estimated $2 in health-care cost savings. Every $1 spent making vegetables cheaper could net $3, and subsidizing whole grains might offer more than a 1,000 percent return on investment.[777] Even a 1 percent decrease in the average price of all fruits and vegetables might prevent nearly ten thousand heart attacks and strokes every year.[778]

From Coke to Coors: Unintended Consequences

Sometimes dietary policy decisions can have unintended consequences. Swapping out sugary cookies for salty chips, for example, might not do the public's health many favors. One field study of a tax on soda found that it can drop soft drink purchases, but households may just end up buying more beer.[779] Another study found that, ironically, calorie labeling of sugary drinks led to an *increase* in consumption, presumed to be because the consumers may have previously overestimated their caloric content.[780]

Stark warnings about the risks of unintended, negative consequences of obesity-targeted health policies are trumpeted by those with ties to the likes of Coca-Cola, Kraft, PepsiCo, Wrigley, Red Bull, the World Sugar Research Organisation, the National Cattlemen's Beef Association, Mars, and corn syrup giant Archer Daniels Midland (and that is just a single scientist's list of funding sources).[781] The concern shouldn't paralyze our efforts, but it should serve up a healthy dose of humility when considering policy proposals.[782]

How about releasing a video game for kids that promotes fruit? Sounds

(continued)

good, right? Well, what do you think happened when kids were seated in front of bowls of fruit and candy, and randomized to play one of three different computer "advergames" (advertising-game hybrids incorporating product placements) that promoted either candy, fruit, or toys? The pro-candy game group ate more candy, but, disappointingly, the pro-fruit group didn't eat more fruit. Then it got interesting. The kids in the pro-fruit group *also* ate more candy. Compared to the pro-toy control group, having a kid play a video game promoting fruit led them to eat more candy. Presumably both the candy and fruit games just made the kids think about food, and they naturally gravitated to their preferred snacks.[783]

Among the most fascinating phenomena I've come across is the boomerang effect of "remedy messaging." One might presume that the advertising of smoking cessation aids like nicotine gum would help make quitting easier. After all, the vast majority of smokers want to quit,[784] so availing them of helpful options couldn't help but help, right? Instead, such remedy marketing can create a vicarious get-out-of-jail-free card that ends up reinforcing risky behavior. Exposure to nicotine replacement product advertising was found to undermine quitting intentions, especially among the heaviest smokers, the very ones who needed it the most. The thought is that smokers may subconsciously interpret the remedy as evidence that the hazards of smoking are more manageable and, therefore, less risky, which thereby helps to justify their habit.[785]

You can see how easily this would translate to the weight-loss arena. We explored how self-licensing could cause those taking slimming supplements to inadvertently eat more, but merely being exposed to an ad for a "fat-fighting pill" appeared to have a similar type of effect. So even when companies are ostensibly selling health rather than disease, they still may be inadvertently making the problem worse. And in the marketplace, there's just no incentive for risk-avoidance messaging. Nobody makes money selling *just say no* unless it can somehow be linked to salable products and services.[786]

A policy in France—where burgers now outsell baguettes[787]—may represent an interesting real-world example of the counterintuitive remedy-messaging effect. Industry lobbying took a valiant effort to ban the advertising of junk and morphed it into a mandate for preventive health messaging on junk food advertisements.[788] On products like Lay's Chips Saveur Poulet Rôti (chicken-flavored potato chips), you'll now see messages like *Pour votre santé, pratiquez une activité physique régulière* (*For your health, practice regular physical activity*).[789] Sounds good, right? Not so fast. Anytime an industry agrees to a regulation, one should get skeptical as to its effectiveness.

To see if such messaging might lead to a boomerang effect, research subjects were randomized to view a Big Mac advertisement with or without the preventive health message *For your health, eat at least five fruits and vegetables per day.* (After all, wouldn't it be great if McDonald's were forced to advertise healthy food?) The subjects then filled out a general questionnaire and, before they left, were allowed to choose one of two McDonald's coupons as a reward for their participation: a free sundae or a free bag of fruit.[790] Guess who was more likely to pick the fruit?

Only one in three who had just seen the straight burger advertisement, the one without the preventive health message, chose the fruit over the sundae, but that number fell to only about one in six among those who had been prompted to eat healthier.[791] Isn't that wild? The *absence* of the healthy message doubled the number of people choosing the healthy snack. The health message made things worse. This may be the remedy-messaging boomerang effect in action. Simultaneously offering a temptation with a reminder about how they can dig themselves out justifies the excuse to indulge. Subconsciously, it may give the chicken-y chip eater the rationalization that they can just work it off the next day at the gym, even if that day never comes.

The recommended antidote to avoid justification effects is to instead use negative framing.[792] That is, instead of offering a way out to compensate for indulging "just this one time," cautionary messages may be more effective. For example, imagine reading *Pour votre santé, évitez de manger trop gras, trop sucré, trop salé* (*For your health, avoid foods that are too fatty, too sweet, or too salty*) on your next chocolate-filled or ham-and-cheese croissant. That's a message for which I doubt Le McDonald's would be quite as enthusiastic.

Truth in Advertising

A tried-and-true method used by alcohol, tobacco, and food-related corporate interests to deflect attention away from health is to reframe something like a fat tax or soda tax as an issue of freedom, railing against the "nanny state" for restricting consumers' rights.[793] However, those complaining about the governmental manipulation of people's choices hypocritically tend to be fine with corporations doing the very same thing.[794] Case in point: former New York City mayor Michael Bloomberg's attempt to cap soft drink sizes. How dare he try to manipulate consumer choice! But isn't that just what the industry's done? In 1950, a twelve-ounce soda was the "king-sized" option.[795] Today, it's marketed as a child's portion. "King-sized" became "kid-sized."

The tobacco industry's classic "personal responsibility" trope does have a certain philosophical appeal.[796] As long as people understand the risks, shouldn't they be free to do whatever they want with their bodies? Sure, risk-taking affects others, but if you have the right to put your own life at risk, shouldn't you have the right to aggrieve your parents, widow your spouse, and orphan your children?[797] There is a social cost argument: People's bad decisions can cost society as a whole, and our tax dollars may have to care for them. As some health law scholars eloquently put it, "The independent individualist [motorcyclist], helmetless and free on the open road, becomes the most dependent of individuals in the spinal injury ward."[798]

For the sake of argument, though, let's forget these spillover effects. If someone understands the hazards, shouldn't they be able to do as they please? This assumes consumers have access to accurate and balanced information. How could smoking be a fully informed choice when tobacco companies spent decades *deliberately* suppressing, manipulating, and undermining the scientific evidence?[799] "Don't worry your pretty little head," said the nanny companies.

Is the food industry any different? We are bombarded with conflicting nutrition messages.[800] People love hearing good news about their bad habits, so clickbait headlines like "Butter Is Back" may sell a lot of magazines, but they sell the public short.

"It is not just Big Tobacco anymore," declared the director-general of the World Health Organization.[801] "Public health must also contend with

Big Food, Big Soda, and Big Alcohol. All of these industries fear regulation, and protect themselves by using the same tactics . . . front groups, lobbies, promises of self-regulation, lawsuits, and industry-funded research that confuses the evidence and keeps the public in doubt." It's like that infamous tobacco industry memo that read: "Doubt is our product since it's the best means of competing with the body of fact that exists in the mind of the general public."[802] The tobacco industry didn't have to convince the public that smoking was healthy to get people to keep consuming its products. It just needed to establish a controversy: Some science says it's bad, some says it's not so bad.

Conflicting messages in nutrition cause people to become so frustrated and confused they may just throw their hands up in the air and eat whatever's put in front of them, which is exactly what the industry wants.

No purveyor of unhealthy products wants the public to know the truth. An extraordinary example of this is the tobacco industry's 1967 response to the Fairness Doctrine. A court ruled that TV and radio stations had to run one health ad about smoking for every four tobacco ads they ran. Rather than risk the public being informed—even on a one-to-four basis—the tobacco companies withdrew all their own advertising from television.[803] They knew they couldn't compete with the truth. They needed to keep the public in the dark.

Now there are health warnings on each pack of cigarettes. Global travelers will notice, though, that while the U.S. mandate is met with simple, black-and-white text, other countries plaster evocative images, such as rotting gums, on their cigarette packs.[804] Canadian smokers are forced to look at a drooping cigarette with the caption TOBACCO USE CAN MAKE YOU IMPOTENT. Similarly, U.S. food packaging just has the inscrutable bring-your-calculator-to-the-grocery-store nutrition facts label on the back. I don't expect pictures of flaccid frankfurters, but other countries have tried to impose clear and simple front-of-package graphics to convey the health risks of fattening foods.[805]

"Signpost labeling" offers easy-to-understand traffic-light symbols alerting shoppers to the salt, sugar, and saturated fat content of products right on the front of every package.[806] When it's been tried, investment analysts at Citibank concluded, "The magnitude of the sales impacts is such that we are left with the inescapable conclusion that the increased prevalence of front-of-pack signposts may lead to marked changes in consumer buying habits." It works so well that green, yellow, and red traffic-light labeling poses "dire consequences" for certain food categories.[807] No wonder the food industry fought it fiercely, spending more than a billion dollars to defeat it in Europe, an amount that's ten times more than the drug industry lobby spends annually in the United States.[808]

It's in the food industry's interest to have the public confused about nutrition.

Vicarious Goal Fulfillment

What about labeling menus with calorie counts? Just as one might divine the significance of front-of-pack signpost labeling from the ferocity of the industry response, one could probably gauge the futility of calorie labeling by the ease at which such regulations have been passed. McDonald's voluntarily started doing it nationally in 2012[809] after a labeling mandate in New York City was found to have no overall effect on consumer behavior.[810] Studies suggest such voluntary labeling could boost "perceptions of the restaurant's concern for customers' well-being,"[811] while not stopping any Big Mac attacks.

At the same time, McDonald's announced plans for adding seasonal produce to its menu.[812] How cynical do you have to be to not at least recognize that as a good thing? Well, ironically, adding a healthy option can actually sway people to make even worse choices.

If you offer people with high self-control a choice of side dishes—something unhealthy like french fries or something more neutral like a baked potato—only about 10 percent of them will splurge for the fries. French fries are so unhealthy, though, that as a public health do-gooder, you add a third option, an even healthier one—a side salad—to appeal to their better natures. Even if they don't choose the salad, perhaps more will elect the middle-ground baked potato. So how much further does french-fry fancying fall by adding the salad option to the mix? It shoots *up* to more than 50 percent. Without the salad option, only one in ten chose the fries over the baked potato, but it jumped to more than half of the people just at the *sight* of salad.

The same thing happens when you offer people the choice of a bacon cheeseburger, a chicken sandwich, or a veggie burger. In a "No Healthy Option" scenario where people were offered the bacon cheeseburger, a chicken sandwich, or a fish sandwich, 17 percent chose the burger. When the fish sandwich was replaced with a veggie burger, however, the bacon cheeseburger preference more than doubled, up to 37 percent. How can just *seeing* a healthy option push people to make unhealthier choices? The title given to the paper describing these series of experiments is "Vicarious Goal Fulfillment: When the Mere Presence of a Healthy Option Leads to an Ironically Indulgent Decision." The thinking is that just by seeing the salad or plant-based option, people make the mental note to choose that the *next* time, thereby giving them the excuse to indulge now. Remember the self-licensing effect, where people making progress toward a goal rationalize making decisions that undermine it? These experiments suggest that even merely *considering* making progress can have a similar licensing effect.[813]

Note that the study participants weren't just moved to make the unhealthier choice, but the *unhealthiest* one. Even if people don't go for the salad or veggie burger option, you'd think that the presence of a healthier alternative might, at the very least, encourage people to choose something in between. Instead, it moved people in the opposite direction altogether. Compared to the "No Healthy Option" scenario of chocolate-covered Oreos, regular Oreos, or golden Oreos, adding a "lower-calorie" Oreo option doubled the likelihood study participants would go straight for the most indulgent chocolate-covered option. This is attributed to another illogical quirk of human psychology, the indelicately named *what-the-hell effect*. This is when one forbidden cookie can lead dieters to eat the whole bag. Once you've already strayed from your goals, why not go all the way? So once people decide they are going to get the salad the next time and spoil themselves "just this once," they might as well go for the most indulgent choice.[814]

The halo of healthy foods can even warp our perceptions. When weight-conscious people were shown a burger on its own and asked to estimate its calories, the average answer was 734 calories. What happened when people were shown the exact same burger, but this time, it was accompanied by three celery sticks? The estimated number of calories dropped to 619. Did they think the celery had negative calories? No, most knew the celery had calories, too, but just the juxtaposition made the burger seem healthier. The same thing happens when you add an apple next to a bacon-and-cheese waffle sandwich, a side salad to beef chili, or

(continued)

some carrots next to a cheesesteak. About one hundred calories appear to disappear.[815] Health halo effects may explain why people are more likely to order a dessert and more sugary drinks with a "healthier" sub at Subway versus a Big Mac at McDonald's, even though the sub used in the study (filled with ham, salami, and pepperoni) had 50 percent more calories than the Big Mac.[816]

Even just a reference to healthy foods can cause this unhealthy behavior. Remember that crazy Big Mac study where the eat-your-fruits-and-veggies message steered people toward the sundae instead of the fruit? The findings get even wackier. When asked to estimate the calorie content of the burger pictured in the ad without any health messaging, people guessed 646 calories.[817] What happened when the text *For your health, eat at least five fruits and vegetables per day* was added to the ad? All of a sudden, the same burger in the same ad appeared to only have 503 calories. So offering and even promoting salads and fruit can bring McDonald's accolades and bolster consumer loyalty without, ironically, helping their waistlines.[818]

Ad Nauseam

The third strategy taken from the anti-tobacco playbook, after taxes and front-of-pack labeling, is restricting advertising to children.[819] The food industry spends more money on advertising than any other industry,[820] with more than $10 billion in ads targeting American children and teens every year.[821] As a case study example, allow me to profile the number-one food advertised to kids: breakfast cereals.

There have been calls for nearly a half century to ban the advertising of sugary cereals to children, which Harvard nutrition professor Jean Mayer referred to as "sugar-coated nothings."[822] In a Senate hearing on nutrition education, he said, "Properly speaking, they ought to be called cereal-flavored candy, rather than sugar-covered cereals."[823]

The Senate committee had invited the major manufacturers of children's cereals to testify. They initially agreed to participate—until they heard the kinds of questions that were going to be asked. One cereal industry representative candidly admitted why he decided to boycott the hearing: He simply didn't have "persuasive answers" for why the industry tries to sell kids candy for breakfast.[824]

In the *Mad Men* age before the consumer movement was in bloom, advertising company executives were more willing to talk frankly about the purpose of their ads and how they felt about aiming them at the "child market."[825] For example, consider this 1965 quote from an ad executive for Kellogg's and Oscar Mayer:

> *Our primary goal is to sell products to children, not educate them. When you sell a woman a product and she goes in to the store and finds your brand isn't in stock, she will probably forget about it. But when you sell a kid on your product, if he can't get it, he will throw himself on the floor, stamp his feet and cry. You can't get a reaction like that out of an adult.*[826]

To preempt federal regulations, the industry pledged to self-regulate and launched the Children's Food and Beverage Advertising Initiative, in which all the big cereal companies promised they would only market healthier dietary choices to kids.[827] The candy industry signed on too. How did that go? Well, how do you think it went? They pledged not to advertise to children, yet after the initiative went into effect, kids actually saw *more* candy ads. Hershey, for example, more than doubled its advertising to children, while, at the same time, pledging not to advertise to children at all.[828]

The cereal companies got to decide for themselves their own definitions of "healthier dietary choices," and what they chose should give a sense of how serious they are about protecting children: They classified Froot Loops and Reese's Peanut Butter Puffs, which consist of up to 44 percent sugar by weight, as "healthier dietary choices."[829] In that case, what are their *unhealthy* choices?! Rather than base it on what might be best for children, they basically set the limit based more on the sugar content of everything they were already selling.[830]

The industry has since revised the "healthier dietary choices" criteria to allow only cereals that are below 38 percent sugar by weight.[831] Even if they're "only" one-third sugar, that means kids effectively are eating at least one spoonful of sugar in every three spoonfuls of cereal.[832] I wouldn't call that a healthy dietary choice.

The Federal Trade Commission (FTC) tried stepping it back in 1978, but industry poured in millions to fight it, and, with enough campaign contributions, Congress essentially threatened to yank the entire agency's funding if it continued to pursue industry regulations.[833] This demonstrated to a former CDC nutrition director "just how powerful market forces are compared to those that can be mobilized on behalf of children."[834] The political post-traumatic stress induced by the industry backlash delayed further federal efforts to rein in food marketing aimed at children for decades.

But then, enter the Interagency Working Group.[835] In 2011, FTC, CDC, FDA, and U.S. Department of Agriculture (USDA) all came together to propose *voluntary* principles designed to encourage stronger and more meaningful self-regulation. Their radical suggestion? Don't market cereal that is more than 26 percent sugar to children.[836]

Not a single one of the top ten breakfast cereals marketed to children would meet that standard.[837] General Mills shot back that the proposed nutrition standards were "arbitrary, capricious, and fundamentally flawed." After all, it pleaded, "literally *all* cereals marketed by General Mills would be barred from advertising."[838] One grocers' association called the proposed nutrition principles the "most bizarre and unconscionable" it had ever seen.[839] Cereal manufacturers charged that the suggested recommendations for voluntary self-regulation would unconstitutionally violate their "free speech rights" under the First Amendment,[840] to which the FTC basically offered to get them a dictionary so they could look up the meaning of the word *voluntary*.[841] All this gives you a sense of how freaked out the food industry got at even the *notion* of meaningful guidelines.

So what happened? Again, agency funding was put into jeopardy, so the interagency proposal was called off.[842] "We just got beat," one of the child advocacy organizations said. "Money wins." It apparently took $175 million of Big Food lobbying to buy the White House's silence as the interagency proposal got killed. As one Obama adviser put it, "You can tell someone to eat less fat, consume more fiber, more fruits and vegetables and less sugar. But if you start naming foods, you cross the line."[843]

"I'm upset with the White House," the chair of the Senate Health Committee said.[844] "They went wobbly in the knees, and when it comes to kids' health, they shouldn't go wobbly in the knees."

How We Won the Trans Fat Fight

In 2012, a prize-winning[845] exposé on corporate lobbyists found that the food and beverage industries had never lost a significant political battle in the United States, winning fight after fight at every level of government.[846] That all changed in 2018 with the successful ban on added trans fat in the American food supply. Trans fat, found largely in vegetable oils partially hydrogenated to mimic the qualities of animal fats in snack foods, was implicated in the deaths of tens of thousands of Americans every year.[847] So how did the public health movement finally triumph?

There are three broad approaches to mediating the ruin of risky choices: inform people (such as through labeling), nudge people (perhaps with financial incentives), or directly intervene to make the activity less harmful.[848] Which do you think prevented more car fatalities: mandating driver education, labeling cars about crash risk, or removing the human element by just making sure airbags are installed?[849] There are public education nutrition campaigns—from "sugar pack" ads on public transit informing consumers how much sugar there is in soft drinks[850] to "Hot Dogs Cause Butt Cancer" billboards educating people about the link between processed meat and colorectal cancer.[851] But just warning people about trans fat wasn't working.

We learned about the dangers of trans fat in 1993, when the Harvard Nurses' Health Study reported that high intake of trans fat may increase the risk of heart disease by 50 percent.[852] That's where the trans fat story started in Denmark—a story that ended a decade later with a ban on added trans fat in 2003.[853] It took another ten years before the United States even started considering a ban.[854] All the while, trans fat continued to kill the estimated tens of thousands of Americans every year,[855] resulting in as many years of healthy life lost as conditions like meningitis, cervical cancer, and multiple sclerosis.[856] If so many people were suffering and dying, why did it take so long for the United States to even *suggest* taking action?

One can look at the fight over New York City's trans fat ban for a microcosm of the national debate. Opposition came down hard from the food industry, complaining about "government intrusion" and likening the city to a "nanny state."[857] The livestock industries echoed[858] the everything-in-moderation argument made by the Institute of Shortening and Edible Oils[859] (since trans fat is present naturally in meat and dairy).[860] Another argument went: If "food zealots" get their wish in banning added trans fat, what's next?[861] Critics styled proposals for a trans fat ban as the "rise of food fascism,"[862] but it was really the restaurant and food industry that was limiting consumer choice, by so broadly fouling the food supply with these dangerous fats.[863]

Vested corporate interests tend to rally around these kinds of "slippery slope" arguments to distract from the fact that people are dying.[864] What if the government tries to make us eat broccoli? Unbelievably, that actually came up in a Supreme Court case over Obamacare. Chief Justice Roberts suggested Congress could start "ordering everyone to buy vegetables," a fear Justice Ginsburg dubbed "the broccoli horrible." Technically, Congress could compel the American public to eat more plant-based, Justice Ginsburg wrote, yet one can't "offer the 'hypothetical and unreal possibilit[y]' . . . of a vegetarian state as a credible [argument]."[865] As one legal scholar put it, "Judges and lawyers [may] live on the slippery slope of analogies; [but] they are not supposed to ski it to the bottom."[866]

But New York City eventually won its trans fat fight in 2006, preserving its status as a public health leader. New York, for example, banned lead paint eighteen years before federal action was taken despite decades of unequivocal evidence for harm.[867] Comparing stroke and heart attack rates before and after the rollout of the trans fat ban in different New York counties, researchers estimate the ban successfully reduced cardiovascular death rates by about 5 percent.[868] This then became the model for the nationwide ban in 2018.

How was public health able to triumph when past attempts to regulate the food industry failed? If you would have asked me back then about the odds of a trans fat ban, I would have answered: *Fat chance.*

In Denmark, as a leading Danish cardiologist put it, "Instead of warning consumers about trans fats and telling them what they are, we've simply removed them." The cardiologist continued, "As they say in North America, 'You can put poison in food if you label it properly.'"[869] And in America, things do seem to work differently. The belief is if people know the risks, they should be able to eat whatever they want—but that's assuming they're given all the facts. Unfortunately, this isn't always the case, especially given the food industry's "model of systemic dishonesty," as one health ethics professor put it.[870]

Because of the predilection for predatory deception and manipulation, government intervention was deemed necessary when it came to trans fat. But how did the ban get passed? First there was a labeling requirement. Manufacturers had to start adding trans fat content to the nutrition facts labels. This ostensibly was to influence consumers, but it may have had a bigger impact on producers. Now that they had to divulge the truth, companies scrambled to reformulate their products to gain a "no trans fat" competitive edge.

Within a year of the mandatory disclosure, more than five thousand products were introduced touting low or zero trans fat on their labels.[871] Kentucky Fried Chicken went from being sued for having some of the highest trans fat levels[872] to running an ad campaign where the mom tells the dad in front of the kids that KFC now has zero grams of trans fat. The father yells, "Yeah, baby! Whoooo!"—and begins eating fried chicken by the bucketful.[873] That was the secret to passing the ban. Once the major food industry players had already reformulated their products and bragged about it, once there wasn't so much money at stake, then there was insufficient political will to block the ban.

Leveling the Playing Field

Even without regulations, the market can be rapidly responsive, but only within certain parameters. The gluten-free craze is a great example. Ten years ago, how many people had even heard the word *gluten*? And now, some surveys suggest as many as 25 percent of the population is trying to avoid it.[874] This has led to an explosion of more than ten thousand products labeled as gluten-free,[875] including ones from major players, such as Tyson Foods launching gluten-free bacon and lunch meat.[876] Ironically, gluten-free products may be less healthy, with more sugar and salt, less fiber, and fewer nutrients, so they're mostly just different shades of the same processed junk.[877] A gluten-free donut is still a donut. And a nutritional analysis of foods marketed to children found that about 90 percent of products—both gluten-free and not—were classified as "unhealthy."[878]

That's the limit of the market. The invisible hand is more than happy to hand us any kind of junk we want—from SnackWell's to keto cookies. The industries can make money off any fad, except real food. Shareholders can profit off any kind of Funyuns but can't do much with real onions. Within a narrow scope of commodity components and chemicals, endless reformulations can fit any fashionable flavor of the month, but produce will never be as profitable.

The market even prevents food manufacturers from taking small steps to make their products less detrimental, such as lowering salt or sugar content. Any deviation from the levels perfectly engineered for maximum craveability could get you immediately undercut by your competitors. How then was England able to so successfully lower sodium intake, which has been associated with dramatic drops in stroke and heart disease deaths?[879] Because it was done across the board. McDonald's Chicken McNuggets have two and a half times more salt in the United States than in the United Kingdom, but that's because Burger King UK was cutting down too.[880]

In the best-documented population-level sodium reduction to date,[881] the British government formed public-private partnerships with major food manufacturers, retailers, and restaurant chains to simultaneously reduce sodium levels so slowly over the years that no one would notice.[882] The secret sauce may be the level playing field, so no company could gain a commercial advantage by outsalting competitors.[883] Analogous proposals have called for the stepwise, gradual, unobtrusive reduction in sugar in soft drinks to effect a similar shift in taste preferences on a population-wide scale.[884]

If this all sounds a bit Big Brother-y, realize that people can still season and sweeten to their heart's desire (or rather, detriment). Salt your nuggets all you want. Dump the whole shaker on them and wash it down with a bottle of corn syrup—it's still your body, your choice. It's like the proposed cap on soft drink sizes. You can still drink all the soda you want. The idea is just to try to make the default options a little healthier. It's easier to add salt to food on your plate than it is to remove it.

The lifesaving success of the trans fat ban and society-wide sodium reduction may lie in the convenience of improving consumers' diets without them having to change their behaviors.[885] Some view this as government overreach, but the slipperiest slope may be that of inaction. As the director of the Rudd Center for Food Policy and Obesity has pointed out, governments initially defaulted to business interests in the case of tobacco to try to counter all the industry lies with weak and ineffective attempts at consumer education. And look what happened: "The unnecessary deaths could be counted in the millions," he wrote. "The U.S. can ill afford to repeat this mistake with diet."[886]

Until the political will is summoned to make industry-wide changes in our food supply, we need to take personal responsibility for our own health and for our families' health because it looks to be a matter of life and death. So what does that best personal solution look like in the interim? That's what the rest of this book is all about.

II. Ingredients for the Ideal Weight-Loss Diet

INTRODUCTION

Fad Diet du Jour

The $50 billion weight-loss industry has been fed by an endless parade of fad diets offering quick-fix solutions. Dr. David L. Katz said it well, as he so often does: "In a market where buyers reject the tried and true in favor of false promises and pixie dust and in a culture where scapegoats and silver bullets are preferred over a prosaic blend of science and sense, the sellers respond accordingly."[887] Indeed, Amazon now lists more than thirty *thousand* weight-loss books.[888]

One of the defining characteristics of fad diets is their reliance on testimonials rather than scientific evidence,[889] but what's particularly insidious, beyond the nonsense and nonscience, is the pseudoscience—when the trappings of science are used to gain a false air of legitimacy. Confident, perhaps, that no one will actually check, some diet book authors (or likely their ghostwriters) cite scientific studies that either don't support their thesis or, at the very least, fail to accurately represent the best available balance of evidence.

When people have taken the time to check the primary sources, it is often to devastating effect.[890] See, for example, Seth Yoder's footnote-by-footnote review of *The Big Fat Surprise* on his blog, *The Science of Nutrition*.[891] Similarly, when researchers looked through *The South Beach Diet,* they didn't just find a few mistakes: Two-thirds of the nutrition "facts" they checked did not appear to be supported by peer-reviewed science.[892] You can always sell more books offering people good news about their bad habits, but at what human cost?

It's worth repeating that every penny I receive from all my books is donated directly to charity. It's written right into my publishing contracts. My overriding motivation is to provide the most accurate information possible. I'm such a stickler for veracity that I hired nine fact-checkers to go through every citation of the *How Not to Die* manuscript, and I committed to the same rigor with this book.

My original intention with *How Not to Diet,* consonant with the title, was to have chapters offering critical analysis on each of the leading popular diets, but I realized that would be like playing a game of Whac-A-Mole. I'm a member of the *U.S. News & World Report* Best Diets expert panel, tasked with scoring dozens of trending diets based on set criteria, and so I'm especially aware how many new diets pop up every year. I didn't want this book to be out of date before it even came out.

Thus, rather than taking a reactionary tactic and wasting page space on Dr. Quack's here-today-gone-tomorrow *New Snake Oil Diet* (now with added tricksy pixie dust!), I decided upon a more timeless, proactive approach: build an optimal weight-loss diet from the ground up. Based on the most compelling evidence my research team and I could find, I sought to generate a list of dietary attributes and components most effectual for weight loss. The best ingredients, if you will.

I've distilled this research into a list of seventeen key ingredients for an ideal weight-loss diet, which we'll explore one by one over the course of part II. These components can then be used to construct a portfolio of dietary changes to attack excess body fat on multiple fronts, as well as offer a template by which to compare any new diet that comes down the pike.

Many popular diets exist in an evidence-free zone powered by personal biases and aggrandizement, free from the bonds of scientific accountability.[893] A few large proprietary programs have been put under scientific scrutiny, though. So before we build an ideal weight-loss diet from scratch, let's briefly assess the current state of affairs.

Anecdotes as Evidence

Most Americans have tried to lose weight at some point in their lives, and as many as around one in three is actively making the attempt at any given moment.[894] This has spawned a massive weight-loss industry valued at more than $50 billion.[895] With so much money at stake, it comes as no surprise that there are so many different flavors of snake oil on tap. The history of weight-loss quackery includes everything from body jigglers to suction-cupped rolling pins. There was the Relax-a-cizor, an ironic name for a device that delivers electric shocks,[896] and wearing the Fat-Be-Gone ring promised the "same benefits as jogging up to six miles per day"![897] "Unwanted pounds and inches scrub right off" with the Amazing Seaweed Weight Loss Soap,[898] and don't forget the "amazing new super-formula" that will "overwhelm fat like Cary Grant overwhelmed your grandmother!"[899]

A major conclusion of congressional hearings on fraud in the diet industry was that the entire sector was characterized by deceptive and misleading advertising, rife with puffed-up promises.[900] In an analysis of hundreds of weight-loss advertisements, the FTC found that most ads made at least one claim that was very likely to be false or, at the very least, lacking adequate substantiation. Some were "grossly exaggerated," "obviously false claims" that were simply not "physiologically possible," like the product that guaranteed weight-loss efficacy comparable to "running a 20 mile marathon while you sleep." And it appears to be getting even worse. Compared to a similar analysis of ads in the 1990s, the FTC noted a "downward spiral to deception in weight-loss advertising."[901] The FTC has recovered millions for conned consumers, but a law journal article described the agency's actions as a "mere slap on the wrist" for an industry worth billions.[902]

By 2001, nearly 80 percent of all ads for weight-loss products or programs featured at least one testimonial.[903] Who doesn't love a good story?[904] Scientists often assert "anecdotes aren't data," but human nature may favor the opposite view—numbers are nice, but narratives can carry more meaning. Fund-raisers know this. They know to tug at the heart, not the head. It may not be surprising that people are more willing to donate to an African relief program after hearing a story of a starving little girl rather than give to an appeal outlining the dry statistics of the millions in need. But what *is* surprising is that when both the story and the stats are put together in the same appeal, people donate *less* than if they had heard just the anecdote.[905] We are notoriously prone to embracing anecdotal evidence,[906] and dietary hucksters rarely fail to exploit this hardwired human instinct.[907]

Researchers have compared the weight-loss claims of commercial programs to the actual results obtained from randomized controlled trials. Weight Watchers, for example, featured a testimonial of a woman who lost more than two hundred pounds after two years on the program[908]—but when Weight Watchers was actually put to the test, the average weight loss after two years was more like six pounds.[909] The Weight Watchers watched a lot more weight stay on than come off.

The Atkins website boasted a three-hundred-pound weight-loss testimonial, and Jenny Craig a four-hundred-pounder. The average advertised testimonial weight loss across twenty different programs was about fifty pounds, a number far in excess of what even the programs' own published trials have shown.[910] Even if the rare testimonial were true, we almost never hear what happens next. When researchers actually followed up on some of the people portrayed in the before-and-after pictures, only about one in four had sustained their success.[911] The commercial diet program that participated in this study must have suspected as much, as its cooperation with researchers was predicated on the stipulation that the program never be identified.[912] This is consistent with the findings of the Deception and Fraud in the Diet Industry hearings in Congress that concluded most programs actively suppress facts about what to expect regarding chances of success.[913]

Programmed to Fail?

Many real-world diet trials are small in size and short in duration, and most lack control groups and fail to follow through on weight loss over time.[914] However, there are exceptions. Americans spend billions a year on commercial weight-loss programs, such as Weight Watchers, Nutrisystem, and Jenny Craig, and to their credit, these companies have spent some of their largesse on efficacy research to try to promote their respective programs.[915] Nevertheless, the results of their own studies are underwhelming.

A systematic review was conducted of randomized controlled trials of commercial weight-loss programs that used exchange-based meal plans like Weight Watchers, prepackaged meals like Jenny Craig, or meal replacements like SlimFast. All in all, the majority of people enrolled in these commercial weight-loss programs failed to achieve even a modest weight loss, defined as a 5 percent reduction of their initial body weights (for example, a ten-pound loss for someone weighing two hundred pounds).[916]

On average, so little weight was lost on these types of programs that cost estimates range up to nearly $200 per pound lost.[917] Most people don't chalk up that high of a bill, though, because most don't stick with the program for very long. For example, a study of more than sixty thousand men and women enrolled in Jenny Craig found that fewer than 7 percent remained at the end of one year.[918] The largest, longest, best-designed randomized trial of a commercial program was funded by Weight Watchers,[919] and after two years, the best it could show was an average weight loss of only about 3 percent compared to a "self-help" control group given informational resources and a couple of nutrition counseling sessions.[920] Imagine all that time and energy spent in weekly Weight Watchers meetings to lose only an average of about three pounds a year.

Programs that include group sessions offer the advantage of social support and accountability,[921] but since some of the plans from leading companies seem to result in similar weight loss,[922] one might as well choose the least expensive. Take Off Pounds Sensibly (TOPS) is a nonprofit, peer-led weight-loss program that has been publishing its results for more than fifty years.[923] Not having to siphon off money for shareholders, TOPS is five times cheaper than Weight Watchers and may be fifty times less expensive than other leading programs such as Nutrisystem or Jenny Craig.[924]

TOPS was the first national program to publish data on all its completers. Only a tiny percentage stayed enrolled over the entire seven-year study period, but the thousands who did maintained about an eighteen-pound weight loss.[925] Still, that only amounts to a few pounds a year. Is that the best we can do? Sadly, as one obesity research pioneer once put it, "Most obese persons will not stay in treatment for obesity. Of those who stay in treatment, most will not lose weight, and of those who do lose weight, most will regain it."[926]

As a physician, my priority is getting (and keeping) people healthy, but when people are surveyed about their motivation for dieting, disturbingly, "health" may come in last.[927] Dieters want results—they want weight to come off.

So that became my challenge. If I were to construct the ideal weight-loss diet, what characteristics would it have? My research team and I dove head-first into the nearly half-million papers published in the English-language peer-reviewed medical literature on weight management and certainly ran into some surprises on the way. What follows is our distilled list of seventeen key ingredients—dietary attributes that could be used to create the most effective eating plan for losing weight.

ANTI-INFLAMMATORY

Meta-Inflammation

One of the most important medical discoveries in recent years was the realization that inflammation appears to play a role in many of our chronic diseases, including at least eight of our top ten leading causes of death.[928] The significance of this new understanding has been compared to the discovery of the germ theory, which, centuries ago, revolutionized our prevention and treatment of infectious diseases.[929] Throughout most of human history, however, inflammation was considered to be a good thing. When you get a splinter in your finger and it gets red, hot, painful, and swollen, that's inflammation. It's your body's natural reaction to tissue damage or irritation. So if the point of inflammation is to trigger the healing process, not a disease process, what's going on?

That splinter reaction is an example of acute inflammation, a short-term, localized, specific response to infection or injury aimed at resolving a problem. In contrast, chronic inflammation, also called *metabolic inflammation,* or *meta-inflammation* for short, is persistent, systemic, and nonspecific, and it appears to perpetuate disease.[930] It has a low-grade, smoldering quality—it's not as though we're red, hot, pained, and swollen all over. Simple blood tests, however, can detect abnormally high levels of inflammatory markers like C-reactive protein so that we can gauge our level of chronic inflammation.

C-reactive protein levels in the blood are ideally under 1 mg/L,[931] but in the presence of an infection, they can jump to 100 mg/L or more within hours.[932] Now that we have highly sensitive C-reactive protein blood tests that can measure levels to a fraction of a point, the medical community has realized that walking around with baseline levels of even just 2 or 3 mg/L appears to set us up for increased risk of catastrophes like heart attacks and strokes.[933] Having a C-reactive protein level under 1 mg/L denotes low risk, yet the levels of most middle-aged Americans exceed this,[934] suggesting most suffer from chronic inflammation.

This widespread meta-inflammation appears to be our immune systems' reaction to many unhealthy aspects of our lives—from the broader environment like traffic pollution and toxic chemicals to our day-to-day lifestyle choices, such as cigarettes, chronic stress, and too little physical activity and sleep.[935] The primary driver of meta-inflammatory chronic disease, however, may be the portions of the outside world we introduce into our bodies multiple times a day: what we eat.[936]

The Dietary Inflammatory Index

It's easy to tell if a food is pro-inflammatory or anti-inflammatory: Feed it to people, and see what happens to their levels of C-reactive protein and other markers of inflammation. With this method, you can check the impact of individual nutrients, whole foods, meals, or entire dietary patterns.

To rate people's diets, researchers developed a Dietary Inflammatory Index by scouring thousands of such experiments to come up with a scoring system.[937] The more pro-inflammatory foods you eat on a daily basis, the higher your score, and the more anti-inflammatory foods you eat, the lower your score. If you eat more anti-inflammatory than pro-inflammatory foods overall, you could end up with the goal—a net negative score, an anti-inflammatory diet.

Broadly speaking, components of processed foods and animal products, such as saturated fat, trans fat, and cholesterol, were found to be pro-inflammatory, while constituents of whole plant foods, such as fiber and phytonutrients, were strongly anti-inflammatory.[938] No surprise, then, that the Standard American Diet rates as pro-inflammatory and has the elevated disease rates to show for it.

Higher Dietary Inflammatory Index scores are linked to a higher risk of cardiovascular disease[939] and lower kidney,[940] lung,[941] and liver function.[942] Those eating diets rated as more inflammatory also experienced faster cellular aging.[943,944] In the elderly, pro-inflammatory diets are associated with impaired memory[945] and increased frailty.[946] Inflammatory diets are also associated with worse mental health, including higher rates of depression, anxiety, and impaired well-being.[947] Additionally, eating more pro-inflammatory foods has been tied to higher prostate cancer risk in men[948,949,950] and higher risks of breast cancer,[951,952] endometrial cancer,[953] ovarian cancer,[954] and miscarriages in women. Higher Dietary Inflammatory Index scores are also associated with more risk of esophageal,[955] stomach,[956] liver,[957] pancreatic,[958] colorectal,[959] kidney,[960] and bladder[961] cancers, as well as non-Hodgkin lymphoma.[962]

Overall, eating a more inflammatory diet was associated with 75 percent increased odds of having cancer and 67 percent increased risk of dying from cancer.[963] Not surprisingly, those eating more *anti*-inflammatory diets appear to live longer lives.[964,965,966,967] But how does the Dietary Inflammatory Index impact body weight?

Obesity and Inflammation: Cause or Consequence?

Pro-inflammatory diets are also associated with obesity, especially abdominal obesity.[968] When researchers followed thousands of normal-weight adults over time, they found those eating more pro-inflammatory foods have higher annual weight gain and those on the most inflammatory diets have a 32 percent greater risk of becoming overweight or obese during about an eight-year period.[969] The researchers were able to control for such nondietary factors as smoking and exercise—but is it possible that higher Dietary Inflammatory Index scores are just a reflection of a poor diet in general? The concept that diets with fewer fruits and vegetables and more meat and junk might lead to more weight gain isn't exactly revelatory. How do we know the connection has anything at all to do with inflammation?

Dozens of studies have shown that obesity is strongly associated with increased levels in the blood of inflammatory markers like C-reactive protein,[970] but is that inflammation a cause or a consequence of obesity?

We used to think fatty tissue was just a passive depot for the storage of excess fat,[971] but we now know it actively secretes inflammatory chemicals. Fatty tissue can expand so quickly it may outpace its blood supply and become starved of oxygen.[972] (You can insert an electrode directly into an obese belly and measure how low the oxygen levels fall compared with healthy-weight individuals.[973]) This is thought to contribute to fat cell death, which draws out inflammatory cells like macrophages, a type of roaming white blood cell present in pus, to try to clean up the mess. If you take a belly biopsy of an obese individual, you can see that the fat is swarming with macrophages.[974] The macrophages then appear to get stuck and fuse into giant cells, a hallmark of chronic inflammation seen in resistant infections like tuberculosis or around foreign bodies the body can't clear.[975] All the while, inflammatory compounds spill out into general circulation.[976]

Obesity, then, appears to lead to systemic inflammation, rather than the other way around.[977,978] And even if inflammation had no role in the cause of obesity, you'd still want any weight-loss diet to be anti-inflammatory to mediate the inflammatory consequences of the excess body fat. But there is a way inflammation seems to play a cause-and-effect role in the obesity epidemic: inflammation in our brains. To understand how inflammation in the brain can lead to obesity, we must first understand how our brains regulate our appetites.

Obesity is widely viewed as a neuroendocrine (nerve and hormone) disorder caused by damage to the appetite-regulating circuits in our brains.[979] Wait—isn't it caused by indulgence in the cheap and easy overabundance of aggressively marketed fatty, sugary, high-calorie foods? Well, if that's all it was, wouldn't even more people be overweight? Maybe 90 percent instead of just 72 percent?[980] The question that perhaps most intrigues obesity researchers is not *Why are so many people fat?* but rather, given how obesity-inducing our food system is, *Why isn't everyone fat?*[981]

I know this is going to sound odd in a book about the obesity epidemic, but our bodies are actually remarkably good at regulating our weight. Think about it. We eat about a million calories a year, yet most of us only fluctuate by a few pounds. Without even thinking about it, our bodies maintain our energy balance with a precision exceeding 99.5 percent.[982] You couldn't even count calories that effectively. Literally. When put to the test, the calorie labeling on packaged foods was sometimes found to be so inaccurate that one investigation discovered up to a quarter of foods sampled failed to even comply with the 20 percent error allowed by the FDA.[983] How do our bodies do better?

The master regulator of metabolism is the hypothalamus,[984] an almond-sized part of our brains near eye level in the middle of our skulls. Just like your hypothalamus regulates body temperature by causing you to shiver when you get too cold and sweat when you get too hot, it also regulates body fat, causing you to eat more when you get too thin and less when you get too fat. It's our "satiety center," carefully controlling our appetites so we eat just the right amount over time and don't gain or lose too much weight. But how exactly does the hypothalamus know how fat we are?

Our fat cells release a hormone called *leptin,* from the Greek *leptos* for *thin.* The more fat we have on our bodies, the higher the levels of leptin in our blood. The hypothalamus uses leptin levels as our fat thermostat and downregulates our appetites when leptin levels get too high.

"Experimental Obesity in Man," a classic set of prisoner experiments published in the 1970s, showed how difficult it was to perturb this system of appetite regulation when it is working properly. Lean inmates in a Vermont prison were fed up to ten thousand calories a day in closely supervised meals with a goal of increasing their weights by up to 25 percent.[985] This turned out to be surprisingly difficult. Most started dreading breakfast and sometimes involuntarily threw it up.[986] Most powered through, though, and achieved the excess weight target. But as soon as they were released from the experiment, they tended to rapidly shed all those extra pounds and get back to around their original weights.[987]

This all makes sense based on what we now know about the leptin-hypothalamus fat thermostat. All that extra body fat led to extra leptin production, and in response, their hypothalami profoundly depressed their appetites until they got back down to baseline. When their fat volumes dropped back to normal, their leptin levels presumably dropped back to normal, too, and so it seems their hypothalami made their normal appetites return. How, then, do people become obese—and what does it have to do with inflammation?

Inflammatory Brain Damage as a Cause of Obesity

People can gain weight—and keep it on—when there is damage to this leptin-hypothalamus circuit. Extreme cases of so-called hypothalamic obesity date back to 1840, when an "uncommonly obese" woman was found on autopsy to have a tumor near her hypothalamus.[988] Anything that harms the hypothalamus can cause obesity—head trauma, aneurysms, brain surgery.[989] Once the damage occurs and that feedback loop is broken, the hypothalamus can no longer respond adequately to rising leptin warning signals. As a result, people can develop out-of-control appetites, even to the point of having to be locked up for stealing food.[990]

You can imagine how the same thing could happen if a baby were born with congenital leptin deficiency, a condition in which their fat cells couldn't produce leptin at all. Their hypothalami would never get the too-much-fat signal to turn down their appetites—and indeed, such children eat constantly, tragically becoming so obese some can hardly walk, sometimes exceeding one hundred pounds by age four.[991]

But inject these children with leptin, and the weight comes off. The first child this was tried on was a nine-year-old girl weighing more than two hundred pounds. Within days of the leptin administration, there was a marked change in her eating behavior. For the first time in her life, she felt satiated eating the same quantity of food as her siblings, in effect proving the importance of leptin in appetite regulation.[992]

Want to guess how eager the drug industry was to start injecting people with leptin as the next new miracle weight-loss cure? But remember: Obese individuals are already awash with excess leptin secreted by all their extra fat. The problem is that the leptin just isn't working.

An analogy can be made with diabetes. In type 1 diabetes, blood sugars get too high because people can't make enough insulin. Inject them with insulin, and their blood sugars come right back down. That's like the kids with the rare leptin birth defect: Their body weights get too high because they can't make enough leptin, but if you inject them with leptin, their body weights come right back down. In contrast, type 2 diabetics *can* make enough insulin, but the target tissues are resistant to the effects of the insulin. There's already enough insulin in the body—in fact, there's often excess insulin, as the pancreas tries to pump out more to overcome the resistance. The body just isn't responding properly.

Similarly, obesity is thought to be caused by leptin resistance. Overweight individuals produce enough leptin—excess leptin, actually—but the target tissue, the hypothalamus, is resistant to its effects. So what can we do about it? Well, what do we do to treat insulin resistance?

Broadly, there are two ways to approach type 2 diabetes: The traditional medical model tries to overwhelm the system by injecting even more insulin, whereas the lifestyle medicine model instead treats the cause, attempting to reverse the insulin resistance itself so the body's own natural feedback loop can start working again. Similarly with obesity, attempts have been made to try to overwhelm the system by injecting even more leptin, but why not instead treat the underlying problem by reversing the leptin resistance?[993]

Interestingly, insulin resistance and leptin resistance may share a common cause: lipotoxicity, from the Greek *lipos,* meaning *animal fat.* Lipotoxicity is caused by eating a diet high in calories with too much saturated fat and can result in inflammation.[994]

Out of the Frying Pan and Into the Fire

If you feed lab animals saturated fat, the fat crosses the blood-brain barrier and accumulates in the hypothalamus within hours, causing inflammation, leptin resistance, and overeating.[995] You can re-create this scenario right in a petri dish. If you drip the main saturated fat from the American diet (found mostly in meat and dairy)[996] onto hypothalamic neurons, inflammation can be turned on like a light switch.[997] The original animal studies were done with lard-based diets, but butterfat seems to work just as well.[998] The good news is that when the lab animals were switched back to eating their regular low-fat food, their hypothalamic inflammation disappeared.[999]

So what about in humans? Extrapolating data from lab animals is infamously fraught with difficulty,[1000] and obesity research is no exception.[1001] For one, the diets between lab animals and humans are incomparable. Lard-based, high-fat rodent food may be around 60 percent fat.[1002] But bacon is only about 40 percent lard,[1003] so you could eat a 100 percent bacon diet and still not get the kind of fat intake that the rodent was receiving.

Because of the difficulty of extrapolating from animals, we didn't know if the same kind of hypothalamic inflammation occurred in obese humans until researchers were able to use high-resolution MRI brain scans to put it to the test.[1004] Subsequent comparisons with brain slices obtained on autopsy confirmed that what researchers were seeing on the MRIs was indeed the same hallmarks of hypothalamic inflammation.[1005] The nerves were inflamed, but not destroyed, suggesting the whole process could be reversible. (No improvement in hypothalamic inflammation was seen about ten months after bariatric surgery,[1006] but this is perhaps because stomach stapling can force a change in diet quantity but not necessarily diet quality.)

Randomized crossover trials show that by covertly increasing saturated fat intake, you can reversibly induce negative changes in brain function, mood, inflammation, and resting metabolic rate, and even, apparently, undercut motivation to exercise.[1007,1008] Study subjects become 12–15 percent less physically active on high–saturated fat diets compared to low–saturated fat diets.[1009] And note that researchers used a saturated *plant* fat—palm oil—found in some nondairy cheeses, vegan spreads, and other processed junk, so an anti-inflammatory diet is not just a move toward a more plant-based diet in general but specifically one centered around whole, unprocessed plant foods.

If Memory Serves

The hippocampus is the seat of memory in the brain. Structurally, it's composed of two upside-down, seahorse-shaped ridges nestled deep in the temporal lobes. In Alzheimer's, it's one of the first areas to be hit. If saturated fat–induced inflammatory damage to the metabolic center of the brain may be contributing to obesity, what might that same damage be doing to the memory center?

When lab animals are fed saturated fat (lard), neurons in their hippocampi exhibit stress within seventy-two hours.[1010] Subsequent memory problems and obesity suggest a vicious cycle, where saturated fat harms the hippocampus, causing memory impairments that result in even more lard being eaten—it's as if they had forgotten how much they'd already had—and then goes on to cause more brain damage, cognitive dysfunction, and weight gain.[1011] This finding inspired human investigations. MRI imaging scans taken of people's brains approximately four years apart found that those eating junky, meat-centered diets experience a significant shrinkage of their hippocampi compared to those eating more healthful diets.[1012] Saturated fat consumption is also associated with accelerated cognitive decline, but you don't know if any of this is cause and effect until you put it to the test.[1013]

Researchers put people on a high-fat, ketogenic diet and confirmed a blunting of cognition, including impaired reaction times and attention, within seven days.[1014] Another research team found that a high-fat diet impaired brain function in just five days: "Deficits were found in the speed of retrieval of information from memory, the ability to intensely focus attention, and performance of a complex higher order task involving working memory and attention."[1015]

Even one bad meal a day for four days can impair our brain function. Australian researchers randomized men and women to eat either a breakfast high in saturated fat and added sugars or a healthier breakfast for four consecutive days. That's all it took to cause a significant loss in hippocampus-dependent learning and memory. People were instructed to repeat a list of twelve words over and over, for example, and then try to recall them twenty minutes later. Most were able to remember about 90 percent of them. For those randomized to eat one fatty meal a day for four days, their recall dropped down to around 75 percent. Although the high-fat breakfasts also had added sugar, overall sugar intake didn't change over the four days or differ from the control group, but their intake of saturated fat was double.[1016]

The fatty breakfast group also appeared to suffer a hit to their *interoception,* the ability to perceive internal body states. In other words, they had to eat more food, about seventy calories' worth, to feel the same sensation of satiety and fullness. The impaired hunger sensitivity, combined with the poorer memory retention, would seem to be a setup for weight gain. The hippocampal injury should be reversible, though. The researchers suggest that the recovery period to repair the damage done by those four fatty meals may be as short as four to six weeks.[1017]

Even though overall sugar intake didn't change, the researchers suspect the breakfast "burst" of saturated fat and added sugar was the most plausible cause.[1018] A single meal high in saturated fat (equivalent to a quarter-pound cheeseburger and large fries) has been shown to increase whole-body insulin resistance by 25 percent.[1019] That, combined with the added sugars, could spike blood sugars high enough to contribute to the hippocampal dysfunction. As the accompanying medical journal editorial put it, a single load of saturated fat "packs a punch."[1020]

FOOD FOR THOUGHT

By choosing to eat more anti-inflammatory foods and fewer pro-inflammatory foods, we may be able to both prevent and treat the damage to the appetite-regulating apparatus in our brains that can lead to—and sustain—obesity.

In the Dietary Inflammatory Index, the single most anti-inflammatory food is the spice turmeric, followed by ginger and garlic, and the most anti-inflammatory beverage is green or black tea. The two most anti-inflammatory food *components* are fiber and flavones.[1021] Dietary fiber is found in all whole plant foods, but it is most concentrated in legumes, such as beans, split peas, chickpeas, and lentils.[1022] Flavones are plant compounds concentrated in herbs, vegetables, and fruits,[1023] and the leading sources in the U.S. diet are parsley, bell peppers, celery, apples, and oranges.[1024] The most flavone-filled beverage is chamomile tea.[1025]

The most pro-inflammatory food components are saturated fat and trans fat. Essentially, the top five sources of saturated fat in the United States are cheese, desserts like cake and ice cream, chicken, pork, and then burgers.[1026] Thankfully, with the ban on added trans fat, the only remaining sources in the food supply will be the small amounts found naturally in meat and dairy and created in the refining of vegetable oils.[1027]

Ultimately, an anti-inflammatory diet in clinical practice first and foremost "focuses on eating whole, plant-based foods."[1028] As I mentioned, not all plant-derived foods are anti-inflammatory (like the tropical oils), just as not all animal foods are pro-inflammatory. Omega-3 fatty acids found in fish, for example, score as an anti-inflammatory component in the Dietary Inflammatory Index.[1029] Though fish oil may not affect systemic inflammation in healthy individuals,[1030] it can reduce inflammatory markers in those with chronic disease.[1031] Curiously, unlike plant-based omega-3 sources like nuts, fish consumption is not associated with lower inflammatory disease mortality.[1032] Perhaps the benefits of the omega-3s are offset by the industrial toxins that now contaminate much of the aquatic food chain.[1033]

CLEAN

Obesogenic Pollutants

The notion that we are being exposed to obesogenic pollutants—that is, obesity-generating chemicals—went from mere speculation in an alternative medicine journal in 2002[1034] to strong scientific plausibility within a decade.[1035] The supposition started out on pretty shaky ground, pointing out, for instance, that recent national surveys appear to show our weight exceeds what we report eating.[1036] Therefore, the argument went, something else must be going on beyond just calories in and calories out. But it is notoriously difficult to get an accurate calorie count from dietary recall surveys, especially from overweight individuals, who tend to underreport their intakes.[1037]

Theoretically, though, the obesogen concept was not that much of a stretch. All sorts of synthetic chemicals cause obesity in humans: They're called *medications.* Multiple classes of drugs are infamous for contributing to weight gain, such as certain types of antidepressants, antipsychotics, and diabetes medications.[1038] The animal agriculture industry has made fattening into a science, utilizing a whole array of chemicals, hormones, and pharmaceuticals to pack on the pounds.[1039] An analysis of chicken feathers found that the poultry industry appears to feed the birds everything from arsenic[1040] to Prozac.[1041] (Poultry producers say feeding caffeine "keeps the chickens awake so that they eat more and grow faster."[1042])

So what evidence do we have that chemicals are making *us* grow fatter too?

Early on, the purported link between chemical pollutants and obesity was based in part on the observation that the rise in chemical production seemed to coincide with the rise of the obesity epidemic.[1043] Yes, but how many other millions of changes have there been over the last half century? Why jump to pollution when there are so many other easier explanations, everything from couch potatoes to fried potatoes?

One clue that pollutants may be playing some role is that our pets are also getting fatter.[1044]

Fido isn't drinking more soda. Of course, the more *Seinfeld* reruns we watch, the less we may walk the dog, but what about our cats? Are we just giving them—and our kids—a few too many treats? That would seem a simpler explanation than imagining pervasive, obesity-causing chemicals building up in the pet and person food chains. It's not just our kitties and kiddies, though. A remarkable paper was published in 2011 entitled "Canaries in the Coal Mine: A Cross-Species Analysis of the Plurality of Obesity Epidemics."[1045] It was a study of more than twenty thousand animals from twenty-four distinct populations, including feral animals, lab animals, and even urban and rural rats. The researchers found "large and sustained" increases in body weight nearly across the board, not just among pampered pets.

We're all getting fatter. The odds that every single population studied would be getting heavier just by chance are around eight million to one. Given that evidence, it's hard to blame our collective weight problem just on things like dwindling phys ed classes, the advent of video games, or junkier food. And our infants are heavier too. There's been an alarming rise in obesity rates among young children under two years of age.[1046] It's hard to argue that today's six-month-olds are eating more or exercising less than they were in previous generations.

These are the kinds of data that piqued serious interest into the search for obesogenic chemicals, and to date, about twenty different purported obesogens have been found.[1047] The most well-studied thus far is a group of tin-based biocides known as *organotins*.[1048]

The Case of the Sex-Change Paint

Organotins were used in "antifouling" paint applied to the outer hulls of ships and other submerged structures like fish farm cages and oil rigs to prevent barnacles from attaching. But once this chemical was being used widely, scientists began to notice that female sea snails started to grow penises.[1049] As a result of a variety of hormone-disrupting effects, organotins were banned from the maritime industry in 2008.[1050] Disrupting hormones isn't the only thing these compounds do, though. Organotins also activate peroxisome proliferator-activated receptor gamma, or PPAR-γ, which is the master regulator of adipogenesis, the process of creating new fat cells (known as *adipocytes*).[1051]

Once activated, PPAR-γ recruits connective tissue stem cells to turn into new fat cells. PPAR-γ stimulation can also cause fat cells to swell up even larger with fat. In other words, contact with this chemical leads to more, and bigger, fat cells,[1052] and exposure in the womb to organotins may permanently establish an elevated fat cell count throughout our lives.[1053]

By the time we hit early adulthood, the total number of fat cells in our bodies remains fairly stable.[1054] When we gain or lose weight, we are pretty much just enlarging or shrinking our existing fat cells. Starting out with a higher number of fat cells or gaining more later in life may make it easier to put on pounds, harder to lose them, and more difficult to maintain weight loss.[1055]

What's more, each fat cell we make may be at the expense of one fewer bone, cartilage, or muscle cell.[1056] The connective tissue stem cells recruited by PPAR-γ to become fat cells could have otherwise become any of those other types of cells, so excess PPAR-γ activation could potentially set us up not only for obesity but also osteoporosis.[1057] The swiss cheese–like holes in osteoporotic bone are often filled with fat.[1058] Perhaps this is why the PPAR-γ-activating diabetes drug rosiglitazone (sold as Avandia) not only causes weight gain as a side effect but appears to increase the risk of bone fractures as well.[1059]

How are we exposed to PPAR-γ-activating organotin compounds? Mainly through food, especially from fish and other seafood.[1060] Even though organotins were banned on boats and other marine vessels years ago, they persist in our waterways, and contamination levels in fish fillets remain comparable to those obtained worldwide before the ban.[1061] Some fish are worse than others. Halibut, swordfish, and canned tuna have been recorded as having the highest levels,[1062] and a sampling of U.S. market-bought seafood found that farm-raised fish was generally worse than wild-caught.[1063]

Are the contamination levels high enough to be of concern? Researchers calculated the "tolerable average residue levels" for tributyltin, a common organotin, in seafood products around the world, defined as the levels in seafood tolerable for the average adult consumption pattern. Of the eighty-four U.S. seafood samples examined, seven products exceeded this level, or about 8 percent.[1064] Note this is for the average adult consumer, so the percentage would be higher in children or those who ate more seafood than average. The percentage violating the tolerable average dose exceeds 30 percent in Japan, for example, but that is because the Japanese tend to eat more seafood, not because their fish is any more contaminated.

Everybody's Plastic

Persistent pollutants have blanketed the world and now are found even in the Arctic, thousands of miles from known sources. Fortunately, many have been regulated strictly since the Stockholm Convention in 2004,[1065] but unfortunately, there continue to be hormone-disrupting chemicals that are underregulated or not regulated at all. DDT, the banned pesticide now found mostly in meat, particularly fish,[1066] is a "presumed" human obesogen[1067] responsible for perhaps thousands of annual childhood obesity cases.[1068,1069,1070] Meanwhile, the number attributable to the plastics chemical bisphenol A (BPA) may be in the *tens* of thousands.[1071]

BPA was first developed more than a century ago as a synthetic estrogen.[1072] It wasn't until the 1950s, however, that the manufacturing industry realized BPA could also be used to make polycarbonate plastic. Despite having long been recognized as having hormonal effects,[1073] BPA rapidly became one of the most widely used chemicals worldwide.[1074] It's currently one of the highest-volume chemicals produced globally, with more than six billion pounds made each year.[1075]

In a petri dish, BPA was shown to accelerate the formation of new fat cells[1076] and increase fat accumulation within fat cells, but that was at doses many thousands of times the concentration found in most people's bloodstreams.[1077] Though more than 90 percent of Americans tested in a national survey had BPA circulating in their bodies,[1078] it was at concentrations down around 10 nM.[1079] In contrast, those early studies were using 25,000–80,000 nM. We knew there were estrogenic effects even at those low, real-world doses,[1080] but it wasn't discovered until recently—in part using fat samples taken from children[1081] and adults[1082] undergoing abdominal surgery—that fat cell formation could also be affected by BPA at as little as 1 nM.[1083] Even once metabolized by the liver, which destroys the estrogenic effects, BPA retains the ability to promote adipogenesis, the process of creating fat cells.[1084,1085]

BPA exposure at all life stages tends to correlate with increased weight,[1086] and population studies in the United States, Canada, China, and South Korea have found it to be associated with various body fat measures.[1087] Six out of seven BPA studies on general obesity and five out of five studies on abdominal obesity have found a link. Putting together all the studies, those with the highest BPA levels had 67 percent greater odds of obesity compared to those with the lowest.[1088] In men, BPA may also be associated with lower lean body mass.[1089] Those in the highest quarter of BPA urine levels averaged about three pounds less lean mass than those in the lowest quarter, suggesting BPA may have negative effects on muscle as well. (BPA exposure is also associated with declining male sexual function, but that's a whole other book.[1090])

How can we stay away from BPA? A small amount of exposure comes from handling thermal paper, such as cash register receipts and printed tickets,[1091] especially if our hands are greasy or wet after the application of lotion or sanitizer.[1092] Ninety percent of exposure, however, appears to be from our diets.[1093] How can you tell? When people fast for a couple of days, their BPA levels drop as much as tenfold.[1094]

Fasting isn't very sustainable, though. Researchers had families try a "fresh foods intervention," where the families switched away from canned and processed foods. (Why canned? BPA is used in the epoxy that lines most canned goods, since it costs companies about 2 cents more per can to use non-BPA material instead.[1095]) Simply by avoiding canned and processed foods, the highest BPA levels dropped 76 percent within three days.[1096]

Alternately, you can conduct the experiment by adding a serving of canned soup to people's daily diets. Compared to serving soup prepared with fresh ingredients, five days of a daily serving of canned soup led to a 1,000 percent rise in BPA levels in the urine.[1097] It could have been even worse had they used cans of condensed soup, which may have about 85 percent more BPA than cans of ready-to-serve soup. Otherwise, the highest BPA levels have been found in canned green beans and canned tuna.[1098] The only fresh food found contaminated with BPA in the United States was sliced turkey.[1099]

Take-Home Tip: BPA is why I specify in *The How Not to Die Cookbook* to choose beans and tomato products in jars, aseptic packaging (Tetra Paks), or BPA-free cans. Eden Foods, for example, has a line of BPA-free canned beans. You can also BYOB: Boil Your Own Beans. It's cheaper, and they end up with a better texture. My favorite way is to use an electric pressure cooker (like an Instant Pot).

Phthalates are another class of plastics compounds associated with weight gain.[1100] A European consensus panel of obesogen experts gave a 40–69 percent probability of phthalate exposure causing more than fifty thousand cases of obesity annually in older women.[1101] Rapid plunges in phthalate levels upon fasting implicated dietary sources,[1102] and significant drops within days of having people eat a vegetarian diet gave researchers a clue as to where to look.[1103]

Indeed, high concentrations of phthalates have been found consistently in some meats (particularly poultry), fats, and some dairy products.[1104] The fact that egg consumption is also associated with elevated phthalate levels suggests that the chickens themselves are contaminated even before they're wrapped in plastic for sale.[1105] The phthalates in dairy, though, appear to be from the plastic tubing in milking machines, as dairy from hand-milked cows can have ten times less.[1106] Diets high in meat and dairy can sometimes contain up to four times the Environmental Protection Agency's recommended daily phthalate safety limit.[1107]

This is what makes population studies linking pollutants and obesity so difficult.[1108] Phthalate levels just may be an indicator of fried chicken intake, and BPA levels a sign of SPAM consumption. Similarly, just as exposure to plastics chemicals may be an indicator of a diet bereft of fresh foods, DDT exposure may be a marker for the foods that frequently contain the highest levels of DDTs identified by the Endocrine Society: "meat, fish, poultry, eggs, cheese, butter and milk."[1109] Pollutants like DDT are just one of many reasons why diets rich in those foods might be associated with obesity risk.

Take-Home Tip: BPA and phthalate metabolites are detectable in 95 percent of the U.S. adult population.[1110] BPA is already banned from baby bottles and sippy cups in the United States,[1111] but for other plastic containers, keep an eye out for recycle codes 3 and 7, as those indicate items that are more likely to contain high levels of BPA.[1112] Certain phthalate levels are now banned from toys for children,[1113] but not from "toys" for adults. Jelly-based sex toys are often made from a plasticized vinyl material packed with phthalates. Sticking to water-based lubricants may reduce phthalate transfer a hundredfold, but such adult toys may still have opposite the intended effect.[1114] Women with the highest levels of phthalates flowing through their bodies report more than twice the odds of lack of interest in sexual activity.[1115]

Up in Smoke

In 2015, when meat was officially classified as a "known carcinogen" or a "probable carcinogen" depending on whether or not it was processed, the focus was on substances generated during cooking, curing, or smoking, rather than on pollutant contamination.[1116] Given this, we could just follow recommendations to keep cooking temperatures under 260°F, thereby avoiding broiling, roasting, pan-frying, or any other cooking method that causes a crust to form, and instead stick to boiling or microwaving to keep the outside "pale and soft."[1117] But even just being around a barbecue may be hazardous, based on the recognition that light clothing probably provides little protection from gaseous carcinogens.[1118]

Polycyclic aromatic hydrocarbons (PAHs), a class of combustion by-products found in cigarettes, car exhaust, and grilled meat,[1119] may explain why the Long Island Breast Cancer Study Project found a 47 percent increase in breast cancer risk among postmenopausal women with a high lifetime intake of grilled, barbecued, or smoked meats.[1120] These contaminants may be more than just carcinogenic—they may be obesogenic as well. A nationwide study of thousands of young people found that the more children are exposed to PAHs, the fatter they tend to be. And prenatal exposure to these chemicals may cause a higher subsequent risk of childhood obesity.[1121]

If you look at one of the most common of these toxins, smokers get about half their exposure from food and half from cigarettes. For nonsmokers, however, 99 percent may come from diet. The highest levels are found in meat, with pork apparently worse than beef.[1122] Even dark green leafy vegetables like kale can get contaminated by pollutants in the air, so don't forage your dandelion greens next to the highway, and make sure to rinse your broad-leafed greens well under running water.[1123]

PAHs are fat-soluble, so absorption may be diminished with eating lower-fat foods,[1124] but importantly, they don't appear to build up in your body. Unlike persistent pollutants like PCBs, a particularly toxic class of man-made chemicals that may take fifty to seventy-five years to clear from the body after regular (even monthly) meals of farmed Atlantic salmon,[1125] PAHs can pass in and out of you in a day. If you have people eat a meal of barbecued chicken, you can see a big spike in these chemicals in their systems—up to a hundredfold increase—but the body can detoxify most of them away within about twenty hours.[1126] Rather than detoxing, though, perhaps it would be better not to "tox" in the first place—at least not on a daily basis.

Prepackaged Pollutants

Industrial chemical contaminants come prepackaged regardless of cooking method in "diary [sic] products, meat and fish."[1127] (Although dioxins are created when paper pulp is bleached, I have a feeling "diary" was an autocorrect error.) The Food and Drug Administration has regulations about toxic chemicals in the food supply, determining the "action levels" of contaminants above which foods must be removed from the market, but those levels tend to be far higher than the levels based on health standards set by the Centers for Disease Control and Prevention (CDC). For example, a glass of milk tainted with the amount of DDT permitted by FDA's action level would expose a consumer to nearly ten times the daily exposure considered "safe" by the CDC, and a single serving of fish could be sold with fifty times the daily limit.[1128] Presumably, the reason the commercial standards are so lax is because too much food would have to be pulled from the shelves.

The USDA determined that, based solely on dioxin levels, American children consuming average servings of meat, including poultry (which regularly contained the highest levels they found), could be ingesting in excess of the daily safety limit.[1129] Taking all thirty-three chemical pollutants in meat shown to be potentially carcinogenic into account, some European toxicologists suggest limiting children's consumption of beef, pork, and chicken to no more than five servings a *month,* an average of no more than one serving every six days or so.[1130] In Europe, lamb is the most contaminated and the recommendation calls for adults to eat no more than a single serving every four or five months.[1131]

In the United States, if there was any standout, it would be chicken and PBDE flame-retardant chemicals—not only compared to other meats but also to other countries. U.S. chickens are about ten to twenty times more contaminated than chickens tested from other countries.[1132] Sadly, the newer flame-retardant chemicals introduced to replace the original PBDEs also[1133] activate adipogenesis, diverting stem cell development away from bone building and toward the formation of fat.[1134]

Meat is certainly not the only source of flame-retardant exposure, though, as those eating vegetarian diets only have about 25 percent lower levels in their bloodstreams.[1135] For other chemicals, meat may play a larger role. Studies dating back over thirty years looking at the pollutants in the breast milk of vegetarians have found the average vegetarian levels of some pollutants were only 1–2 percent as high as the national average.[1136] For six out of seven pollutants reviewed, there wasn't even an overlap in the range of scores; the highest vegetarian value was lower than the lowest value obtained in the general population. This is presumed to be because these pollutants concentrate *up* the food chain, so by eating more from all the way *down* the food chain, those eating more plant foods may have an edge.[1137]

The problem with studies just comparing populations is that you can't single out the diet. Maybe vegetarians have other lifestyle behaviors that protect them. You don't know until you put it to the test by changing people's diets and seeing what happens. That's hard to do with persistent pollutants like PCBs, which may take literally decades to detoxify from the body, but we can get rid of heavy metals like mercury in a matter of months. And, indeed, within three months of the exclusion of eggs and meat, including poultry and fish, from people's diets, there was a significant drop in their levels of mercury, cadmium, and lead. Within just a few months of changing their diets, the levels of toxic heavy metals in their bodies dropped by up to about 30 percent.[1138]

What About Organic Meat?

What if we just stick to organic meat? Certified organic meat comes from livestock fed organically produced feed free of pesticides and animal by-products. Therefore, you would assume there would be less chemical residue accumulation, but there hadn't been any studies measuring the chemical contamination in organic meat until recently. Researchers acquired seventy-six samples of different kinds of meat, both organic and conventional, and quantified their levels of contamination with thirty-three different persistent toxic pollutants. No sample was completely free of industrial toxins, which is to be expected given how polluted our world has become. What was surprising, though, was how minimal the differences were between organically and conventionally produced meats. In some cases, organic was inexplicably worse. Whether choosing conventional or organic meat, the researchers concluded that the current pattern of meat consumption exceeded the maximum tolerable safety limits either way.[1139]

Given that 90 percent of persistent pollutant exposure comes from animal-derived foods,[1140] it's no surprise that those eating more low-carbohydrate, high-protein-type diets have higher levels of pollutants circulating in their systems. This included PCBs 118 and 153, trans-nonachlor (a component of the banned pesticide chlordane), hexachlorobenzene (a banned fungicide), DDE (from DDT), mercury, and lead.[1141] Mediterranean diet scores were correlated with elevated levels of PCBs (118, 126, 153, and 209), trans-nonachlor, and mercury, presumably because of the focus on fish consumption.[1142]

Any increase in body fat caused by obesogenic chemicals could potentially serve as a reservoir for further chemical accumulation, possibly setting up a vicious cycle.[1143] Our fat stores—like those of farm animals—harbor toxic pollutants. How do we know this? Because we see a surge in these chemicals in people's bloodstreams as they lose weight.[1144] After bariatric surgery, for example, certain pollutant levels can rise more than 300 percent.[1145]

The release of these compounds trapped in our body fat may then affect our metabolisms, slowing down the rate at which we burn calories during sleep, which could frustrate additional weight loss.[1146] To help break this cycle, a reduction in animal fat is suggested to reduce further accumulation of pollutants, along with an increase in whole grains, as the fiber may help draw toxins out of the body.[1147]

What About Organic Produce?

A recent expert review on obesogens suggests that doctors can help patients reduce their exposure by advising them to choose organic fruits and vegetables "insofar as possible."[1148] What evidence is there that the pesticides used on produce may play a role in the obesity epidemic? Just as the link between asbestos and disease first became apparent when studying those with the greatest exposure—miners and shipbuilders—public health researchers set out to study more than eight thousand licensed pesticide applicators to see if there was any connection between crop pesticides and weight gain.[1149] One pesticide stood out, atrazine, the weed killer commonly used in corn production that was found to induce complete feminization of frogs—as in total sex reversal, with male frogs ending up laying eggs.[1150] Agricultural workers spraying lots of atrazine had about 50 percent greater odds of being overweight and obese.[1151]

Just because levels in the field may predispose people to obesity doesn't mean levels in the grocery store are high enough to have any effect, though. To see if buying organic makes a difference, can't we just compare the body weights of those who choose organic to those who don't? A study of more than fifty thousand consumers did exactly that, and those who chose organic "most of the time" only had about half the obesity rates of those who "never" chose organic.[1152] Your critical thinking alarm bells should have started ringing instantly. Think of all the other attributes of organic shoppers. Indeed, those choosing organic were better educated and better off financially, both of which in and of themselves have been associated with lower obesity risk,[1153,1154] and, more to the point, exercised more and had better diets.

Those who chose organic ate more whole plant foods and less meat, dairy, and junk. No surprise they had a healthier weight.

The researchers controlled for each of these other factors, however, and still found dramatically lower obesity rates in "most of the time" organic consumers, though not necessarily in those who just chose organic "occasionally."[1155] Still, this was just a cross-sectional study, meaning a snapshot in time. Rather than conventional foods contributing to weight gain, maybe weight gain led people to throw up their hands and care less about how their food was grown or produced.

In 2017, we got a prospective study where people were followed over time. Sixty thousand French consumers were followed for about three years to see if those choosing organic gained less weight. After controlling for such factors as education, income, physical activity, and overall dietary quality, those who reportedly ate more organic foods were significantly less likely to become overweight or obese.[1156] Note, though, that this was only for those choosing healthier diets in general. Eating organic Oreos and Pop-Tarts doesn't do your body any favors.

Take-Home Tip: Personally, I try to choose organic whenever I have the option, but I never let pesticide concerns prevent me or my family from indulging in as many fruits and vegetables as possible regardless of how they were grown.

Microplastics in Seafood

In 1869, a patent was taken out on a new substance to replace elephant ivory in the production of billiard balls, and the plastics industry was born.[1157] What started as a conservation-minded measure has turned into an environmental calamity.[1158] Trillions of little plastic particles now float on the surface of the sea.[1159] Plastic objects like water bottles get worn down into tinier and tinier pieces, and plastic microbeads in personal care products like facial cleansers flow from our sinks down into the

(continued)

waterways. Up to ninety-four thousand microbeads are flushed down the drain in a single rinse.[1160]

The plastic then accumulates toxic compounds from the water and shuttles them, along with any chemicals originally in the plastic, into marine life, concentrating up the food chain and eventually ending up on our plates.[1161] This may explain how fresh cod can sometimes end up with higher BPA levels than canned tuna.[1162]

It is inevitable that we'll ingest at least some microplastics when we eat seafood, particularly when the entire animal is consumed, such as with sardines.[1163] Researchers sampled twenty brands of canned sardines and sprats from thirteen countries over four continents and found plastic particles in about one in five.[1164] They suggested the disparities may have been due to improper gutting in the contaminated samples, but in mammals, at least, ingested microplastics can get through the gut wall, circulate throughout the body, and even cross the placental barrier.[1165]

When researchers compared the level of microplastics in eviscerated flesh versus the guts of fish, the meat sometimes actually contained higher microplastics loads than the excised organs.[1166] Some studies have detected microplastics in all fish muscle samples tested.[1167] The average intake of microplastics from eating fish like flathead, grouper, shrimp scad, or barracuda may be in the hundreds per serving or in the dozens of plastic particles in a two-ounce, child-sized serving.[1168] As the particles travel through our bodies, they may then release any absorbed pollutants or plastics additives—some of which may play a role in the obesity epidemic.[1169] Because of this, some have suggested weekly servings of these kinds of fish may threaten the health of consumers, especially vulnerable groups, such as children and women who are pregnant or breastfeeding.[1170]

FOOD FOR THOUGHT

The obesogen field is still in its infancy but continues to gain scientific support.[1171] The American Medical Association, American Public Health Association, and the Endocrine Society, the oldest and largest association of hormone specialists, have all called for improved regulatory oversight of hormone-disrupting chemicals.[1172] We don't have to wait to make simple diet and lifestyle changes to reduce our exposure, though. We can make a difference now by prioritizing plant foods, opting for fresh or frozen vegetables over canned, and, if eating or drinking out of polycarbonate and PVC plastics, choosing not to microwave them, put them in the dishwasher, leave them in the sun or in a hot car, or use them once they're scratched,[1173] as that can increase the release of the chemicals.

HIGH IN FIBER-RICH FOODS

Feeding Our Forgotten Organ

We used to think of food simply as a source of nutrients and energy, but we now know there are components in what we eat that can act as signaling molecules that bind to specific receptors within the body and trigger drug-like effects to regulate our metabolisms, among other things. Ironically, one of the food components that produces the most dramatic effects is something that initially appeared to be the most inert of dietary constituents: fiber.[1174] In fact, telling people to increase their intakes of fiber-rich foods may actually be one of the single most effective pieces of advice for weight loss.

Fiber seems so, well, boring. By definition, fiber is indigestible. Since it can't be absorbed into the body, it just stays in our gut to bulk up our stool. This is not to belittle the importance of bowel regularity. If just half the adult population ate three additional grams of fiber a day—only a quarter cup of beans or a bowl of oatmeal—we could relieve enough constipation to save billions in medical costs a year.[1175] But it's not as if we thought fiber really *did* anything beyond helping to keep us regular.

While it's true *we* can't technically digest fiber, that's only applicable to the part of us that's actually human. But most of the cells in our bodies are bacteria.[1176] Our gut flora, which weigh more than one of our kidneys and are more metabolically active than our livers,[1177] have been called our "forgotten organ."[1178] And our good gut bacteria don't just digest fiber—they thrive on it. Fiber is like comfort food for your colon. So we *can* digest fiber, just not without a little help from our little friends.

What do the bacteria do with the fiber? They make short-chain fatty acids (SCFAs) with the fiber that can then be absorbed from the colon into our bloodstreams, circulate throughout our bodies, and even end up in our brains.[1179] In this way, these fiber-sourced SCFAs can potentially have wide-ranging effects on everything from immune function and inflammation[1180] to mental health[1181]— and, as you'll see, may play a key role in regulating our appetites, metabolisms, and body fat.[1182]

Crowding Out Calories

The first major review, "Dietary Fiber and Weight Regulation," included a dozen interventional studies in which people were randomized into higher- or lower-fiber diets. The additional consumption of fourteen grams of fiber a day led to an average weight loss of 1.9 kilograms over 3.8 months.[1183] That's only about a pound a month, but the weight loss was greater among those who needed it; overweight and obese study subjects lost triple the weight compared to lean individuals. How much is fourteen grams of fiber? Not much. Fourteen grams would barely bring the average American's diet up to the recommended *minimum* average adequate daily fiber intake.[1184]

The increased fiber intake appeared to lead to about a 10 percent drop in daily caloric intake.[1185] Why would more fiber mean fewer calories? Well, conventionally, fiber is considered to have zero calories, so it adds bulk to food without adding extra calories. To illustrate, let's compare a food to its fiber-depleted equivalent. Consider a bottle of cold-pressed apple juice, which is basically an apple with its fiber removed. You could chug a regular 15.2-ounce bottle of juice in a matter of seconds, but to get the same number of calories, you would have to eat nearly five cups of apple slices.[1186,1187] Which do you think would fill you up more? Obviously, the apple slices. But why?

First, you'd need to chew every apple slice. Fiber-rich foods require more chewing, slowing down eating rate, which itself can improve satiety.[1188] This also allows for more secretion of saliva and stomach juices. In one study, researchers spread a barium paste onto slices of different kinds of bread and found that, upon x-ray, the stomach shadow was larger after eating whole-wheat compared to white bread, showing how much fuller you physically get.[1189] So, in our cold-pressed apple juice versus apple slices scenario, we have the extra fluid secretion on top of the five cups of slices pushing on the walls of the stomach, which has nerves with stretch receptors that can send fullness signals directly to the brain.[1190]

One type of fiber in apples is pectin, the gelling agent used to make jams and jellies. Imagine how eating all those apples would not only add a lot of extra bulky volume but could start to form a gel to further slow the rate at which those five cups of slices left your stomach. This would keep you feeling fuller for longer compared to consuming the same number of apple calories in fiber-depleted juice form, which would pass right through you much more rapidly. Other gummy fibers like those found in oats can have the same gelling effect. Five grams of a highly gelling fiber can hold approximately one quart of water as it passes through the stomach and small intestine, so that's like having an extra two pounds of zero-calorie food mass filling you up.[1191]

Obviously, juice is going to drain out of your stomach faster than apples, but even the same volume of fiber-depleted solid food exits more quickly. In a study entitled "Gastric Emptying of a Solid Meal Is Accelerated by the Removal of Dietary Fibre Naturally Present in Food," researchers compared how long it took for a meal that included higher-fiber foods—whole-wheat pasta with puréed fruits and vegetables—to leave the stomach compared to a meal with the same volume and same calories, but made from white pasta and fruit and vegetable juices. The fiber-depleted meal was out of the stomach forty-five minutes earlier than the meal with the fiber intact.[1192]

It's Not the Calories You Eat but the Calories You Absorb

Now imagine what happens next: The apple juice would get rapidly absorbed as soon as it spilled out from the stomach into the small intestine and spike our blood sugars, whereas sugar trapped in the mass of apple slices would be absorbed more slowly along the length of the intestine. Our bodies can only absorb nutrients when they come in physical contact with our intestinal walls, so fiber, which never gets absorbed, can act as a carrier to dilute and even eliminate calories out the other end. Fiber doesn't just trap sugars; it can act as a fat-[1193] and starch-blocker[1194] too. There are drugs on the market that can do this, but eating fiber-rich foods can do it more safely—and naturally.

What if you dipped those apple slices in peanut butter? Everything would get mixed together, and some of the peanut oil calories would make it all the way through the intestines, trapped in the middle of a gelled mass of apple fiber. In contrast, if you ate a spoonful of peanut butter and then washed it down with apple juice, the juice would get absorbed right off the bat, leaving the peanut butter to coat the walls of the intestine and all the calories to get absorbed. This has been demonstrated in experiments measuring fecal fat excretion dating back nearly a half century.

What happens if you feed people white bread with butter versus whole-wheat bread with butter, along with lots of fruits and vegetables, and measure how much butter comes out the other end? The higher-fiber whole-wheat group poops out more than twice as much fat as the white-bread group,[1195] since some of the butter calories get trapped in all that fiber. Even if you just drink a third of a cup of oil on a high-fiber diet, you'd excrete twice as much fat as you would on a low-fiber diet.[1196] The same goes for the calories of starch. Eat whole-grain bread as opposed to white bread, and stool analyses will find that you flush out nearly ten times as many carb calories.[1197]

It's not what you eat but what you absorb, so you can lose more weight on a high-fiber diet eating the exact same number of calories simply because some of those calories get trapped and never make it into your system. Those on a Standard American Diet lose about 5 percent of the calories they eat in their waste,[1198] but a higher-fiber diet can double that.[1199] It's not simply that the calories in high-fiber foods are less available. High-fiber foods trap calories across the board. So eat a Twinkie on a high-fiber diet and absorb fewer Twinkie calories! It's like every calorie label you read instantly gets discounted on a high-fiber diet.

We learn in school that a gram of protein has four calories, a gram of fat has nine calories, and a gram of carbs has four calories—but that's only on a typical, low-fiber diet. On a higher-fiber diet, up around the average of those eating completely plant-based diets,[1200] the effective calorie counts drop from 4-9-4 to around 3.5-8.7-3.8.[1201] That may not seem like a lot, but if Americans just reached the minimum recommended fiber intake, that might decrease calorie absorption by more than one hundred calories a day,[1202] which may be enough to prevent that average, gradual, annual weight gain most experience through middle age.[1203] Even a small, consistent change in daily calorie absorption could potentially have long-term significance for weight management.[1204]

Putting On the Brakes

A review entitled "Food Fibre as an Obstacle to Energy Intake" summarized what I call the Four Ds by which dietary fiber results in reduced caloric intake:[1205] *dilution* of calories by expanding the volume of food, *distention* of the stomach through fluid absorption, *delay* in stomach emptying of the gelled mass, and *dumping* of calories by blocking the absorption of other macronutrients, such as carbs and fat. That fourth *D* triggers a fifth phenomenon known as the *ileal brake*.

The ileum is the last part of the small intestine before it empties into the colon. When undigested calories are detected that far down our intestines, our bodies put the brakes on eating more by curbing our appetites. This can be shown experimentally. If you insert a nine-foot tube down people's throats and drip in protein, fat, or sugar, you can activate the ileal brake. Then, if you sit them down to an all-you-can-eat meal, they will eat at least one hundred fewer calories than those in the placebo group who had only gotten a squirt of water through the tube.[1206] Activating the ileal brake can make people feel full up to nearly two hundred calories earlier.

Ever since its discovery, the ileal brake has been considered a medical target for appetite control. So did doctors simply advise patients to eat lots of whole, unprocessed plant foods so that the fiber would drag calories down to activate the brake? Not quite. Instead, they developed the first major bariatric surgery, the jejunoileal bypass.

Fiber-depleted foods get absorbed quickly and never make it all the way down to the ileum, but instead of having people eat foods in their natural form, some doctors decided just to cut out the intervening twenty or so feet of intestine. By attaching the end of the ileum right up to within about eighteen inches of the stomach, the ileal brake is activated no matter what you eat. It's like your emergency brake is always on. You can still drive, but not as fast. So, with the jejunoileal bypass, you can still eat, but not as much because you're already feeling full.

More than twenty-five thousand patients underwent the procedure in the United States before it was realized that cutting out 90 percent of the intestines wasn't such a good idea. The jejunoileal bypass resulted in long-term progressive liver scarring in 38 percent of patients.[1207] That's nearly two out of every five patients. Though the surgical approach failed, the medical mindset still prevails, with researchers teaming up with drug companies and the food industry to exploit the ileal brake for weight loss with "dietary en-capsulation or slow release strategies,"[1208] failing to recognize that Mother Nature already designed a natural strategy in the form of fiber-rich food.

Intestinal Workout

There are many ways eating more fiber means eating fewer calories, but the "Dietary Fiber and Weight Regulation" review found that study subjects ran-domized to consume higher-fiber diets lost more weight even when caloric intake was fixed.[1209] Think about it: more weight loss even when prescribed the same number of calories. So if it wasn't the calories-in side of the equa-tion, could it be the calories-out side? Normally, *calories out* means things like exercise, but, in the case of high-fiber diets, there are literally calories out—as in out the other end and flushed down the toilet. But the same-calorie, higher-fiber groups were losing more weight even after taking into account the excess calorie dumping. Where were the calories going?

To solve the mystery of the missing calories, researchers fed people dif-ferent amounts of fiber and sealed them in an airtight chamber called a *whole-body calorimeter* to closely monitor their metabolic rates.[1210] Those with more fiber in their systems burned more calories—even in their sleep. Though it was only about 2 percent more, that translated into about fifty more calories burned a day without getting out of bed. What was going on?

For people on long-term, fiber-rich diets, the researchers figured that all that fiber might bulk up their intestinal linings, which are highly metaboli-cally active tissues. The gut may only represent 5 percent of body weight, but it might burn 25 percent of daily calories.[1211] Why were the research subjects spontaneously burning off more energy even while they were sleeping? It turns out all that extra fiber may be giving their gut a workout.

Our intestines are muscular tubes, so our small intestines are essentially twenty feet of muscle, which contract in waves to move food along. But fiber-depleted foods don't offer much resistance. Wonder Bread and apple juice get absorbed almost immediately without much effort. It's like pumping iron with barbells made out of Styrofoam.

Researchers had people swallow long strings of electrodes to measure the electrical activity of the muscular contractions of the intestines of those eating low-fiber meals versus high-fiber meals.[1212] Those eating more fiber sometimes not only had stronger, faster, and longer contractions, but they had also reduced the periods of intestinal inactivity. Turns out our gut can be sedentary too. But if you eat lots of fiber-rich foods, your gut could be exercising all night long while you sleep.

Discovering the Keys to Weight Loss

This laundry list of mechanisms for fiber-induced weight loss included the best explanations we had back in 2001 when the "Dietary Fiber and Weight Regulation" review was published, but that was two years before a discovery was to change our ideas about fiber forever.[1213]

Cells are the fundamental unit of life. We're composed of trillions of them,[1214] and they communicate with each other through receptors on the cell surface. That's how many hormones work: Like a lock and key, hormones are signaling messengers, and each has a unique shape. When released into the bloodstream, they circulate throughout the body until they find a receptor they can fit into. Once the key is in the lock, a whole series of reactions can be turned on or off in the target cell. For example, cells in our adrenal glands release adrenaline when we get scared, and there are receptors on our hearts, called *beta receptors*, into which adrenaline fits that can trigger an increased heart rate. That's how beta-blocker drugs work to lower our heart rates—by gumming up this lock so adrenaline can no longer fit.

The largest family of cell receptors is known as *G protein–coupled receptors*. G proteins are molecular switches inside the cells that transmit the receptor signal.[1215] More than one-third of the drugs currently on the market work by plugging into these receptors,[1216] from antihistamines to heroin overdose drugs that block opioid receptors. We've discovered hundreds of different G protein–coupled receptors, but remarkably, we don't know what many of them do.[1217] We have the lock, but we just don't know which key fits into them. Accordingly, these are called *orphan* receptors.

Two of these mystery receptors, known only as *G protein–coupled receptor #41* and *G protein–coupled receptor #43*, were found heavily expressed throughout the body in our gut, on our nerves, and in our immune, muscle, and fat cells.[1218] We knew they must be vital, but we didn't know what activated them until 2003 when they were "deorphanized." (That's actually what scientists call it.) And the keys that fit into those important locks were the short-chain fatty acids that our gut bacteria make when we feed them fiber.[1219]

This may be how our gut bacteria communicate with us.[1220] Renamed *free fatty acid receptors,* their existence gives us crucial insight into how fiber could play such a critical role in so many of our chronic diseases.[1221] They may explain why fiber is so anti-inflammatory.[1222] So, for example, how can a single high-fiber meal improve lung function in asthmatics within a matter of hours? The fiber we eat is turned into SCFAs by our good gut bacteria, which then are absorbed into our bloodstreams, where they are thought to dock with these free fatty acid receptors found on inflammatory immune cells in our airways, turning them off.[1223]

Hormones are defined as signaling messengers that are produced in one organ, circulate through the bloodstream, and have a regulatory effect on another organ. So these SCFAs could be considered hormones. It's just that the organs producing them are our microbiomes, the bacteria that populate our gut. They can't make these hormones without fiber, though. Just like our bodies need iodine to make thyroid hormones and our thyroid function suffers when we eat iodine-deficient diets, our bodies need fiber to make short-chain fatty acids and can suffer the consequences if we eat fiber-deficient diets.

Hacking Hunger Hormones

Short-chain fatty acids also stimulate the production of leptin,[1224] the hormone produced by fat cells to tell our brains to trim us down. Leptin is an *anorectic* hormone, so called because it generates a loss of appetite and weight, but it does so over the long term. Leptin levels slowly rise as the volume of body fat gradually increases. In contrast, there are other anorectic hormones that work rapidly, signaling our brains on more of a meal-to-meal basis.[1225] Two of these short-term appetite suppressants are PYY and GLP-1, both of which are secreted by specialized *L cells* that line our colons (named for their release of large packets of hormones).[1226] Guess which receptors are crowded all over the surface of L cells? Free fatty acid receptors.[1227]

Drip some SCFAs onto L cells, and they start churning out PYY and GLP-1. You can do this in a petri dish[1228] or in a person, either by infusing their rectums with an SCFA enema[1229] or the old-fashioned way of feeding people fiber[1230] or, even better, fiber-rich foods.[1231] These hormones then get released into the bloodstream where they can shoot right up into the appetite center of the brain and turn down our cravings.[1232]

The flip side to PYY and GLP-1 is ghrelin, the so-called hunger hormone.

Ghrelin levels rise in our blood before a meal to stimulate our appetites and fall right down once we eat, before slowly building back up again to propel us once more to the fridge.[1233] But feed people twenty-four grams of fiber, and four hours later, ghrelin levels are suppressed as much as if they had just eaten five hundred calories' worth of food.[1234] Over the longer term, overweight eleven- and twelve-year-olds who had been randomized to increase fiber intake for sixteen weeks ended up eating hundreds of fewer calories at a buffet meal challenge compared to a placebo control group.[1235]

One of the most fascinating studies that has been done in this area involves putting people into an fMRI machine that measures real-time brain activity. Subjects were shown a high-calorie food such as a donut, and the reward centers in their brains instantly lit up compared to when they were shown a low-calorie food like cucumber slices. What happens if you repeat the experiment, but this time, after secretly delivering SCFAs directly into their colons? The subjects reported the high-calorie foods seemed less appealing, and this was matched by decreased activity in some of the reward centers in their brains, whereas their brains continued to react about the same to the less-craveable foods.

The researchers figured this was due to PYY and GLP-1 secretion, but that wasn't the case: The effect was independent of hormone release. The researchers speculated that perhaps they had directly stimulated free fatty acid receptors on nerves in the gut that travel straight to the brain.[1236] Similar results were not found with psyllium supplements (like Metamucil),[1237] which makes sense since psyllium is nonfermentable, meaning our gut bacteria can't eat it—so although it can improve bowel regularity, it cannot be used to make the key ingredients for appetite suppression.[1238] Eat fiber-rich foods, though, and our good gut flora take the fiber we eat and churn out molecules that calm our cravings.

Putting Fiber to the Test

The evidence for the role of fiber in weight control started with so-called ecological studies.[1239] These involve comparing population averages, noting that populations with extraordinary fiber intakes tend to have negligible obesity rates. The problem with dealing with population averages is that we don't know if the individuals eating the higher-fiber diets are themselves necessarily the ones protected from obesity. In cross-sectional studies, you can confirm in both adults[1240] and children[1241] that those who eat more fiber are indeed significantly less likely to be obese. A problem with these types of studies, however, is that they represent only a snapshot in time, so you don't know which came first, the obesity or the poor eating habits.

This brings us to cohort studies, where individuals and their diets can be followed over time. A cohort study of overweight youth found that the amount of fiber in a single, half-cup, daily serving of beans over about a two-year period was associated with a "profound" 25 percent difference in abdominal obesity.[1242] In about the same time frame, in middle-aged women, each two-gram increase in daily fiber was associated with a weight decrease of about a pound.[1243] The postpartum period places women at risk for retaining baby weight,[1244] and a study of hundreds of new moms followed for the first five months found that inadequate fiber intake during the postpartum period appeared to increase obesity risk by 24 percent. And the benefits of fiber are not limited to women.[1245] A cohort that included tens of thousands of men who were followed for years concluded that a daily ten-gram increase in fiber consumption might be expected to prevent about 10 percent of weight gain within the population.

Overall, the evidence is strong from these kinds of observational studies that "increasing consumption of dietary fiber with fruits, vegetables, whole grains, and legumes across the life cycle is a critical step in stemming the epidemic of obesity."[1246] These studies can control for nondietary influences like physical activity by equipping people with gadgets to measure their movement, but there may be uncontrolled confounding dietary factors. Think about that list of high-fiber foods—fruits, vegetables, whole grains, and beans. Maybe fiber intake is just a marker for the intake of healthy foods. There are many reasons why eating whole plant foods could facilitate weight loss that have nothing to do with fiber. To know if there's a cause-and-effect relationship between fiber and weight loss, you need to put it to the test in interventional trials.

This is where rectal infusions come in handy.

In a randomized, double-blind, placebo-controlled crossover study, researchers showed that by infusing SCFAs into people's rectums, you can boost their metabolisms within thirty minutes.[1247] They used the amounts you'd expect to create yourself from eating a high-fiber diet. Not only did the subjects' resting metabolic rate go up (that is, the amount of calories burned just by being alive), but specifically, their fat oxidation jumped up, too, increasing the amount of fat they were burning by more than 25 percent.[1248] This translates into about an extra third of a pat of butter's worth of fat burned off their bodies within two hours of the infusion.[1249]

Colonic catheters aside, you can feed people SCFAs directly and get the same little bump in resting metabolic rate and whole-body fat breakdown,[1250] in addition to decreasing appetite. So, again, fiber may work on both sides of the energy-balance equation.[1251] But does that decreased appetite actually result in people eating less? Given the equivalent of about ninety grams of fiber worth of SCFAs, study subjects consumed about two hundred fewer calories at an all-you-can-eat meal.[1252,1253]

Can't you just feed people some beans? Indeed you can. Researchers in Sweden fed people beans for dinner, and, by the next morning, after their friendly flora had also had a chance to feast, their satiety hormones like PYY were up, their hunger hormone ghrelin was down, and they reported feeling less hungry.[1254] The researchers didn't measure subsequent food intake, but a similar study with whole-grain rye for dinner led to a decreased food intake at lunch the next day. Those who had eaten the fiber-rich whole grain the night before felt fully satiated about one hundred calories sooner at a meal more than twelve hours later.[1255] So, by eating fiber-rich foods on a daily basis, you can set yourself up for success.

What About Fiber Supplements?

Reduced caloric intake at a single meal or even over the course of a whole day doesn't necessarily translate into long-term weight loss, though, as our bodies may find ways of compensating.[1256] Experimentally delivering SCFAs directly to the colon every day for months showed that it does reduce abdominal fat, liver fat, and overall weight gain,[1257] but what about getting SCFAs the old-fashioned way, by taking fiber by mouth?

To isolate out the effects of fiber, studies have tried using straight fiber supplements. A 2017 systematic review and meta-analysis compilation of a dozen randomized controlled trials of various fiber supplements versus placebo powders found that the groups taking the actual fiber lost an average of about five and a half pounds more than the control groups.[1258] These were studies ranging in duration from two to seventeen weeks, though there have been fiber supplementation trials that have lasted up to a year that have shown significantly superior weight changes in both young adolescents[1259] and adults.[1260]

Many of the fiber supplement findings were inconsistent,[1261] though, presumably because dozens of different isolated fiber types had been tested.[1262] There are all sorts of newfangled fibers on the market with names like *IQP G-002AS*. (The *IQP* stands for *InQpharm*, the drug company that came up with it.[1263]) After all, how much money can you make selling beans?

Real Fiber FTW

Using isolated fiber extracted from plants or made in a lab can be useful in experimentally proving fiber's effectiveness apart from all the other healthy components in whole foods, but, if anything, you might expect even greater benefits from getting fiber the way nature intended: by eating intact plant foods.[1264]

Published in the prestigious *Annals of Internal Medicine,* a study entitled "Single-Component Versus Multicomponent Dietary Goals . . ." randomly assigned hundreds of people into one of two weight-loss regimens:[1265] One simply encouraged people to get at least thirty grams of fiber each day, which is about the recommended minimum adequate intake, and the other advised people to also follow the far more complex weight-loss program recommended by the American Heart Association. So, in addition to also hitting that thirty-grams-of-fiber target, study subjects in the second group were prescribed carefully calculated caloric intake goals and were told to switch from red meat to white, moderate their alcohol intakes, cut down on sugary beverages, and reduce sugar and sodium intake across the board.[1266]

Even though both groups were told to reach the same fiber target, the group whose focus was solely on fiber intake ended up eating more than twice as much extra fiber as the multicomponent intervention and, surprisingly, similarly improved the quality of their diets. For example, the group focused only on fiber intake ended up reducing their saturated fat intakes as much as the group who was explicitly instructed to do so.[1267] Simply telling people to eat more whole plant foods seems to naturally crowd out some of the less healthy options by default. With similar dietary improvements, both groups lost similar amounts of weight,[1268] suggesting if you could give only one piece of weight-loss advice, eating more fiber might not be a bad choice. Of course, it only works if you actually do it.

There was one study that reported favorable results when eating a low-carb diet compared to a "high-fiber" diet. But just how high was this so-called high-fiber diet? The subjects started out at a pitiful 17.4 grams of fiber a day. Sadly, that's about typical for the United States,[1269] but it's only about half the average recommended minimum daily intake of 31.5 grams.[1270] The low-carb study subjects started out at 17.4 grams a day and, on their "high-fiber" diets, shot up to . . . 18.6 grams a day. Seriously. In no universe is that a high-fiber diet. Nevertheless, the low-carb study researchers used their findings to conclude "previous claims of the benefits of fiber for weight loss may have been overstated."[1271]

Eating the Way Nature Intended

Fewer than 3 percent of Americans reach even the recommended *minimum* daily adequate intake of fiber.[1272] There's so much fuss about protein, but for that, the stats are reversed: More than 97 percent of Americans get enough protein, but more than 97 percent of Americans don't get enough fiber. Nearly everyone is suffering from a fiber-deficient diet, and that's just based on the wimpy federal recommendations of fourteen grams per thousand calories, which comes out to be about twenty-five grams per day for women and thirty-eight daily grams for men.[1273] That's a far cry from the hundred grams our bodies were designed to get,[1274] based on the diets of modern-day, isolated, hunter-gatherer tribes[1275] and an analysis of coprolites, human fossilized feces—paleopoo![1276]

For perhaps more than 99 percent of our existence as a distinct species, the natural state of affairs was having our guts literally packed with fiber-filled foods all the time.[1277] Before the gristmills and certainly for the millions of years before the first stone tools and evidence of butchering, our physiology evolved eating huge amounts of unprocessed plants.[1278] That's the nutritional landscape upon which our bodies developed.

This could explain why our bodies centered this whole elaborate system of body fat regulation around short-chain fatty acids, the microbial by-product of fiber. Indeed, for most of our time on Earth, fiber equaled food.[1279] In fact,

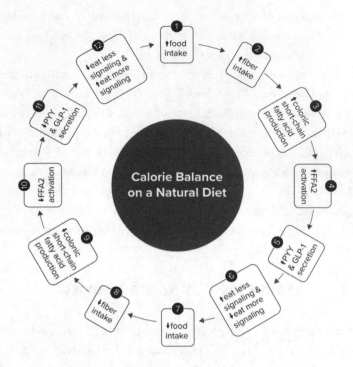

one of the theories used to explain the obesity epidemic is that the body's mechanisms for controlling appetite evolved to match our ancestral diet.[1280] It's like a classic negative feedback loop (adapted from Sleeth et al.).[1281]

Follow along in the diagram above, starting at the top (1). Imagine if we ate too much of the foods we were designed to eat. Since, essentially, food meant fiber, (2) our fiber intake would go up. The body would detect that change because of (3) all the extra SCFAs flooding the system, which would (4) activate the free fatty acid receptors all over the body, with direct effects on our fat cells and brains, and indirect effects by (5) stimulating the release of those anorectic hormones that (6) suppress our appetites. With fewer cravings and less hunger, our (7) food intake would drop, which is beneficial because, remember, we were (1) eating too much.

On our original, natural diet, a drop in food necessarily meant (8) a drop in fiber intake, which our bodies would pick up on, because, all of a sudden, there would be (9) less signaling by SCFAs and (10) less activation of those free fatty acid receptors, which means (11) less of those anorectic hormones circulating throughout our bodies, (12) perking up our appetites once again. That may be how our bodies were meant to work to keep our body weight stable.

Okay, but now, fast-forward past the Industrial Revolution and time-machine drop the human body into the middle of bologna-on-Wonder-Bread country. The figure above shows what happens when food doesn't equal high fiber anymore. When calories are divorced from fiber, we may just keep getting these signals to eat, eat, and eat some more. We're always hungry because our bodies aren't getting the signal that we've eaten enough, even though we're piling in the calories. If we haven't eaten our hundred grams of fiber for the day, our bodies may be like, *What? Are we starving here?*

Sadly, the average fiber intake in the United States has failed to improve in recent years despite ongoing public health messaging about its importance.[1282] One problem may be that people just don't know what fiber is. More than half of Americans surveyed think steak is a significant source of fiber.[1283] However, literally by definition, fiber is only found in plants.[1284] There is zero fiber in meat, dairy, or eggs and typically little or no fiber in junk food.

Therein lies the problem.

Ninety-six percent of Americans don't eat the minimum recommended daily amount of beans, 96 percent don't eat the measly minimum for greens, and 99 percent don't get enough whole grains.[1285] Nearly the entire U.S.

population fails to eat enough whole plant foods—the *only* place fiber is naturally found in abundance. You know things are bad when french fries make it into the top ten sources of fiber in the American diet,[1286] and donuts, cookies, and cake come in at number thirteen. In comparison, sweet potatoes are down at number forty-seven. And what's the number-one source of fiber in the American diet? Ironically, it's white bread. Even though it's severely fiber-depleted, we eat so much of it and so few whole grains and beans that white bread is Americans' top fiber source.

You'd think the discovery of the free fatty acid receptor mechanism for appetite control would reignite the public health push to get us all to eat healthier food, but instead, Big Food and Big Pharma view it as an opportunity to market new products. Since "large amounts of dietary fibre (>30g/day)"—in other words, the recommended *minimum* adequate intake—"are required for these beneficial effects,"[1287] researchers conclude, "alternative ways of optimising colonic SCFA production may be needed."[1288] The measly minimum represents "unpalatably high levels,"[1289] according to these drug industry–funded researchers. Thus, there are calls for "pharmacological manipulation of appetite using a GPR43 agonist [stimulator]."[1290] Their conclusion is that "activation of colonic [free fatty acid receptor] FFA2 by . . . pharmacological mimetics [mimickers] is a promising candidate in the fight against the current obesity onslaught."[1291]

Or we could just eat as nature intended.

FOOD FOR THOUGHT

What are the best sources of fiber? The American Medical Association published a patient summary about fiber-rich foods listing an array of whole, unrefined plant foods.[1292] Those of us who may be a little smug about our hearty intake of fruits and vegetables need to realize that fruits and leafy veggies are the *poorest* whole-food sources of fiber. Why? Because they're 90 percent water. Root vegetables have about twice as much on a per-weight basis, but the fiber superstars are whole grains and legumes, which include dried or canned beans, split peas, chickpeas, and lentils.[1293]

HIGH IN WATER-RICH FOODS

Mouthwatering

Like fiber, water adds bulk to foods without adding calories. A prune and a plum are pretty much the same—one just has more water. You could eat a whole handful of prunes as a snack, but the same number of plums would be an armload. In a famous experiment, dozens of common foods were scored for their ability to satiate the appetites of individuals for hours, and the characteristic most predictive of satiety in general was water content.[1294]

Grapes, for example, have less fiber than bananas but were significantly more satiating—perhaps in part because of their greater water content.[1295] Apples and oranges, which have even higher water content, beat out both grapes and bananas, but researchers fed people up to twice as much to match them calorie for calorie. So, in effect, they found that four oranges were more satiating than two bananas, which seems kind of obvious, but the size difference is exactly the point. Because apples and oranges are about 85 percent water, you have to eat a lot more of them to get the same number of calories.[1296]

People tend to eat a fairly consistent weight of food on a day-to-day basis, and serving weight is largely determined by water content.[1297] The more water-rich the food, the fewer calories are being taken in overall. Higher-volume foods also take longer to eat, which slows the rate of consumption and increases "oropharyngeal stimulation,"[1298] the sensation of food in our mouths and throats. The more we chew, taste, and feel food in our mouths, the more our brains get tipped off that we're filling up. Stomach tube studies in which food bypasses the mouth show that the body has difficulty regulating appetite when we don't experience those oral sensations.[1299]

Which foods have the most water? On the next page, I've put together a ranking for you of the water content of common foods.[1300]

As you can see, vegetables top the charts, with most being more than 90 percent water by weight, followed by most fruit coming in around the 80s. Starchier vegetables, whole grains, and canned beans are in the 70s, meaning about three-quarters of their weights are pure water. Pasta and most unprocessed meat, including seafood, fall down to the 60s. Most dried

Water Content of Foods

100–90%

asparagus, beets, bell peppers, broccoli, cabbage, cauliflower, celery, cucumber, grapefruit, green beans, greens, lettuce, melons, mushrooms, okra, onions, pumpkin, strawberries, summer squash, tomatoes, zucchini

89–80%

apples, apricots, artichokes, bean sprouts, brussels sprouts, carrots, cherries, grapes, jello, kiwifruit, mangoes, oatmeal, other berries, other citrus, pears, peas, pineapples, plums, tofu, winter squash, yogurt

79–70%

avocados, bananas, canned beans, corn, couscous, edamame, eggs, millet, oysters, pomegranates, potatoes, pudding, quinoa, rice, sweet potatoes

69–60%

barley, beef, boiled beans, canned tuna, hummus, ice cream, lobster, lunch meat, pasta, pork, poultry, salmon

59–50%

cream cheese, frankfurters, tempeh

49–40%

cheesecake, french fries, sausage

39–30%

bagels, bread, cheese, dried apples, dried apricots, figs, prunes

29–20%

cake, croissants, dates, pepperoni

19–10%

brownies, cookies, energy bars, goji berries, jerky, raisins

9–0%

breakfast cereals, candy bars, chocolate, crackers, nuts, oils, popcorn, potato chips, pretzels, seeds, tortilla chips

fruits, cheeses, and breads are in the 30s. Cake crumbles into the 20s, cookies into the teens, and candy and most common snack foods are all the way at the bottom with less than 9 percent water by weight. In general, when it comes to water-rich foods, most whole plant foods float up near the top, most animal foods fall somewhere in the middle, and most processed foods sink to the bottom.

Trapped vs. Free Water

Can't you just drink a few glasses of water while you eat a steak and make up for the meat's low water content that way? If you drank ten gulps of water with every bite, wouldn't you end up with the same 95 percent water stomach contents you'd get eating, say, cucumbers and lettuce? This scheme works for fat cats—adding water to dry kibble can help our pet cats lose weight[1301]—but it doesn't seem to work for dogs.[1302] So are we more like dogs or cats?

If you have people drink two glasses of water with a meal, their subjective feelings of hunger and satiety can be affected. This led researchers to suggest that drinking extra water could decrease food intake in a manner "far more simple and cheaper than installing an intragastric balloon."[1303] Drinking water with meals would certainly be safer, but it doesn't appear to actually cut down on food intake.[1304] People tend to feel fuller when they drink water with a meal, but that doesn't appear to actually translate into eating less.[1305]

Why does water *inside* a food reduce intake, but not water *alongside* a food? It all just ends up in the same place, right? What appears to be happening is a phenomenon known as *sieving*.[1306] When water is outside the food, the stomach simply siphons it off from the solid chunks and strains it right out, which leads to a rapid drop in stomach volume. On the other hand, when water is part of a food, it all forms a homogenous mass that more slowly empties from your stomach over time.[1307]

If you give people a casserole for lunch, they eat the same amount whether or not they're also given a glass of water, about four hundred calories' worth. But if that same casserole and that same water are blended into a soup, they only eat three hundred calories' worth before feeling full.[1308] You can do real-time MRI scans of people's stomachs and witness the sieving process in action. A half hour after eating, the stomach volume remained 36 percent greater after eating the same meal in soup form.[1309] Blended together, the same meal components served as a soup left people significantly fuller even three hours later.[1310]

Even though the soup was puréed in a blender, its thickness from all the little suspended particles prevented the stomach from separating out the water and draining it off.[1311] It even works with thinner liquids.[1312] If you give people a milkshake followed by a glass of water, the body is able to layer out the water and empty the stomach twice as fast than if you had preblended in the water to make a more dilute, thinner shake. This helps explain observational data showing that, compared to water consumed separately, the intake of water in foods is more closely related to a slimmer waist.[1313]

Does Dried Fruit Make You Gain Weight?

Some dried fruit is as dry as beef jerky. Drying concentrates the calories. Compared to dried fruit, fresh fruit gives us more volume, more weight—more *food*—for the same number of calories.[1314] Drying also concentrates the sugars, which could drive overeating. The raisin industry is quick to point out that raisins don't cause any more of a sugar spike than when consuming the same number of calories of grapes, but with grapes, that means eating about four times as much food.[1315] On the other hand, in dried fruit, the fiber also gets more concentrated, which could potentially aid satiety. So which is it?

In population studies, those who eat dried fruit tend to be slimmer than those who don't,[1316] but they also tend to eat better diets overall. This is one reason interventional studies are so important to prove whether there's a cause-and-effect relationship. Leave it to the California Raisin Marketing Board to dream up a study entitled "An After-School Snack of Raisins Lowers Cumulative Food Intake in Young Children."[1317] Sounds good, right? Well, what did they compare raisins to? Potato chips and chocolate chip cookies. They gave kids raisins, grapes, chips, or cookies and told them to eat as much as they wanted. Surprise, surprise, the kids ate less fruit and more junk. To be fair, I guess naming the paper "Kids Prefer Cookies" would not have garnered the same kind of sponsor approval.

Give people fresh fruit, and they end up eating less at subsequent meals. Give people strawberries, raspberries, blackberries, and blueberries, and they eat less pasta an hour later compared to those given the same number of calories in the form of gummy bears, which have about the same water content as raisins.[1318] The same effect can be found with other kinds of fresh fruit,[1319] and this can translate into greater weight loss. Give people apples or pears every day instead of the same calories in cookies, and they lose significantly more weight.[1320] The only way to know if *water* content played the critical role, though, is if the researchers had included a third group in the study who had been given *dried* pears and apple rings.

There have been experiments directly comparing raisins to grapes.

Although grapes appear to suppress appetite better than raisins,[1321] raisins beat out grapes when it came to reducing pizza intake a half hour later. I know as parents there's a concern that if our kids eat snacks, it might spoil their dinners, but when the snacks are fruit and the meal is "pepperoni and 3 cheese pizza,"[1322] perhaps the more we can ruin their appetites, the better.

Does the satiating effect of raisins translate into weight loss, though? Prunes can also cut down on appetite[1323] and subsequent meal intake,[1324] but feed people about nine prunes a day and they don't appear to lose any weight, at least in the short term (though their bowel habits did improve).[1325] Similarly, replacing about four hundred to five hundred calories of someone's diet with raisins every day may not lead to weight loss. However, you can imagine how adding the same caloric load in the form of grapes every day—four or five cups—might have more of an effect.[1326] Bottom line: Although eating dried apples,[1327] figs,[1328] dates,[1329] prunes,[1330] or raisins[1331] may not lead to inordinate weight gain, they don't appear to actively promote weight loss. That makes fresh fruit the better choice.

FOOD FOR THOUGHT

Take a deep dive into the Water Content of Foods chart so your diet swims in water-rich vegetables and juicy fruit (though not the gum!).

LOW GLYCEMIC LOAD

Chew on This

One of the major dietary shifts from the ancient to the modern world has been the increased consumption of fiber-depleted processed carbohydrates—sugars and starches.[1332] The impact of carbs on the body depends on their source. Kidney beans and jelly beans are both rich in carbs but can have diametrically different impacts on our bodies. Bread made from the exact same ingredients as pasta causes nearly twice the blood sugar spike, leading to nearly three times the insulin release as the same number of carbs consumed in noodle form.[1333] That's because bread is filled with tiny bubbles, allowing digestive enzymes easy access to more surface area to more rapidly digest starch into sugars compared to pasta, which is more compact. The more solid nature of pasta forces the enzymes to have to work their way in from the edges, slowing the rate at which pasta can be broken down.

You can try this experiment at home: Take a bite of a piece of bread, and chew, chew, and chew some more without swallowing. Gradually, that piece of bread will taste sweeter and sweeter, thanks to the starch-digesting enzyme in our saliva. Next, try it with cooked spaghetti. Sore jaw alert! It may take two hours of chewing pasta to get the same sweetness in your mouth that you'd get from chewing bread for only ten minutes. You probably won't want to try it with the whole intact grain—wheat berries—because it might take all day.[1334]

Why do we care how quickly carbohydrates are digested? Because it can affect our appetites, our metabolic rates, and how much fat we burn.

You can measure the impact different carbohydrate-rich foods have by feeding people a certain amount and seeing what happens to their blood sugar levels over the next few hours. Then you can compare the size of the blood sugar bump from the carbs in bread form to the same number of carbs in pasta form, or fruit form—or cotton candy form, for that matter. This is how the glycemic index of foods is generally calculated. Then, based on the

Glycemic Load Per Serving

Low ≤ 10	Medium 11–19	High ≥ 20
beans	oatmeal	corn flakes & rice krispies
chickpeas & split peas	spaghetti	dates
fruit	brown rice	white rice
lentils	sweet potato	white potato
whole-grain bread	white bread	raisins

number of carbs per serving, we can come up with the glycemic load of a food. The higher the glycemic load, the higher our blood sugars tend to spike when we eat them. A breakdown of some common sweet and starchy foods appears on page 142.[1335]

Lighten Your Load

If you feed people two types of meals matched for calories, nutrition, and taste, but one has a high glycemic load and the other low, what happens when you put them in a brain scanner? The high-glycemic-load meal causes significantly greater activation in the regions of the brain associated with reward and craving, along with increased hunger four hours later.[1336] This may help explain why most of the top dozen problematic foods identified in a study entitled "Which Foods May Be Addictive?" were high-glycemic-load foods. (I expand on this study in the Low in Addictive Foods section.) Rather than the *quantity* of refined carbs, such as white flour and sugar, it was the speed at which they were absorbed in the system that was more predictive of being "addictive."[1337]

What do you think happened when kids ate Corn Flakes, Coco Pops, or Rice Krispies for breakfast versus a lower-glycemic-load food like oatmeal with a spoonful of sugar? After the high-glycemic breakfast, the kids went on to eat more of a buffet-style lunch than when they had started their day eating about the same number of calories of the lower-glycemic breakfast. Even with the extra sugar added to their oatmeal, they ended up eating about one hundred fewer calories of the all-you-can-eat lunch, compared with after the high-glycemic breakfast.[1338] In this case, the difference in fiber intake also could have played a role, but in general, these types of short-term satiety studies have shown that lower-glycemic carbohydrates may make one feel fuller longer.[1339]

Beyond appetite regulation, lower-glycemic-load foods can also cause you to burn more fat. If you feed people a low-glycemic meal (All-Bran cereal and fruit) and put them on a treadmill three hours later, they burn more fat than they would after having eaten the same number of calories of a high-glycemic meal (for example, Corn Flakes and white bread).[1340] This enhanced fat loss can occur not only during brisk walking[1341] or running[1342] but can happen even when doing nothing.

One of the reasons it's so hard to maintain weight loss is that our bodies try to defend themselves against losing fat by slowing down our resting metabolic rates, the number of calories our bodies burn every hour just by existing.[1343] That's one of the reasons weight loss can stall on a diet. But put people on a low-glycemic-load diet, and metabolic rate doesn't slow down as much—their metabolisms slow by 96 calories a day after losing about twenty pounds, compared to a metabolism that is 176 calories slower on a higher-glycemic-load diet.[1344] An 80-calorie-a-day difference might not seem like a lot, but those calories are burned automatically without an ounce of additional effort on our parts. Eighty calories is about how much we'd burn walking an extra mile a day (or eating about two fewer bites of a donut).

This process can work the other way too. If you overfeed people on a high-glycemic diet, then they store more fat than those eating the same number of calories of a low-glycemic diet. If you eat 50 percent more calories than needed, you add about a quarter pound of pure fat to your body each day on a high-glycemic diet. However, if you eat the same number of extra calories on a low-glycemic diet, you gain about 40 percent less,[1345] which comes out to a difference of about a pound of fat a week while eating the same number of calories.

Putting Lower-Glycemic Eating to the Test

Between the satiating power and metabolic benefits of low-glycemic foods, it's no wonder that those randomized to be given lower, rather than higher, glycemic meals appear to lose more body fat.[1346,1347] What did surprise me was how underwhelming the evidence was for significant or long-term weight loss with low-glycemic-load interventions. A review prepared by the Cochrane Collaboration, historically considered to be the evidence-based gold standard, concluded that "lowering the glycaemic load of the diet appears to be an effective method of promoting weight loss" but only found the benefit to be a few extra pounds of weight loss after weeks or months on lower-glycemic-load diets.[1348]

The DIOGENES trial is held up by advocates of lower-glycemic eating as evidence of its efficacy.[1349] Hundreds of overweight individuals were advised to eat either higher- or lower-glycemic index diets after losing an average of twenty-four pounds to see who could keep off the weight better. Those on lower-glycemic diets regained less weight at six months compared to those on the high-glycemic-index diet, but it was only two pounds less,[1350] and the benefit appeared to effectively vanish by the one-year mark.[1351] In retrospect, this is unsurprising given how unsuccessful they were at convincing people to change their eating habits.

Anytime findings in controlled feeding studies don't seem to translate into real-world results, the first question you always have to ask is: *Did the subjects actually follow the prescribed diet?* In a controlled setting like in that metabolic rate study, the glycemic load can be dropped 70 percent, from a total daily glycemic load of 287 down to 82. In the case of the DIOGENES trial, where people were randomized not to different diets but to different dietary *recommendations,* the difference in daily glycemic loads between the "high" glycemic group and the "low" glycemic group differed by less than 3 percent.[1352] No wonder the demonstrated benefits were slim to none. Foods only work if you eat them.

Even in the most successful studies, it's hard to separate out the specific effects of the glycemic change. Many high-glycemic foods are highly processed and fiber-depleted, so when you swap them for low-glycemic foods like beans and fruit, you're doing more than just changing the glycemic load. The big drop in glycemic load in the metabolic rate study was accompanied by a similar-sized boost in fiber intake—so how do we know it was the glycemic load and not the fiber?[1353] That's the problem with diet studies: It's hard to change just one thing. With drug trials, it's easy—just give the drug or a sugar pill and if there's a change, you know it was the drug that caused it. If only we could stuff the change in glycemic load into a pill. Well, it turns out we can.

Acarbose is a drug that partially blocks our sugar- and starch-digesting enzymes in the digestive tract, slowing their absorption into the body.[1354] When taking the drug with a meal, you can effectively transform a high-glycemic meal into a low-glycemic meal without changing the foods at all.[1355] Weight-loss trials with acarbose offer the strongest case that simply lowering dietary glycemic load may indeed be beneficial for weight management.[1356,1357]

FOOD FOR THOUGHT

As you can see in the Glycemic Load Per Serving chart, the simplest way to stick to a lower-glycemic diet is to try to stick to foods that were grown, not made. If you are going to eat high-glycemic foods, though, there are ways to help blunt the blood sugar spikes. I explore a few options in part IV, where I cover a series of weight-loss boosters, including the use of vinegar in the Amping AMPK section and choosing intact grains over whole ones in the Wall Off Your Calories section.

You can also eat berries with your meals, which can act as starch blockers by inhibiting the enzyme that digests starch.[1358] This slows the absorption of blood sugars into your system. So, if you are going to sit down to a high-glycemic breakfast, put a raspberry spread on your toast, add strawberries on your cornflakes, or make your pancakes blueberry, for example, to help mediate the glycemic rush.

Some starch is naturally resistant to digestion. Prior to the discovery of this "resistant starch" in 1982, we thought all starch could be broken down by the enzymes in our small intestines.[1359] Now we know there are indeed starches that resist digestion, which not only lowers their glycemic impact but, since they make their way down to our large intestines, can act as prebiotics to feed our good bacteria, just like fiber does. (*Probiotics* are live bacteria; *prebiotics* are the fuel that feeds them.) Resistant starch is found naturally in many common foods, including beans, grains, vegetables, seeds, and some nuts—but in small quantities, just a few percent of the total.[1360] There are ways, though, to get more resistant starch into your diet.

When regular starches are cooked and then cooled, some of the starch recrystallizes into resistant starch. For this reason, pasta salad can be a bit healthier than hot pasta, and potato salad sometimes healthier than a baked potato. But the effect isn't huge. The resistant starch goes from about 3 percent up to 4 percent. So rather than relying on cold starches, the best source of resistant starch is legumes—beans, split peas, chickpeas, and lentils—which start out at 4–5 percent and then go up from there.[1361]

LOW IN ADDED FAT

The Fat Wars

Dueling *Time* magazine covers, one depicting an egg-and-bacon frowny face and another exhorting people to eat butter, exemplify the two battlefronts in the contentious issue of dietary fat's role in disease. On one side, all sources of fat are villainized, while on the other, lard is lauded. As is so often the case with fervent partisan positions, both could stand a dose of science.

A common trope of the pro-fat faction is that the obesity epidemic was fueled by government calls to reduce fat intake. This presupposes the American public actually followed that advice. In fact, fat intake has not fallen; it's gone from an estimated average of 743 daily calories of fat in the 1970s to 747 in the latest national survey.[1362] The availability of added fats and oils rose more than 50 percent, from 52.5 pounds per person in 1970 to 82.2 in 2010.[1363] America presumably got fat because we ate more of everything—more carbs, more protein, and more fat.[1364] We now eat about 500 more calories every day and gained about an extra 500-calories-a-day's worth of weight.[1365] So there's no great mystery there.

The percentage of calories from fat decreased from about 37 percent to 34 percent, but that's just because the increase in carbs and protein exceeded the increase in fat. At no time in recent history has America eaten a low-fat diet.[1366] The pro-fat faction is right about one thing, though: The food industry's response to the call to reduce fat may have made things worse.

The low-fat diet recommendation, as proposed in the original *Dietary Goals for the United States,* was intended, for example, to "decrease consumption of meat"[1367] and increase consumption of naturally low-fat foods, such as fruits, vegetables, and whole grains.[1368] But how much money can be made on millet? Not nearly as much as bastardized "low-fat" junk foods. Enter SnackWell's Fat-Free Devil's Food Cookie Cakes.

The packaged-food industry is happy to hop on any bandwagon and sell us any kind of junk food we want: low-fat junk, low-carb junk, gluten-free organic junk, and even, ironically, processed paleo junk. But low-fat doesn't necessarily mean low-calorie.[1369] A systematic comparison of different foods and their low-fat versions found that items with reduced-fat claims tend to have more sugar.[1370] Instead, we can dismount the processed food industry's sugar-fat seesaw by opting for whole, natural foods.

Researchers have shown that overfeeding people with either fat or sugar can cause the same weight gain.[1371] The debate is often framed as fat versus carbs, but health-wise, the term *carbs* is practically meaningless, as it could refer to black beans or Blow Pops. If, for weight loss, you replace fatty foods in people's diets with sugary foods, nothing happens, but if you replace fatty foods with starchy foods, they lose weight.[1372] Presumably, this is because the researchers started feeding people more real food (as inferred by increased fiber intake), rather than just processed foods with either added fats or added sugar.

The Halo Effect

Akin to the way people evidently tend to start doing more laundry when they get energy-efficient washing machines and thereby undercut their savings,[1373] low-fat claims can lead consumers to eat larger portions and take in more calories.[1374] When M&M's candies were labeled as "low-fat," for example, overweight study participants ate 47 percent more of them.[1375] Consumers tend to overgeneralize specific claims and arrive at overreaching conclusions. Many people see the words *low fat* and assume that means the product is healthy overall.

Taken from the social psychology literature, the halo effect theory helps explain these types of leaps. Positive personality traits, for example, are inexplicably attributed to people who are more physically attractive.[1376] Cereals use this ploy all the time with nutrient-specific claims like "good source of vitamin D." Lucky Charms can produce a positive "health halo" impression to distract the purchaser from the incongruity of feeding their children multicolored marshmallows for breakfast.

Deliberately distracting attention away from negative qualities or the overall vacuity of nutritional content has a name: *nutri-washing*.[1377] Ironically, cereal boxes bearing low-calorie claims have been found to have *more* calories on average than those not asserting to be low-calorie, so nutrient claims can be misleading even when understood correctly.[1378]

Food, not nutrients, is the fundamental unit in nutrition.[1379] The *source* of fat is likely more important than the *amount* of fat. And let's not forget that the healthiest foods don't have any nutrition labeling on them at all. In the grocery store, you're more likely to see "healthy" claims adorn Apple Jacks than apples.[1380]

What Do Losers Eat?

To bolster their position, low-fat diet proponents often point to the National Weight Control Registry. The largest study of those who have successfully lost weight,[1381] the registry followed thousands of individuals who on average reportedly lost sixty-nine pounds and kept it off for more than six years.[1382] The hope of the study was to identify behaviors associated with the most successful losers. What were their secrets?

Most reported being physically active (primarily walking)[1383] and weighing themselves at least a few times a week.[1384] In terms of diet, at both time of entry into the registry and after ten years of successful weight maintenance, they were said to have "low calorie and fat intake." However, only a third of the participants ate what you might consider truly low-fat diets (no more than 20 percent of their calories from fat).[1385] In general, though, they did eat relatively low fat, coming in at 26 percent calories from fat[1386] compared to the current national average of 34 percent.[1387]

Although the average registrant dropped from severely obese (BMI 35) to normal weight (BMI 24) and kept off the weight for years, several hundred of the participants began adding back some of the weight at follow-up. This offered the researchers an opportunity to study the factors associated with the flip side of the coin, weight gain, and the same finding arose: Those who started gaining back the weight were significantly more likely to report an increase in fat intake.[1388]

Together, the National Weight Control Registry studies provide suggestive evidence that lower-fat diets may help with weight loss and maintenance, but because it's not a random sample, the findings can't be generalized to the entire population.[1389] Maybe those on lower-fat diets are just more likely to submit their medical records and apply for a spot on the registry. You don't know until you put low-fat diets to the test.

Is Fat Fattening?

A review of "low-fat" diets for "long-term" weight loss found they resulted in about twelve pounds greater weight loss compared to people's usual diets.[1390]

Why the quotation marks? The tested diets were rarely low in fat in actuality, and just a single year counts as "long-term" in many weight-loss research circles.

A major limitation of such studies is that the control groups often don't receive the same amount of attentiveness as the group given the diet being tested.[1391] Any intervention that focuses greater attention on food intake and dietary instruction, regardless of the specifics, may facilitate weight loss. Simply being in an obesity study and knowing you have to go in and get weighed regularly can motivate people to watch what they eat and cause them to lose weight even if they're in the control group and not told to do anything.

There have been low-fat studies that weren't about weight loss at all and instead aimed to reduce cancer or cardiovascular disease risk. A compilation of thirty-two such randomized controlled trials involving more than fifty thousand participants found that dietary fat reduction was consistently shown to induce body fat reduction even when that wasn't the intention of the intervention.[1392] That's more promising, but there were often other lifestyle changes as well, such as exercising or quitting smoking, so you can't separate out the effects of the dietary component.[1393] What's more, at least five long-term weight-loss trials failed to show low-fat diets offer the same or superior weight loss compared to other diets,[1394] adding to the debate. But what were these researchers considering "low-fat"?

A Big Fat Low-Fat Fail?

To define *low fat,* you first need to figure out what a normal-fat diet is. Not surprisingly, the "normal" intake of dietary fat varies widely by cultural cuisine around the world, from 6 percent of calories on the traditional Okinawan diet[1395] to 66 percent among indigenous Arctic people.[1396] But what's normal for us as a species?

For millions of years, we may have evolved getting approximately 10 percent of our calories from fat.[1397] There was no butter or oil, nuts were trapped inside hard shells, and animals hadn't yet been bred to be extra juicy. The flesh of some wild game, like moose and elk, is less than 2 percent fat by weight and less than 15 percent calories from fat.[1398] Even the "lean" ground beef of today can have nearly half of its calories from fat.[1399] What about "extra lean"? That comes in at 28 percent fat calories,[1400] which is about double that of the extra, extra, *extra* lean meat of many wild animals eaten by our ancestors.

Some low-fat proponents have used our evolutionary legacy to support their case. After all, the argument goes, what's the ideal fuel for a motor? The fuel it was designed and built for.[1401] Our metabolic physiology was essentially genetically programmed by our ancestral fat intake, but just because 10 percent fat may be normal doesn't mean it's best. Natural selection is more about getting us to reproductive age intact than it is about optimal health and longevity. So while we may not be able to use our prehistoric diets to argue for the ideal, we can use them to define normalcy for our species.

It's been argued that for about 99.8 percent of our time on Earth, it was virtually impossible for us to regularly consume more than 15 percent of calories as fat.[1402] If it's the case that 10 percent is a normal fat intake for humans, less than 10 percent could be defined as low-fat. Given that context, let's review the five studies I could find that purported to show "low-fat" diets failed.

One study published in *The New England Journal of Medicine* claimed to put people on a low-fat diet, but their fat intakes didn't budge significantly, drifting only from 31 percent fat to 30 percent fat.[1403] The "low-fat" groups in three other studies also ended up at 30 percent fat, far from actually being low in fat.[1404,1405,1406] A study in Tehran did claim that a 30 percent fat group beat out a 20 percent fat group for weight loss, but the lower-fat group had zero change in fiber intake and no significant change in protein, saturated fat, or cholesterol consumption.[1407] To get a bump in fiber-depleted carb intake without adding fruits, vegetables, whole grains, or beans, or without removing meat and dairy would presumably mean giving people the Iranian equivalent of SnackWell's. Regardless, even 20 percent fat may be high by evolutionary standards.

So if 10 percent of calories from fat is normal for us as a species and less than that can be considered to be low-fat, why are these studies of so-called low-fat diets allowing double and even triple that? You can't tell if a low-fat diet works unless you test a diet that's actually low in fat.

You Can't Win If You Don't Play

If you put people on a specific diet and nothing happens, then either the diet didn't work or the people didn't follow it. Adherence to prescribed diets in weight-loss studies is poor even when researchers provide all the meals[1408] and truly abysmal when the subjects are left to fend for themselves.[1409] Just as medications never work if you don't take them, diets don't work if you don't eat them.

The accompanying editorial to a meta-analysis of "low-fat" weight-loss studies that showed little to no benefit was entitled "Prescribing Low-Fat Diets: Useless for Long-Term Weight Loss?"[1410]—with the key word *prescribing*. One could imagine a similar editorial called "Prescribing Smoking Cessation: Useless for Preventing Lung Cancer?" because the failure rate of physician advice to quit smoking is 98 percent.[1411] It's not that quitting smoking doesn't help; it's just that people often don't comply. If smokers are able to stop, they can see dramatic improvement in their health, but it may take them an average of thirty attempts to quit before they're successful and stop lighting up.[1412] Even with a dismal 2 percent success rate, we physicians are still urged to advise our patients to stop smoking because we know it works if they actually do it. Is that the same with low-fat diets? You don't know until you put *actual* low-fat diets to the test.

In a remarkable study out of Hawaii that I detail further on pages 188 and 189, subjects achieved seventeen pounds of weight loss in twenty-one days eating unlimited quantities of fruits, vegetables, whole grains, and beans.[1413] That diet was 7 percent fat, similar to the traditional Okinawan diet. But what about longer term? Some of the heart disease reversal studies got people's diets down to 10 percent of fat or less, which can lead unintentionally to a sixteen-pound weight loss in three months.[1414]

In the famous Lifestyle Heart Trial, Dr. Dean Ornish motivated people to reduce their fat intakes to 6 percent with a diet centered on whole plant foods for a year.[1415] The participants were also told to exercise, but they failed to become any more significantly active than the control group. Even though weight loss wasn't the intention of the study and people could eat as much as they wanted, by the end of the year, those randomized to the low-fat lifestyle intervention got a twenty-four-pound weight loss as a side benefit to reversing their heart disease. At five years, their fat intakes were still low at 9 percent and they had sustained a thirteen-pound weight loss.[1416]

The Leaking of Alli's (Orlistat's) Spotty Record

Like studies involving changes in glycemic index, low-fat interventions involve myriad dietary changes, such as changes in meat, junk food, and fiber content. With so many factors, how do you know what role the change in fat itself played? You may remember that in the case of the glycemic index, there was a starch- and sugar-blocking drug that could effectively change the glycemic index of a meal without actually altering the meal itself, which allows us to isolate the effect. Well, there's a fat-blocking drug too.

Orlistat inhibits the enzyme in your intestines that digests fat and can effectively block the absorption of up to 30 percent of the fat you eat.[1417] Researchers were able to track people on similar diets, with half on the drug and the other half on a placebo, to see if reducing the absorption of fat in our bodies really does lead independently to weight loss. So does it work? Yes,[1418] but it may result in only about a half pound of weight loss a month.[1419] But half a pound is still half a pound. Orlistat's serious potential side effects like severe acute kidney[1420] and liver[1421] failure are rare, so why aren't more people taking the drug?

As I mentioned before, orlistat—sold as Alli—causes "unpleasant symptoms such as anal leakage."[1422] Well, the fat that doesn't get absorbed has to go somewhere. For the oily discharge, the drug company apparently prefers the term *fecal spotting* over *anal leakage*,[1423] but soiled clothes by any other name would smell as (not so) sweet.

The drug company's website offered some helpful tips, such as "it's probably a smart idea to wear dark pants, and bring a change of clothes with you to work."[1424]

How did this drug even get approved? A Freedom of Information Act inquiry unearthed more than a thousand adverse events the drug company effectively hid from regulators.[1425] Ironically, though, the "highly visual side effects" actually may have facilitated weight loss by steering users away from fattier foods.[1426]

So how many people actually stick with the drug? Those seeking weight loss are often willing to go to extremes—even major surgery—to lose weight by any means necessary. But crapping your pants at work? The percentage of people still on the drug after two years was found to be only 2 percent.[1427]

The More the Merrier

Is it possible to lower fat intake yet still achieve weight loss even when there is no restriction on portion sizes, no conscious effort to cut calories, and unlimited opportunities to eat? Yes. People lose weight on low-fat diets not because they are eating less but because they are eating more. In the Hawaii study, the subjects lost seventeen pounds in three weeks because their caloric intakes dropped 40 percent. If you were to do that with caloric restriction, you'd have to cut the amount of food you ate nearly in half, but the Hawaiians ate *more* food—in excess of four pounds of food a day.[1428] Natural, low-fat foods tend to be so calorie dilute—that is, have so few calories per bite—that eating the same amount of food inevitably leads to fewer calories. The same, of course, cannot be said of fat-free cookies.

This calorie-density mechanism of low-fat-diet weight loss was illustrated by an elegant study from my medical alma mater, Tufts. Research subjects were switched from a more conventional diet of 35 percent calories from fat down to a diet getting only 15 percent of its calories from fat, but they were forced to eat so much food that they didn't lose any weight. Their weights were monitored closely, and if they started to lose weight, they were made to eat more food. The subjects had to eat more than five pounds of food a day to maintain their weights and "frequently complained of abdominal fullness." Then, after five or six weeks, they were kept on the same 15 percent fat diet but were allowed to eat however much they wanted, the amount of food with which they were comfortable. Over the next ten to twelve weeks, they lost an average of eight pounds. They weren't told to purposely lose weight. They just couldn't help it.[1429]

Normally on a diet, if quantity limits are suddenly removed, you gain weight. But on a low-enough-fat diet, even when most people can eat as much as they want, they lose weight. It doesn't happen for everybody, though. One guy in the Tufts study actually gained weight in the free-feeding phase, and another, who must have gotten used to eating that much more food, stayed the same. But the other twenty-seven out of twenty-nine participants lost weight, one as much as twenty-nine pounds, all eating ad libitum, which is Latin for *at one's pleasure*. That's where the term *ad lib* comes from. In acting, it means going off script. In nutrition research, it means eating without limits on quantity.

It isn't hard to imagine how ad libitum diets might be superior for long-term weight maintenance. To test this, researchers had people lose twenty-eight pounds through a combination of drugs and severe caloric restriction. They then randomized the subjects to an ad libitum low-fat diet or a food exchange–based calorie-counting system to restrict caloric intake to see which group was better able to keep off the weight. One year later, the weight loss was three times higher in the ad libitum group, and they were about 50 percent more likely to maintain a substantial portion of their initial lost weights.[1430] In the short term, most people can force themselves to cut down on the amount of food they eat, but for lifelong weight loss, eating as much as you want may be more sustainable.

Too Little, Too Late

Give people all-you-can-eat buffets of lower-fat foods, and they end up eating hundreds of fewer calories a day than if the buffets contained similar foods containing more fat.[1431] Depending on the fat content of the food, this can then translate into weight loss (at 15–20 percent fat) or weight gain (at 45–50 percent fat).[1432] Researchers offered people essentially the same foods, but with some slight tweaks, such as more or less oil, butterfat, or margarine slipped in. The foods evidently looked and tasted about the same, so people ate about the same amount and spontaneously lost or gained weight depending on the fat content. This is the passive consumption I explore on page 191, an artifact of calorie density.[1433] It's not the fat per se but rather the consequent increase in calories per mouthful because fat can sneak lots of calories into a relatively small space.[1434] However, there may actually be a difference in the appetite feedback loop between fat calories and carb calories.

If I hooked you up to an IV and, unbeknownst to you, dripped 1,300 calories of sugar into your veins, studies show your body somehow "tastes" how sweet your blood has become, does the math, and turns down your appetite so much that you spontaneously eat about 1,100 fewer calories that day.[1435] That's a huge drop in intake, but your body sensed all those extra calories in your system and made you that much less hungry to compensate. Genius!

But if I repeat the experiment with fat, we get a different result. Have 1,300 calories of fat secretly infused into your veins, and your body knows something is going on but doesn't quite get the same picture as it did when you got those extra calories from sugar. So you only end up compensating by eating about 500 fewer calories that day.[1436] Your body just doesn't seem to register fat calories as well as sugar calories. You can demonstrate this with food too.

If you give people a breakfast of yogurt with a few hundred extra calories of sugar mixed in, they eat significantly less of a meal offered ninety minutes later than they do when their morning yogurt doesn't have the added sugar. Not enough to account for all the extra sugar, mind you, but at least their bodies are trying to compensate. But when they're given the same number of extra calories in fat rather than sugar, there is no effect on subsequent meal intake; in fact, they eat a little more.[1437] The fat just didn't seem to induce the same braking effect on their appetites, or at least not in time.

So perhaps our bodies aren't so smart after all? They can only be as smart in the context in which they were designed. Snake a tube down someone's throat and secretly squirt some fat straight into their intestines, and their hunger can be slashed abruptly.[1438] Our bodies successfully sense the fat in our intestines and turn down our appetites. The problem is it happens too late. By the time high-fat foods make it through our stomachs and hit our intestines, we're usually already done eating. So what good are our bodies' detection mechanisms? Well, what kinds of high-fat foods were around during the millions of years our whole system was first evolving? Nuts. How fast can you eat walnuts in a shell? Even with a nutcracker in hand, it's slow going. So, in a natural context, our bodies can pick up on the fact we just stumbled on some nuts and make sure we don't overeat, but by the time our bodies sense we just ate that fat-infused yogurt or a donut, it's too late. We've already swallowed the last bite.

Dumping More Calories

So far, we've only talked about the calories-in side of the equation—how higher fat intakes can unintentionally lead to higher caloric intakes. When you think of calories out, expending energy, you likely think exercise, but the majority of the calories most of us burn is just from existing. That's what's called the *resting metabolic rate,* how many calories we burn every hour just to keep our hearts pumping and everything working. For most people, that's around 65 percent of the calories we burn every day.[1439] Another 25 percent is from movement, and the final 10 percent is the *thermic effect of food,* meaning the calories it takes for us to digest what we consume. Interestingly, what we eat not only constitutes calories in but also can affect all three of these dimensions of calories out.

Eat a low-fat diet (11 percent calories from fat), and you burn more calories in your sleep than when on a high-fat diet (58 percent).[1440] The difference could be as much as sixty-five calories a night, though measurements in this study were taken during overfeeding, which would be expected to exaggerate the effect. People on lower-fat diets may inexplicably start to move more too. Those randomized to a 20 percent fat diet started exercising more, expending eighty-three more calories a day on physical activity, whereas the group randomized to the 40 percent fat group started expending fifty-nine *fewer* calories a day.[1441] Between them, that's a difference of about a two-mile walk a day.[1442] This may help explain why those on the higher-fat diet lost significantly more *lean* body mass, down three pounds in six months compared to a gain in lean mass in the lower-fat group.[1443]

At rest, we burn about one calorie a minute, which is comparable to the heat produced by a seventy-five-watt light bulb. After meals, that bulb burns a little brighter to handle what we just ate.[1444] Fat also appears to be absorbed more efficiently from the digestive tract, meaning it takes fewer calories to process it.[1445] A *really* low-fat diet (3 percent of calories from fat) costs about 65 percent more calories to digest than a high-fat diet (40 percent fat), so, in effect, you're doing more work just by eating low-fat, though the benefit may only come out to be about forty calories a day.[1446]

In addition to the three primary components of calories out, there's actually a fourth component, and it's much more literal: the calories we poop out. Those eating low-fat appear to flush more calories down the toilet. Overeating on an 11-percent-calories-from-fat diet led to 620 more calories down the toilet every week than a same-calorie diet containing 58 percent calories from fat.[1447] That's nearly 2,500 fewer calories a month available for building up fat. Though calories in is the more important side of the equation, all these little benefits on the other side may add up to greater weight loss over time.

The Fat You Eat Is the Fat You Bear

In the Vermont prison studies I mentioned earlier where lean "volunteers" were overfed to study experimental obesity, the researchers made an important discovery: They learned how difficult it is to get people to gain weight on purpose—unless you feed them lots of fat. To get prisoners to gain thirty pounds on a mixed diet, it took about 140,000 excess calories per a certain body surface area. To get the same thirty-pound weight gain just by adding fat to their diets, all the researchers had to do was feed the prisoners as few as 40,000 extra calories.[1448] When the extra calories were in the form of straight fat, it took as many as *100,000* fewer calories to gain the same amount of weight. Why? Isn't a calorie a calorie? Why are our bodies so much more efficient at storing *fat* calories?

The reason our bodies so easily store fat as fat is because it's already fat. Our bodies can turn protein or carbs into fat, but it's costly. To store one hundred calories of dietary fat as body fat, it only takes three calories of energy, but converting one hundred calories of dietary carbs into fat for storage takes twenty-three calories.[1449] So, if your body wanted to store the fat from one hundred pats of butter, it would have to essentially burn three pats to make it happen, so you'd end up only storing ninety-seven pats. But in order to store one hundred sugar cubes as fat, the conversion process alone would burn up nearly a quarter of them. This is why our bodies would rather burn carbs and store fat instead of the other way around. Simply stated, fat may be more fattening.[1450]

When we eat a meal, most of the fat is deposited directly as fat on our bodies, whereas a large proportion of the carbs get stored in our muscles for quick energy.[1451] A study on children found that a high-fat meal deposited nine times more fat onto their bodies than the same number of calories of a low-fat meal.[1452] Where exactly does the fat go? Researchers at the Mayo Clinic tagged the fat in a meal with special isotopes to track its movement throughout the body. They had research subjects eat the tagged fat and then, twenty-four hours later, brought them into the operating room and took fat biopsies from their thighs, belly flab, and deep within their abdomens. Of the fat in the meal they could account for, about 45 percent was burned right off the bat, but most of the fat consumed was simply directed right into their fat stores. The researchers found that about 50 percent went straight into belly flab, 40 percent to their thighs, and most of the remaining went into visceral fat, the fat that's buried around our major organs.[1453] Under normal circumstances, less than 1 percent of ingested carbohydrates suffers the same fate based on similar studies of isotope-labeled sugar.[1454]

Low-fat proponents often point out this fact, that making significant amounts of new fat from scratch from ingested carbs only occurs with "massive overfeeding"[1455] of, for example, a "diet consisted of candy."[1456] If you feed people an extra thousand calories of sugar a day, the equivalent of up to eleven bags of cotton candy,[1457] they do gain about four pounds in three weeks,[1458] but most of the extra carb calories end up being burned off as excess heat.[1459] If, however, you added an extra thousand calories of fat, like a stick or so of butter every day or a half cup of oil, most of that would be directly socked away and stored for a rainy day.[1460]

Under more normal circumstances, even if less than 1 percent of the carbs in a meal end up as fat, that doesn't mean that carbs can't be fattening. Normally, our bodies burn fat around the clock at, interestingly, about the rate at which a candle burns. (Candles, after all, used to be made from animal fat.[1461]) Carbohydrates are the body's preferred fuel, so when we eat them, our bodies switch from burning fat to burning carbs, effectively snuffing out the candle for a few hours. So, while we can certainly gain weight from eating carbs, it's more from sparing our own fat from being used, rather than adding more fat directly.[1462]

Is All Fat Just as Fattening?

If you were surprised to learn that, in some ways, fat calories are handled differently by the body from how carbohydrate calories are, you may be *really* surprised by the data suggesting that some types of fat calories are more fattening than others. I certainly was. There have long been studies linking greater saturated fat intake specifically with greater weight gain,[1463] but I always assumed it was just because it was a marker for poorer diets and lifestyles in general. After all, the top five sources of saturated fat in the United States are essentially cheese, desserts like cake and ice cream, chicken, pork, and then burgers.[1464]

Interventional studies started to make things more interesting. If you switch people from a 38-percent-calories-from-fat diet down to a 28-percent-calories-from-fat diet, they lose body fat. Nothing too surprising there. But if you switch people from a 38-percent-fat diet of mostly saturated fat to a 38-percent-fat diet of mostly monounsaturated fat, like that of a more Mediterranean diet, they *also* lose body fat.[1465] The same number of calories and the same amount of fat—but a different type of fat—meant a different degree of weight loss.

One way researchers have switched people from a diet rich in saturated fat to a more Mediterranean diet is to swap out some meat and dairy for nuts and avocados. In this way, they would be eating the same amount of fat and calories, but suddenly, they'd also be eating significantly more fiber.[1466] In that case, when they lose more weight, how do you know it was the change in fat quality rather than the change in fiber quantity?

To determine if there's really a difference between fats, researchers designed a study where people ate essentially the same foods—different only by the kind of fat. They baked scones. Half were made with sunflower oil, and the other half with butter. The liver fat in the sunflower scone eaters went down, while the liver fat in the butter scone eaters went up.[1467]

Is it possible it was less unsaturated fat versus saturated fat, and more plant fat versus animal fat? Dietary cholesterol may be one of the main factors associated with liver injury and the development of nonalcoholic fatty liver disease,[1468] which helps explain why those who eat even just a few eggs a week were found to have more than triple the odds of fatty liver disease.[1469] So how could you separate out that factor?

Researchers designed a study where people ate essentially the same foods, but, this time, different only by saturated versus unsaturated fat. Instead of scones, this time they baked muffins. Half were made with sunflower oil, and the other half with palm oil, a fat that is saturated, but, like all plant fats, free of cholesterol. Not only did the palm oil muffins result in significantly greater liver and total body fat, they produced twice as much visceral fat, the particularly harmful fat wrapped around our internal organs.[1470] On the saturated-fat diet, they also gained four times as much fat as lean tissue.[1471] So saturated plant fats like coconut oil not only join animal fats in increasing heart disease risk[1472] but may also play a role in the obesity epidemic.

One reason saturated fats may be more fattening is that they appear more likely to be stored immediately rather than burned. This was found in comparisons to both monounsaturated fats (in a match between olive oil and cream)[1473] and polyunsaturated fats (in a match between mostly safflower oil and lard).[1474] Oleic acid, the primary monounsaturated fat found in olives, nuts, and avocados, is burned promptly about 20 percent more readily than palmitic acid,[1475] the predominant saturated fat in the American diet, which is sourced mainly from meat and dairy.[1476] You can drip palmitic acid on muscle cells in a petri dish and openly demonstrate the suppression of fat utilization.[1477] But this difference is too small to account for the pounds of extra weight lost when these fats are switched in randomized controlled studies.

In the five hours following a breakfast with about four teaspoons of olive oil, research subjects burned about sixteen grams of fat.[1478] In the same five-hour period after eating essentially the same breakfast, but with the olive oil replaced with butterfat, only about thirteen grams of fat were burned. A pound of fat is 454 grams, so even if you burned 3 more grams of fat at every single meal, at the end of the month, you might only end up about a half pound lighter. But in a study where saturated fat was swapped for the same amount of mostly olive oil, people lost five pounds of fat in a month.[1479] Something else has to be going on.

Remember that thermic effect of food, the amount of energy spent digesting, absorbing, and storing a meal? Well, it apparently costs 28 percent more calories to process a meal containing walnuts and 23 percent more calories to process a meal containing olive oil than it does to process a meal with the same number of calories and fat but in the form of cheese and butter.[1480] That sounds like a lot, but our bodies are so efficient either way that it doesn't add up to much—maybe as few as twenty or so calories a day.[1481] A similar increase of a few calories a day in resting metabolic rate has been noted in a trial comparing hazelnut oil to palm oil,[1482] but, again, there appears to be a missing piece.

What About Virgin Coconut Oil?

Coconut oil, one of the latest internet sensations, is touted as a weight-loss "miracle" that "ACTUALLY Burns BELLY Fat!"[1483] If rats are given purified, medium-chain fatty acids, one component of coconut oil, they end up eating less food[1484]—but does the same apply to people?

An open-label pilot study was published that suggested coconut oil could facilitate weight loss.[1485] "Open label"? That just means the participants knew what they were eating. They didn't use any kind of placebo control. In fact, there was no control group at all. We've talked about the well-recognized effect in dietary studies where just being in a weight-loss study and under observation tends to lead to a reduction in caloric intake—because you know the researchers are looking over your shoulder and are going to put you on a scale.[1486] So you can't tell from that kind of study what role—if any—the coconut oil played.

(continued)

Enter a non-open-label study. When researchers pitted virgin coconut oil against a placebo control, the coconut oil did worse. Not only was there no difference in fat burning, the study subjects ended up hungrier after the coconut oil meal. Coconut oil was less satiating than the same number of calories of a control oil.[1487] It turns out coconut oil is just as fattening as other oils in terms of total, belly, or butt/thigh fat and may have adverse metabolic effects.[1488] Give people two tablespoons of coconut oil a day, and, compared to two tablespoons of soybean oil, no significant[1489] effect on weight or waistlines was found. What did happen, though, was a worsening of insulin resistance in the coconut oil group (despite being instructed to increase fruits and vegetables, cut down on sugars and animal fat, and exercise three hours a week).[1490] Coconut oil hawkers claim coconut oil is special because it contains medium-chain triglycerides, but MCTs only make up about 10 percent of the product.[1491] Cholesterol-raising saturated fats like those found in beef tallow make up the bulk of coconut oil.[1492]

If no benefit to coconut oil for obesity over placebo has ever been demonstrated, how can coconut oil proponents get away with saying otherwise? They often cite studies of Pacific Islanders who were slimmer eating their more traditional, coconut-based diets than those now eating more modernized diets with fewer coconut products.[1493] Guess what they were eating instead? "The modern dietary pattern [was] primarily characterized by high intake of sausage and eggs and processed foods."[1494]

Solving the Mystery of the Missing Calories

How can people lose five pounds of body fat in a month eating the same number of calories? Well, if calories in are the same, then it must be calories out. If you remember, there are four main components to calories out: resting metabolic rate, physical activity, the thermic effect of food, and fecal losses. We already determined the differences in resting metabolic rate and the thermic effect are insufficient, and there does not appear to be a difference in fecal losses between saturated and unsaturated fats.[1495] That just leaves one other outlet: exercise.

How could a different type of fat make people exercise more? Early studies offered a clue. Those randomized to meals with fat from olives, nuts, and avocados tended to feel significantly "more energetic" than those getting the same amount of fat from meat and dairy, suggesting the weight loss they experienced could have been "enhanced by subtle, unconscious, increases in physical activity."[1496] You don't know, of course, until you put it to the test.

Twenty-nine people were covertly randomized to one of two diets that appeared identical but featured different oil blends, one with palm oil and one with hazelnut oil. Same calories, same amount of fat, same diets, but the palm oil group was secretly slipped saturated fat in place of monounsaturated fat. Researchers then attached activity monitors on all the subjects to objectively measure how much they were moving. The study found that 90 percent of the subjects inexplicably ramped up their exercise when they were unwittingly eating the low-saturated-fat diet, increasing their activity levels 12–15 percent on average. The researchers concluded that a high intake of saturated fat "might dampen motivation for physical activity."[1497]

FOOD FOR THOUGHT

The take-home message is to cut down on fatty meats and dairy, fried foods, greasy snacks like corn chips, and added oils.

At first I was skeptical of oil-free cooking. So many of the dishes I made growing up started with sautéing garlic and onions, and how could you possible bake without fat?

I was delighted to discover that cooking without oil is surprisingly easy. To keep foods from sticking in the pan, you can sauté in wine, sherry, broth, vinegar, or just plain water. The trick is to just use a little liquid at a time. I use dried mushrooms a lot and always make it a habit to save the soaking liquid. I find porcini mushrooms produce an especially rich, dark, savory broth that's perfect for my garlic and onions, and the added umami flavor makes it even easier to leave the salt out completely.

For baking, I've successfully substituted a variety of healthy whole foods in place of oil. Ground flaxseeds blended with water, applesauce, mashed bananas or avocado, soaked prune purée, and even canned pumpkin can provide a similar moistness. Vegetables roast just fine without added oil. I use a silicone baking sheet, but I hear parchment paper works as well. That's how I make my purple sweet potato fries. I spritz the wedges in apple cider or malt vinegar and dredge in coarse blue cornmeal seasoned with sage and smoked paprika. Now I'm getting hungry!

LOW IN ADDED SUGAR

Sugar Daddy

A founding member of Harvard's nutrition department recalled that the "meat, milk and egg producers were very upset"[1498] by the original *Dietary Goals for the United States*—and they weren't the only ones. The *Dietary Goals* encapsulate healthy eating advice from the federal government, and they named names when it came to foods Americans should cut down on. The president of the National Cattlemen's Beef Association explained that his industry "reacted rather violently" because "if these 'Dietary Goals' are moved forward and promoted in the present form . . . entire sectors of the food industry—meat, dairy, sugar, and others—may be so severely damaged that . . . recovery may be out of reach."[1499]

Critics suggested the adoption of the *Dietary Goals* would be costly for taxpayers too. Because of more expensive groceries? No. Because "health care expenditures increase if the lifespan is prolonged." It's like when people quit smoking: "The increase in the expected lifespan would simultaneously increase the cost of care of old people."[1500] In other words, if people eat more healthfully and stop smoking, there may be more seniors, some of whom might need our care.

The president of the International Sugar Research Foundation called the report "unfortunate and ill-advised" and evidently part of an "emotional anti-sucrose [anti-table-sugar] tidal wave." As immortalized in the official record, he said: "Simply stated, people like sweet things, and apparently the [Senate] Committee believes that people should be deprived of what they like. There is a puritanical streak in certain Americans that leads them to become 'do-gooders.'"[1501]

By the time the World Health Organization (WHO) attempted to release a similar report decades later, Big Sugar had graduated from name-calling to flexing its political muscle. The WHO report, entitled *Diet, Nutrition and the Prevention of Chronic Disease,* contained six fateful words: "limit the intake of free sugars" (meaning added sugars). Within days, the sugar industry led a vicious attack, culminating in a threat to get Congress to withdraw U.S. funding to the World Health Organization entirely[1502]—all because of those six words.

The threat from the sugar industry was described by WHO insiders as worse than any pressure they had ever gotten from the tobacco lobby.[1503] As revealed in an internal memo, the U.S. government apparently had a list of demands from Big Sugar that included the removal of all references to the science that WHO experts had compiled on the matter, as well as the call for the "deletion of all references to fat, oils, sugar and salt."[1504] In the United States, the food industry, like Big Tobacco before it, has had a corrosive effect on global public health efforts. When asked why Michelle Obama's childhood obesity programs in the United States should not be modeled around the world, a U.S. official responded that they might harm American exports.[1505]

Sugarcoated Science

At least a dozen interventional studies document adverse metabolic effects of consuming added sugars, though this may be due largely to the accompanying weight gain spurred by sugar consumption.[1506] This has led sugar industry spokespersons, like the head of the World Sugar Research Organisation, to say things like "overconsumption of anything is harmful, including of water and air."[1507] Yes, he compared the overconsumption of sugar to breathing too much.

This is a throwback to the well-worn tobacco industry script: They're simply providing choices; they don't condone the overuse of their products; and, if people fall ill after consuming it, the victims can only blame themselves.[1508] The reason this is disingenuous, of course, is that the tobacco industry works day and night to make their products as addictive as possible, just as the manufacturers of ultraprocessed foods like sugary breakfast cereals engineer their products to be as hyperpalatable as possible to maximize consumption.[1509]

Why won't cereal manufacturers reduce the amount of sugar in their products? A number of explanations have been offered, such as "a product with semi-addictive properties may be a safe way to ensure long-term revenues. . . . Another possibility is that selling cereals high in sugar is a smart technique to sell expansively a cheap commodity product—*sugar.*"[1510] Ultraprocessed foods like breakfast cereals[1511] tend to have the highest profit margins.[1512] Remarkably, the cost of *packaging* may outweigh the cost of *ingredients* in a cereal box by more than ten to one.[1513]

Denying evidence that sugars are harmful to health seems always to have been at the heart of the sugar industry's defense.[1514] When the evidence is undeniable, though—like the link between sugar and cavities[1515]—the industry switches from denial to deflection, such as trying to refocus attention away from restricting intake to finding a vaccine against tooth decay. We seem to have reached a similar point with obesity, as the Sugar Bureau again dodges denial and rushes to deflect. It commissioned research suggesting losing weight was useless for extending life among "healthy" obese individuals[1516]—a stance strongly contradicted by hundreds of studies across four continents involving more than ten million participants.[1517]

The Bitter with the Sweet

The obesity epidemic may just be the tip of the iceberg in terms of excess body fat.[1518] As I noted in the Causes section, more than 90 percent of adults and greater than two-thirds of the children in the United States are estimated to be "overfat"—that is, having excess body fat sufficient to impair health. This can occur even in people of normal weight (often due to excess abdominal fat). Added sugars have been blamed in part for this overfat epidemic.[1519]

A century ago, sugar was heralded as one of the cheapest sources of calories in the diet.[1520] Just ten cents' worth of sugar could furnish thousands of calories. Sugar pushers bristled at the term *empty calories,*[1521] asserting that the calories in sugar were "not empty but full of energy"—in other words, full of calories, of which we now get too many. The excess body weight of the U.S. population corresponds to about 350–500 excess daily calories on average,[1522] which just so happens to be how many calories, on average, Americans failing to stay under the suggested sugar limits of the U.S. Dietary Guidelines get in added sugars every day.[1523] Maybe that's a good place to start cutting calories?

Even the most die-hard sugar defenders—researchers who rely in part on sugary food and beverage industry funding for their livelihoods—agree that not only is it considered indisputable that sugars contribute to obesity but that it is "also undisputable that sugar reduction . . . should be part of any weight loss program."[1524] And that came from someone who was reportedly paid $40,000 a month by the high-fructose corn syrup industry on top of the $10 million it paid for his research.[1525] Of all sources of calories to limit, a "reduction in consumption of added sugars should head the list because they provide no essential nutrients,"[1526] said researchers funded by the Dr Pepper Snapple Group and the Coca-Cola Company, including Richard Kahn, infamous for signing a million-dollar sponsorship deal with the world's largest candy company when he was chief science officer at the American Diabetes Association.

Not surprisingly, randomized controlled trials show that increasing sugar intake increases caloric intake,[1527] which leads to body weight gain in adults, while sugar reduction leads to body weight loss in children.[1528] When researchers randomized individuals to either increase or decrease their intakes of table sugar, the added-sugar group gained about three and a half pounds over ten weeks, whereas the reduced-sugar group lost about two and a half pounds.[1529] A systematic review and meta-analysis of all such ad libitum diet studies—that is, real-life studies where sugar levels are changed but people can otherwise eat whatever they want—found that reduced intake of dietary sugars resulted in a decrease in body weight, whereas increased sugar intake resulted in a comparable increase in weight. The researchers concluded that "considering the rapid weight gain that occurs after an increased intake of sugars," it seems reasonable to advise people to cut down.[1530]

Findings from observational studies have been more ambiguous, though, with an association found between obesity and sweetened beverage intake, but failing to show consistent correlations with sugary foods.[1531] Most such studies rely on self-reported data, however, and obese people tend to underreport consumption of sugar-rich foods, *fudging* their data, if you will. Researchers can, however, measure trace sucrose levels in the urine to get an objective measure of actual sugar intake while excluding contributions from other sweeteners, such as high-fructose corn syrup. Using this method, researchers discovered that sugar intake is indeed not only associated with greater odds of obesity and greater waist size in snapshot-in-time cross-sectional studies but also in a prospective cohort study over time.[1532] Using urinary sucrose as the measure of sucrose intake, those in the highest versus the lowest fifth for table sugar intake had more than 50 percent greater odds of being overweight or obese.[1533]

Not Sweet Nothings

On April Fools' Day 1998, the FDA announced its approval of the artificial sweetener sucralose,[1534] sold as Splenda, aka 1,6-dichloro-1,6-dideoxy-β-D-fructofuranosyl-4-chloro-4-deoxy-α-D-galactopyranoside.[1535] Despite its scary-sounding chemical name, the worst thing about it seemed to be that it was a rare migraine trigger in susceptible individuals,[1536] to which the manufacturer of sucralose responded that you have to weigh whatever risk there may be against the "broader benefits," such as "helping to mitigate the health risks associated with the national epidemic of obesity."[1537]

How's that going?

Large-scale population studies have found that the consumption of artificial sweeteners, particularly in diet sodas, is associated with increased weight gain and abdominal fat over time.[1538] Now, the obvious explanation for this finding would be reverse causation: Instead of drinking more diet soda leading to obesity, it would make more sense that obesity leads to drinking more diet soda. But even when researchers controlled for preexisting differences in body fat, they still found evidence of increased obesity risk.[1539]

However, not all reviews of the science concluded there was a link between artificial sweeteners and weight gain. Can you guess which ones? An analysis of industry bias found that reviews funded by the food industry were seventeen times less likely to suggest unfavorable effects, and in nearly half of the sponsored reviews, the authors failed to even disclose their conflicts of interest.[1540] That's even worse than the sugar industry, whose studies were "only" five times as likely to question the link between sugar-sweetened beverages and obesity.[1541] You don't really know, though, until you put them to the test.

Ironically, many of the interventional studies on artificial sweeteners and weight gain were executed by animal agribusiness, feeding them to farm animals to fatten them faster.[1542] (Is there anything they won't feed to chickens?) Animal agriculture has been feeding artificial sweeteners to farm animals since the 1950s,[1543] boasting their addition "increases . . . body weight gain and . . . optimizes return on investment."[1544] What about in people?

If you give obese individuals the amount of sucralose found in a can of diet soda, for example, they get significantly higher blood sugar and insulin spikes in response to a sugar challenge, suggesting sucralose is not just an inert substance.[1545] The Splenda company emphasizes that sucralose is hardly even absorbed into the body and ends up in the colon to be eliminated.[1546] Therein may lie the problem.[1547] The adverse metabolic effects of artificial sweeteners correlate with "pronounced" changes in the microbiome that occur within a week of daily consumption.[1548]

The good news is that after stopping artificial sweeteners, your original balance of gut bacteria can be restored within a matter of weeks.[1549] The problem is that we may be exposed without even knowing it. Nearly half of study participants randomized to avoid sucralose, for example, still turned up positive, thought to be due to exposure from nondietary sources, such as toothpaste and mouthwash.[1550]

Another way artificial sweeteners can lead to metabolic disturbance is via the disconnect that develops between the amount of sweetness the brain tastes on the tongue and how much blood sugar actually ends up reaching the brain. Your brain may end up feeling cheated by the artificial sweeteners, figuring you have to consume more and more sweetness in order to get enough calories.[1551] For example, researchers slipped people either Sprite, Sprite Zero (a no-calorie, artificially sweetened Sprite), or unsweetened, carbonated lemon-lime water, and then, later on, offered them a choice: They could have M&M's, spring water, or sugar-free gum. Guess who picked the M&M's? Those who drank the artificially sweetened soda were nearly three times more likely to take the candy than either those who had consumed the sugar-sweetened soda or the unsweetened drink.[1552] So it wasn't a matter of sweet versus nonsweet or even calories versus no calories. There appeared to be something about noncaloric sweeteners that tricks the brain into wanting more junk.

The same researchers performed another study in which everyone was given Oreos and then asked how satisfied the cookies made them feel. Again, those who had drunk the artificially sweetened Sprite Zero

(continued)

reported feeling less satisfied after eating the Oreos than either the subjects who had had normal Sprite or sparkling water. These results are consistent with brain imaging studies demonstrating that regular consumption of artificial sweeteners can alter the reward pathways responsible for the pleasurable response to food.[1553]

What about the natural, plant-based sweeteners derived from stevia and monk fruit? Researchers randomized people to drink a beverage sweetened with sugar, aspartame, monk fruit, or stevia. Blood sugars were measured over twenty-four hours, and surprisingly, there was no significant difference found among any of the four groups.[1554]

Wait a second. The sugar group was given sixteen spoonfuls of sugar, the amount in a twenty-ounce bottle of Coke, so the other three groups consumed sixteen fewer spoonfuls of sugar—yet all four groups still had the same average blood sugars? How is that possible? Table sugar causes a big blood sugar spike. Drink that bottle of sugar water with its twenty sugar cubes' worth of sugar, and your blood sugars jump forty points over the next hour. In contrast, after drinking a beverage sweetened with aspartame, monk fruit, or stevia, nothing happens to blood sugars, which is what we would expect. These are noncaloric sweeteners. Since they have no calories, isn't it just like drinking water? How could our daily blood sugar values average out the same? The only way that could happen is if the noncalorie sweeteners somehow made our blood sugar spikes worse later in the day—and that's exactly what happened. In the group who drank the aspartame-sweetened beverage, even though their blood sugars didn't rise *at the time,* they shot up higher an hour later in response to lunch, as if they had just consumed a bottle of soda.[1555]

That was for an artificial sweetener, though. What about the natural sweeteners, stevia and monk fruit? The same thing happened. The same exaggerated blood sugar spike to a regular meal occurred an hour later. So that's how it all equals out in terms of average blood sugars even though, in these three noncaloric sweetener groups, the subjects took in sixteen fewer spoonfuls of sugar. This is at least partly because they ate more. After drinking a Diet Coke, you're more likely to eat more at your next meal than you would if you had drunk a regular Coke. In fact, you'd eat so much more that the calories "saved" from replacing sugar with noncaloric sweeteners would be fully compensated at subsequent meals, resulting in no difference in total daily caloric intake. It's as if the zero-calorie sweetener groups—whether sweetened artificially or naturally—had chugged a bottle of sugary soda. So, when it comes to caloric intake, blood sugars, or insulin spikes, all the other sweeteners appeared just as bad as straight sugar.[1556]

Do we have direct evidence that diet beverages can adversely impact body weight? Yes. If you swap out diet beverages for water, there theoretically should be no difference in weight control since they both provide zero calories, right? Well, when researchers put it to the test, overweight and obese individuals on a diet randomized to replace diet beverages with water lost significantly more weight, about 15 percent more over six months.[1557,1558]

The researchers who demonstrated artificial sweeteners can disrupt our microbiomes and metabolisms recognized the irony of their findings. Though these food additives were introduced to reduce caloric intake and counter the obesity epidemic, they noted their findings suggest artificial sweeteners may have instead "directly contributed to enhancing the exact epidemic that they themselves were intended to fight."[1559]

Long in the (Sweet) Tooth

The industry is quick to point out that a calorie is a calorie, and an excess of calories from Coca-Cola would cause no more weight gain than the same excess of calories from carrots.[1560] While this may be true in a tightly controlled laboratory setting,[1561] it doesn't take into account the appetite-enhancing effects of sugar.[1562] Remember the experiment where children were alternately offered high- or lower-sugar cereals? As I mentioned on page 7, surprisingly, Cheerios has a similar number of calories to Froot Loops (104 calories per cup[1563] versus 110,[1564] respectively). Had the kids eaten more Cheerios than Froot Loops, they could have gotten more calories, but the opposite happened. On average, the children poured and ate 77 percent more of the sugary cereals. So even with comparable calorie counts per serving, sugary cereals may end up nearly doubling caloric intake.[1565]

Millions of years of evolution have genetically hardwired us with both an innate liking of the sweet taste of ripe fruit[1566] and a sugar-induced subversion of some of our satiety mechanisms.[1567] When we eat, desire for salty, fatty, and savory tastes diminishes as we slake our hunger, whereas our desire for sweetness is maintained.[1568] This makes sense. Because fruit is sporadic and seasonal, an overfeeding response upon discovering a berry bush would have triggered our hunter-gatherer ancestors to eat as much as possible to store energy for later.[1569] This may explain why we seem to grow a "second stomach" when it comes to dessert. Children may be especially vulnerable since they have a stronger preference for sweet foods than adults,[1570] and repeated exposures to sugary foods may accustom young children to a lifelong habit of consuming overly sweet foods.[1571]

In recent years, much has been learned about the reinforcing effects of sugar and how it can promote overeating.[1572] Evidence supports the thinking that we don't just overeat sugar because we like its sweet taste.[1573] As I note in the Low in Addictive Foods section, innovations in brain scanning technology have shown that the pleasure-generating reward circuitry in our brains overlaps with the neurocircuitry that mediates the addictive properties of drugs like alcohol and opioids. Sugar consumption has also been shown to inhibit anxiety-induced cortisol (stress hormone) secretion, helping to explain why many "comfort foods" are high in sugar and also why excessive sugar consumption may be such a difficult habit to break.[1574]

How Much Is Too Much?

At the time of the American Revolution, we consumed about an estimated four pounds of sugar per person per year.[1575] Now, we may each average more than fifty pounds annually.[1576] That's the equivalent of about seventeen teaspoons of added sugars every day.

The excessive consumption of added sugar is a systemic problem that extends far beyond just a small group of individuals making poor dietary choices.[1577] In the United States, individuals in every single age bracket exceed the U.S. Dietary Guidelines' recommended limit of no more than 10 percent of calories from added sugars. The average American exceeds the guideline by more than 30 percent,[1578] and adolescents exceed it by 60 percent.[1579]

Though the Sugar Association describes the maximum limit as "extremely low,"[1580] let's not forget that there is no dietary requirement for added sugars at all.[1581] The American Heart Association went further, recommending that most American women should get no more than 100 calories per day from added sugars and most American men no more than 150.[1582] This comes out to be about 6 percent of calories,[1583] with recommendations for some demographics falling as low as 3 percent.[1584] Currently, approximately nine out of ten Americans are exceeding these recommendations.[1585]

In 2017, the American Heart Association released its guidelines for children, recommending they get no more than 100 calories of added sugars per day (and none for those under age two).[1586] For a teenager expending 2,500 calories a day, that represents a limit of fewer than 5 percent of calories from added sugars. Sugary breakfast cereals alone violate these limits in up to 30 percent of toddlers.[1587] An average serving[1588] of every single one of the top ten breakfast cereals marketed to children would take up more than half the daily sugar limit,[1589,1590] and there are nearly one hundred cereals on the market for which a single serving would push kids up and over the limit.[1591]

The United States is one of at least sixty-five countries that have implemented dietary guidelines or public health policies to curb sugar consumption.[1592] In the United Kingdom, the Scientific Advisory Committee on Nutrition made recommendations to reduce calories from added sugars down to 5 percent,[1593] consonant with the American Heart Association and the latest conditional recommendation from the World Health Organization,[1594] whose policy-making process is protected from industry influence.[1595] That means a single can of soda could easily take us over the top for the day.[1596]

FOOD FOR THOUGHT

Note that none of these recommendations to cut down on added sugars applies to fruit. As you'll read in the Rich in Fruits and Vegetables section, fruit can actually facilitate weight loss. If you randomize people to a diet low in all sugars, even the naturally occurring sugars in fruit, they do worse than those randomized to just cut down added sugars. Those who retained fruit in their diets lost nearly 50 percent more weight.[1597]

For those of you who have a sweet tooth like I do, all hope is not lost. The same palate-changing effects on your taste thermostat found after cutting down on salt and fat also work with cutting down on sugar. Put people on a sugar-free challenge for two weeks, removing all added sugars and artificial sweeteners, and by the end of the trial, up to 95 percent said "sweet foods and drinks tasted sweeter or too sweet, and . . . said moving forward they would use less or even no sugar."[1598] Most stopped craving sugar within the first week.

LOW IN ADDICTIVE FOODS

Gut Instincts

Food tastes good for the same reason sex feels good. We wouldn't last very long as a species without both. Without pleasure centers and reward pathways in our brains incentivizing our efforts, we might not have sufficient drive to seek out either. Hunting and gathering take a lot of work. No surprise, then, that our appetites and food cravings are governed in part by the "feel good" messengers in our brains: dopamine (the "reward hormone"), serotonin (the "happiness hormone"), oxytocin (the "love hormone"),[1599] endorphins (our own body's natural opioids), and endocannabinoids (our bodies' natural cannabis compounds—think of the "munchies" effect).[1600]

Dopamine release is such an important motivator of food intake that animals genetically engineered to be unable to make dopamine simply starve themselves to death.[1601] Food just doesn't seem to do much for them. Too much dopamine release, however, may lead to overeating.

Hijacking Our Natural Drives

Not all foods are equally rewarding. If you perform PET scans of people's brains after they eat different meals, you can show that dopamine release is greatest in response to foods people like the most,[1602] which tend to be foods high in salt, sugar, and fat. We evolved for millions of years in an environment where sodium was scarce, so a taste for saltiness used to give us a survival advantage. Calories were sometimes scarce, too, but we didn't need nutrition labels to tell us which foods had more energy. Our taste for sweetness led us to ripe fruit, and our taste for fat drew us to nuts and seeds. Simple survival skills we developed over millions of years. The food industry, however, has hijacked these natural drives and turned them against us.

Ever find yourself eating even when you're no longer hungry and then continuing to eat even when you know you should stop? Taste engineers manipulate the salt, sugar, and fat contents of foods to achieve what's referred to in the industry as the *bliss point,* the peak of craveability.[1603] These days, food is designed so we "can't eat just one." Hyperpalatable foods can overstimulate our reward pathways, not only overriding our normal satiety signals but potentially our better judgment as well.[1604]

Brain areas activated just by the *smell* of foods like potato chips, ice cream, roast beef, and cake are similar to those activated by addictive substances like alcohol.[1605] Drugs, whether illicit or legal, may in effect be co-opting brain circuitry originally designed for seeking healthy foods. The reason we may be so vulnerable to such compulsions is that our brains are just not designed to cope with omnipresent access to drugs, video games, pornography, and snack foods.[1606]

There's been an exponential increase in scientific publications on food addiction in recent years,[1607] spurred by a study entitled "Intense Sweetness Surpasses Cocaine Reward."[1608] Researchers found that when rats were allowed to choose between sugar-sweetened water or intravenous cocaine, nine out of ten chose the sweet taste over one of our most addictive drugs.

People have been chewing coca leaves for at least eight thousand years[1609] as a mild stimulant without any evidence of addiction, but when certain components in the plant were isolated and concentrated into cocaine, it became a different story.[1610] Just like with many drugs of abuse, salt, sugar, and fat are substances found in nature, but they exist naturally in much smaller concentrations and may only become problematic when extracted and concentrated by modern industrial processes.[1611] Only when the coca leaf is processed into a concentrated form for rapid delivery, such as cocaine and crack, does it become highly addictive. Similarly, the sugarcane stem has been chewed for its pleasant taste for ages,[1612] but it only presents a disproportionate reward signal once highly refined into added sugars[1613] with the potential to override our self-control mechanisms and, thus, lead to analogous addictive-type behaviors.[1614] From the medical journal *Current Drug Abuse Reviews:*

First, highly processed foods and drugs of abuse are both capable of triggering cravings. Second, consumption of highly processed foods and drugs of abuse can both be associated with compulsive overuse in the face of severe negative consequences. And finally, in some individuals there is evidence of chronic relapse and an inability to cut down consumption of both substances.[1615]

Certainly, there are lots of people who eat sweet, salty, and greasy foods yet don't exhibit addictive eating behaviors, but the same is true of addictive drugs. Only about one in seven people who try cocaine goes on to develop a cocaine addiction.[1616] Some have contended that food addiction cannot exist because we *have* to eat, but that's like arguing alcoholism can't exist because we *have* to drink.[1617] Yes, we have to drink, but we don't have to drink alcohol. Yes, we have to breathe, but we don't have to breathe tobacco. And yes, we have to eat, but we don't have to eat junk.

The Frosting Effect

The brain-imaging evidence supporting the concept of food addiction is bolstered by data from pharmaceutical trials that manipulate reward pathways. When researchers gave people the opiate-blocking drug naltrexone (similar to the drug Narcan used to reverse opioid overdoses),[1618] the research subjects rated sweets as not tasting as good[1619] and were found to consume fewer cookies.[1620] Narcan itself reduces the consumption of chocolate cookies, but not an unprocessed, whole-food source of sugar (orange fruit segments).[1621] Given over a period of days, opiate blockers can decrease the calories consumed at all-you-can-eat meals by obese individuals by 30 percent.[1622]

These Narcan-type studies suggest sugar consumption causes the release of endorphins.[1623] This would explain the more than one hundred randomized controlled studies on the pain-relieving effects of a little sugar water for infants undergoing painful procedures such as vaccinations[1624] (though it was not found effective enough for the pain of circumcision).[1625]

Fat appears to have a similar effect on the brain as sugar. Feed people yogurt packed with butterfat, and within thirty minutes, they exhibit similar brain activity changes[1626] to those who had just drunk straight sugar water.[1627] In the largest study of food addiction to date, involving more than one hundred thousand women from the Harvard Nurses' Health Study, greasy foods—hamburgers, french fries, and pizza—were the types of fare most linked to food addictions.[1628]

So which is worse: fat or sugar? The answer is *both*. As it turns out, opiate-blocking drugs work best not for sugary foods like jelly beans but for foods that combine sugar and fat.[1629] The combination of sugar with fat creates a "hedonic synergy."[1630] Think ice cream, candy bars, and donuts. Few folks may sit down to enjoy a bowl of straight sugar or a tub of shortening, but put them together and you have frosting! The sugar can act as a vehicle for fat intake and vice versa. Obese compared to lean individuals have similar pleasure responses to sugar solutions like Kool-Aid, but appear to have a heightened response to sweet foods that are also rich in fat.[1631] The "sweet tooth" link to obesity may be more of a "sweet-fat tooth."[1632] If you follow people's chosen diets, the best predictor of overeating and weight gain in children, adolescents,[1633] and adults may be the selection of high-fat, high-sugar foods.[1634]

In nature, while there are foods that contain sugar (like fruit) and foods that contain fat (like nuts), sugar and fat rarely occur in the same food naturally.[1635] There is one, and it's the most natural food of all. Can you think of it? *Breast milk.* Maybe that's why high-fat, high-sugar foods are so addictive. We wouldn't last long as a species if babies didn't crave breast milk. Some have speculated that much of the success of both low-fat and low-carb diets may be from the elimination of these high-fat, high-sugar mixtures that we're programmed to crave.[1636]

It's All in the Process

Why don't we crave trail mix as much?[1637] That's about as sugary and fatty as natural foods get. The key appears to lie in the processing, which increases the dose and speed of absorption of the sugar and fat. Hard liquor is more addictive than beer because of the dose, and crack is more addictive than cocaine because of the speed of absorption. Food processing can increase both simultaneously, delivering high loads of concentrated sugar and fat, while, at the same time, stripping away fiber, protein, and water to maximize the rate of absorption.[1638]

In the landmark study published in 2015 entitled "Which Foods May Be Addictive?" that I mentioned in the Low Glycemic Load section, dozens of foods were ranked based on reports of problematic, addictive-type behaviors from hundreds of individuals. The two most troublesome were high-fat, high-sugar combos: chocolate and ice cream. Most at the top of the list were high in fat, but every single one of the top fifteen was a processed food. In contrast, all the foods least likely to be associated with addictive behaviors were unprocessed. The bottom ten least-addictive foods were strawberries, apples, corn, salmon, bananas, carrots, brown rice, cucumbers, broccoli, and beans.[1639]

This was finally put to the test for weight control in 2019. Study subjects were presented with the same amounts of calories, salt, sugar, fat, carbs, protein, and fiber in processed versus unprocessed forms, such as a breakfast of cereal and a muffin versus oatmeal with fruit and nuts. Over a two-week period, those randomized to eat the processed foods gained two pounds, whereas those randomized to unprocessed foods lost two pounds. The researchers concluded that "limiting consumption of ultra-processed foods may be an effective strategy for obesity prevention and treatment."[1640]

Processed food manufacturers may also insert flavor-enhancing additives like sodium to further manipulate the reward value,[1641] reminiscent of tobacco industry additives to enhance nicotine delivery and flavor[1642]—including added fat, sugar, and salt.[1643] One of the dietary changes noted during opioid detox is an increase in salted foods, perhaps to tap into the same reward pathways.[1644] In one sense, we have no control over most of the sodium we're exposed to since more than two-thirds of sodium intake comes not from the saltshaker at home but from salt added to packaged foods and dishes in restaurants.[1645] In another sense, however, most of us actually have total control, as we can choose to buy fewer processed foods and eat out less.

Eaten Away

The eating habits of Americans have been described as "eat[ing] breakfast in their cars, lunch at their desks and chicken from a bucket."[1646] Most of us eat out at least three times a week[1647] and average an extra two hundred or so calories on the days we do, all while taking in less nutrition.[1648] The blood levels of nearly all examined micronutrients were lower among those who ate more meals out, largely reflecting a drop in the consumption of plant foods.[1649] This may be a particular problem at fast-food restaurants. A modern-day case of scurvy was even diagnosed in someone on a "strict fast food diet."[1650]

Little has changed in recent years to improve the quality of fast-food restaurant menus. (The one exception is the removal of partially hydrogenated oils, thanks to the trans fat ban, but not all trans fat has gone away—cheeseburgers are now worse offenders than fries, due to the inherent trans fat in meat and dairy.[1651]) Those who eat out more often in general tend to be at greater risk of becoming overweight or obese, and this appears to particularly be the case for fast food.[1652] People who eat more fast food also tend to eat more unhealthfully in general, though—more meat, white bread, and sweets—so rather than fast food leading to bad eating habits, bad eating habits may lead people to fast food.[1653]

An estimated three-quarters of adolescents eat fast food on a weekly basis, a dramatic rise over the last fifty years.[1654] What role might this play in the obesity epidemic? Teens were seated in a food court and allowed to eat as much as they wanted of a typical fast-food meal. If you assume three meals a day and a couple of snacks, you would want to stay under about 30 percent of your daily energy requirements in any one meal, which, in the case of these teens, came out to be just under 800 or so calories. Fast food, however, is so high in calorie density, so high in fat and sugar, and so low in fiber that they ended up eating an average of 1,652 calories at that one meal.[1655]

Is it just the supersized portions and rapid eating rate intrinsic to the fast-food business model? The same researchers set up another experiment in which they portioned out a fast-food meal of chicken nuggets, french fries, and cola into smaller servings presented at fifteen-minute intervals to prevent gorging. It didn't work. In the end, the teens ended up eating the same amount, basically filling their stomachs to physical capacity.[1656]

The industry spends nearly $2 billion marketing these kinds of foods to children and adolescents.[1657] Maybe the nutrition profession would be more vocal in their disapproval if they stopped allowing their conferences to be sponsored by the likes of McDonald's and Coca-Cola.[1658] Just a thought.

Buzzkill

Fast-food meals frequently contribute a fourth addictive factor to the salt, sugar, and fat trifecta by adding caffeinated drinks. In response to a proposal to ban the use of caffeine as a food additive, soda manufacturers claimed it was not used to make their products more addictive but rather as a "flavoring agent."[1659] When put to the test, though, even highly trained subjects could not detect a difference in taste between soda with and without caffeine.[1660] Given that, the more plausible explanation is that caffeine is added to produce physical dependence, which in turn encourages repeat purchases by consumers, many of whom are children.[1661]

Caffeine has a well-known reinforcing effect. It creates a Pavlovian connection between whatever behaviors the body associates with it, from experimentally conditioning one's choice of color-coded capsules[1662] to changing flavor preferences.[1663] No wonder the food industry started adding caffeine not just to soda but to everything from ice cream and candy bars to beef jerky and potato chips.[1664] Even bottled water and instant oatmeal have been spiked.[1665]

The phenomenon of caffeine reinforcing whatever behaviors we're up to when we're exposed to it brings up an interesting point: Caffeine is a problem when it's used by the soda industry to hook our kids on liquid candy, but anything that gets people to eat more oatmeal could flip the whole risk-versus-benefit equation. It makes me think we should start drinking our green tea with broccoli. Maybe that will get us to start craving greens!

Change Your Palate's Palette

The obesity epidemic has been blamed on the abundance of "palatable hyper-caloric" foods[1666]—in other words, high-calorie foods that taste good. After all, as one medical journal editorial put it, "Yummy food is made from fat and sugar."[1667] So is the answer to just not eat anything tasty? No. As I detail in the conclusion of *How Not to Die,* you can actually change your taste buds and end up with the best of both worlds: tastes great *and* more filling.

One pharmacology journal review concluded that we "need to find ways to restrain compulsive intake of palatable food."[1668] It suggests opiate-blocking drugs, but you can imagine jaw-wiring or stomach-stapling would have the same desired effect. The underlying assumption is that palatable food equals unhealthy food, which is only true because the food industry has so deadened our palates with hypersalty, hypersweet, hyperfatty foods. The ripest peach in the world may taste sour after a bowl of Froot Loops. The good news is that studies show the more we eat healthy foods, the more we come to like them.[1669]

The original taste-changing studies were done on salt reduction. Switch people to a low-salt diet, and everything may taste like cardboard at first.[1670] You can imagine the study subjects thinking they could never live like that. But then it happened. Over the ensuing weeks, they liked the taste of salt-free soup more and more, and the taste of salty soup less and less. Our tastes physically change. Let them salt their own soup to taste, and they added less and less the longer they were on the low-salt diet and began to prefer it that way. By the end, soup tasted just as salty with half the salt. The longer we eat healthier foods, the better they taste.

Surprisingly, we can change our sixth sense too. You've probably heard of the five basic tastes: sweet, sour, bitter, salty, and savory. It turns out there are indications our taste buds can register the taste of fat as well.[1671] This may help explain why people on low-fat diets start liking low-fat foods more and high-fat foods less.[1672] The less fat we eat, the more sensitive to fat our tongues appear to become, which may translate into people spontaneously reducing their intakes of butter, meat, dairy, and eggs.[1673] Salt may override this effect,[1674] though, so it may be important to cut down on both simultaneously.

It's all about resetting our taste thermostats. The average life span of a taste bud cell may only be about 250 hours.[1675] That means each of our taste buds could get replaced every ten days or so. This makes sense since they are constantly being assaulted by everything from burning-hot liquids to normal everyday abrasion by our teeth, food, and the roofs of our mouths. Though much of the change in taste perceptions is presumably higher up in our brains, it may be helpful to reflect that our taste buds are basically reborn anew every few weeks, giving us another chance for a fresh start.

FOOD FOR THOUGHT

There have been times when someone happens to see me eating something simple like a sweet potato, and they look at me as if I'm some type of ascetic monk. "Good for you," they might say, "but I could never eat that way." They think I'm living a life of deprivation. Far from it. They don't understand that a sweet potato really tastes good to me (and with a little sprinkle of cinnamon, it tastes even better!). Natural foods as grown can be delicious, but only after you've escaped the numbing shackles of industry manipulations to deaden your senses. I realize the thought of eventually savoring something like corn on the cob without butter or salt may sound ridiculous to some. You won't believe it until you try it out for yourself: Cut out processed foods for a few weeks, and you'll be amazed how good healthy can taste.

LOW IN CALORIE DENSITY

Solving the Mystery of the Obesity Epidemic

One of the key questions we've been trying to address is: *What's behind the explosion in obesity rates over the last few decades in the United States?* Well, we know that if we're to believe the food industry, the blame falls on our inactivity. Remember those leaked internal emails that evidently showed that Coca-Cola spent more than a million dollars covertly creating the Global Energy Balance Network to emphasize exercise over consumption to "serve as a 'weapon' to 'change the conversation' about obesity in its 'war' with public health"?[1676] But as I covered on page 13, if anything, physical activity may have actually even gone *up* since the 1980s.[1677] There's little mystery as to the primary cause of the obesity epidemic: We're consuming more calories.[1678]

It's hard to track actual food consumption on a population scale, but you can monitor the food supply and how much is produced per person, taking into account imports and exports, as well as adjusting for food spoilage and waste. When you look at the number of calories produced per capita in the 1970s compared to the 2000s, the difference is more than enough to explain the obesity epidemic.[1679]

Based on how many more calories kids appear to be eating these days, we'd expect them to weigh an average of about nine pounds more now than back when they were riding Big Wheels and banana-seat bikes, and that's exactly the case. The numbers add up. The prediction based solely on estimated increased caloric intake matches perfectly with how much heavier our children have become.[1680]

Grown-ups have grown bigger too. Given the greater number of calories U.S. adults appear to be eating nowadays, we'd expect to weigh an average of about twenty-four pounds more than we did back in the 1970s, but we're actually only about nineteen pounds heavier.[1681] So we're not *as* fat as one might expect based on increased calorie availability estimates, but this may be due in part to us wasting a greater proportion of food these days.[1682] Regardless, the increase in calories we consume could easily account for our expanding waistlines.

To return to the average body weight of the 1970s, American children would need to eat about 350 fewer calories each day, which is about a can of soda and a small order of fries, and adults would need to cut back about a Big Mac's worth, which is about 500 calories (or take a brisk, daily two-hour walk).[1683]

Was America Supersized?

Just because we're eating more calories doesn't necessarily mean we're eating more food. The calories in what we're eating these days may just be more concentrated. Theoretically, the estimated 20 percent more calories we're getting now could simply mean we're getting an average of 20 percent more calories per bite.

Portion sizes have gone up, though. From the 1970s to the 1990s, the average cheeseburger went from 5.8 to 7.3 ounces, the average portion size of salty snacks grew from 1.0 to 1.6 ounces, and the average soft drink increased from about 13 to nearly 20 fluid ounces.[1684] What's more, larger portions do seem to translate into larger intake, even if we don't take that last bite or final sip—so size does matter. Give moviegoers popcorn in a bucket, and they eat about 50 percent more than when they're served the same popcorn in a smaller (but still excessively sized) box.[1685] In a candy experiment, people given one-pound bags of M&M's reportedly ate 120 candies while watching a video compared to those given a half-pound bag who only ate 63.[1686]

On a population scale, the increased portion sizes, along with increased eating frequency throughout the day, do appear to account for most of the national increase in caloric intake.[1687] On an individual basis, however, calorie concentration can trump portion size.[1688] Decrease by 33 percent the *size* of an extra-large serving of pasta, and people eat about 10 percent less, but decrease by 33 percent the calorie *concentration* of the sauce for a broccoli, cauliflower, and tomato purée by replacing some of the cream and cheese, and the decrease in calorie consumption is nearly three times greater.[1689]

Obese individuals don't necessarily eat a greater weight of food, but the foods they choose do tend to have more calories per mouthful.[1690] So excess intake may have more to do with food quality than quantity. Overeating may be less about consuming an abnormal amount of food and more about consuming an abnormal type of food: meals that are unnaturally dense in calories.

How Many Calories Can You Stomach?

Our stomachs are only so big. Once we fill them up, stretch receptors in our stomach walls tell us when we've had enough. Given this limit, if you wanted to gain weight, how could you do it? Well, you could eat more frequently. Alternatively, you could increase the number of calories in each stomachload by changing what you eat—that is, by changing calorie density, the number of calories for a given weight or volume of food.

Some foods have more calories per cup, per pound, per mouthful than others. Oil, for example, has a high calorie density, which means it has a high calorie concentration with lots of calories packed in a small space. Drizzling just one tablespoon of oil on a dish adds 120 calories.[1691] For those same 120 calories, you could eat about two cups of blackberries, a food with a low calorie density.[1692] You could swig down that spoonful of oil and not even feel a difference in your stomach, but eating a couple of cups of berries could start to fill you up.

A handful of jelly beans has about sixteen times more calories than a handful of cherry tomatoes.[1693,1694] So for the same number of calories, you could eat that one handful of jelly beans or about four cups of cherry tomatoes. A large serving of french fries is about the same size and weight as a baked potato but has about four times more calories.[1695,1696] So for the same number of calories, you could have that single serving of fries or around four baked potatoes. Which do you think would be more filling?

The average human stomach can expand to fit about a quart of food,[1697] which is around four cups. A single stomachful of strawberry ice cream, about two pints, could max out our caloric intake for an entire day.[1698] What if you wanted to get those same two thousand or so calories from strawberries themselves? You'd have to eat forty-four cups of berries.[1699] That's eleven stomachfuls. As delicious as strawberries are, I don't think I could fill my stomach to bursting eleven times in a day. Some foods are just impossible to overeat. They are so low in calorie density that you just couldn't physically eat a big enough quantity to maintain your weight.

On the next page is an infographic of how many stomachfuls of food you would need to eat in a day to get two thousand calories.

Zucchini is even less calorie dense than broccoli. You could eat 100 cups of sliced zucchini a day and still lose weight.[1700] The calories in cucumbers are so dilute you'd have to eat more than 150 cups a day to gain weight[1701] and more than 250 cups of chopped kale.[1702] You just couldn't do it. That's the magic of nonstarchy vegetables and fruit. You could be filled to the brim with fresh fruit three times a day and still lose weight because they're mostly water and air. An apple, for example, is 85 percent water by weight and 20 percent air by volume (which is why you can bob for them on Halloween).[1703]

At the other extreme, there are pure fats like butter and oil that are so calorically dense you could exceed your total calorie input for the day filling up your stomach only a quarter of the way just once. So, hundreds of cups of vegetables or a single stick of butter? Hopefully no one is eating butter by the stick—this is just to illustrate how leaning toward the lower-calorie-density foods on average could enable you to eat the same amount of food, or even more, and still lose weight.

Stomachfuls to Fit 2,000 Calories

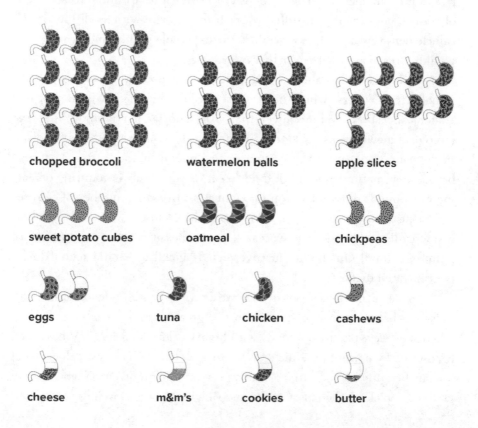

chopped broccoli

watermelon balls

apple slices

sweet potato cubes

oatmeal

chickpeas

eggs

tuna

chicken

cashews

cheese

m&m's

cookies

butter

On average, those who eat low-energy-density diets consume hundreds of fewer calories, yet they eat significantly more food, about three-quarters of a pound more a day.[1704] Most weight-loss diets focus on decreasing portion size, but we know "eat less" approaches can leave people feeling hungry and unsatisfied.[1705] Shifting the emphasis from restriction to positive "eat more" messaging of increasing intake of healthy, low-energy-density foods may offer a more promising strategy.[1706]

Apes vs. Twinkies

It's ironic that the method used to achieve rapid weight gain in malnourished children—frequent, high-calorie-density meals—has become the de facto norm for many children (and adults) today.[1707] In the study about fast food that I explored in the Low in Addictive Foods section, the teens, when presented with an unlimited fast-food lunch, piled in an average of 1,652 calories in just one meal.[1708] The propensity to overeat isn't limited to fast food, of course, but even if you stuffed yourself to the brim with foods low on the calorie density scale—like vegetables, fruits, whole grains, and beans—you wouldn't reach anywhere near that caloric load.

Fast food averages about 1,200 calories per pound,[1709] whereas traditional African diets, which more closely represent the likely diet of our ancient ancestors, average fewer than 500 calories per pound.[1710] So the biological mechanisms our bodies use to regulate our weight likely evolved in the context of eating at least four or five pounds of food a day. That may be the more natural amount of food to eat. If your body is counting on eating five pounds of food but you max out with the same number of calories eating just two pounds of modern convenience food, what do you think happens? It's no wonder we overeat—our bodies are expecting three more pounds of food! Our bodies just weren't designed to handle such calorie-concentrated diets.

It makes evolutionary sense that we crave calorically dense foods. Put kids in a brain scanner, and you can see greater reward center activation when they view pictures of foods with higher calorie density.[1711] We've been hardwired by eons of periodic scarcity to seek out the greatest caloric bang for our foraging buck.[1712] In a primitive setting, that motivation would drive us toward picking the ripest fruits and digging up the starchiest roots, but now, that same biological drive compels us toward processed junk heaviest in added sugars and fats.

Traditional grain-based diets represent what we've been eating for thousands of years before the Industrial Age, but if you go back millions of years to the dawn of humanity, we likely ate more like contemporary great apes, with whom our DNA still differs at most by only a few percent. This means a diet centered around leafy vegetables, shoots, roots, berries and other fruits, seeds, and nuts.[1713] Researchers at the University of Toronto decided to try putting people on just such an ape diet. Even after including higher-calorie-density foods like nuts, research subjects had to eat twelve pounds of food a day to maintain their weights.[1714] So it seems very likely our appetite control mechanisms evolved eating massive quantities of food. Our bodies never expected to meet a Twinkie.

How much food does it take to reach 2,000 calories at different caloric densities? As you can see in the graph below, you would need to eat eight pounds of food a day on a low-calorie-density diet of 250 calories per pound, whereas on a high-calorie-density diet, you'd have to restrict yourself to eating four times less food.

What happens when you go back for seconds? On a low-calorie-density diet, an extra helping might only add a few dozen calories, whereas, at the higher end, the same helping could add hundreds. A second serving of concentrated-calorie foods a few times a week could translate into tens of thousands of excess calories a year.

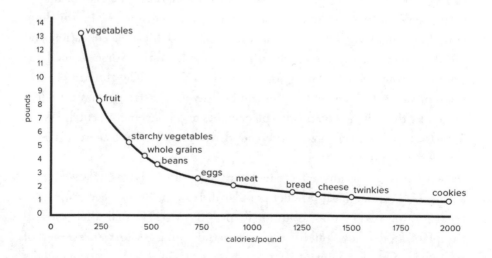

Seventeen Pounds in Twenty-One Days

Given that on a day-to-day basis, we tend to eat a similar amount of food,[1715] it would make sense that if there were fewer calories in the same mass of food, you'd take in fewer calories and lose more weight. Studies in which foods are covertly passed into people's stomachs through a tube have confirmed that the stomach registers volume much more than it does calories in terms of appetite and subsequent food intake.[1716] Researchers were able to cut people's caloric intake nearly in half, from 3,000 daily calories down to 1,570, without cutting portions—just by substituting less-calorie-dense foods.[1717] They replaced meats and sugary foods with lots of fruits, vegetables, whole grains, and beans. Despite the sudden slashing of their caloric intakes almost in half, the research subjects reported equal satiety and enjoyment.

So do people who eat higher-calorie-density diets gain more weight? Apparently so. There is "strong and consistent evidence" that those consuming a diet higher in calorie density do tend to gain weight, while those eating diets lower in calorie density improve both weight loss and weight maintenance.[1718] We can't be sure this is due to calorie density itself, though, since calorie-dilute foods tend to be healthier[1719] in a variety of ways—for example, less processed, more fiber.

Low-calorie-density diets offer the best of both worlds: higher dietary quality and better weight loss.

Portion-controlled diets, often incorporating liquid meal replacements, can be effective in the short term[1720] but may increase the risk of binge-eating episodes[1721] and may actually be counterproductive in the long run. Individuals randomized to a few months of lifestyle education and SlimFast meal replacements actually did significantly worse years later than the group who had just gotten the education.[1722] The thinking is that the motivation to learn and implement healthy eating strategies was undermined by the reliance on meal replacements as a convenient crutch. What if instead of having people eat *less* food overall, you have them eat *more* calorically dilute foods?

Before spam was unwanted email cluttering our in-boxes, it was SPAM, a processed canned meat product popular in Hawaii. Researchers in Hawaii tried putting people on a traditional, pre-SPAM, Hawaiian diet with all the plant foods they could eat.[1723] The study subjects lost an average of seventeen pounds in just twenty-one days. Caloric intake dropped by

40 percent, but not because they were eating less food. The subjects lost seventeen pounds in three weeks eating *more* food, in excess of four pounds of food a day.

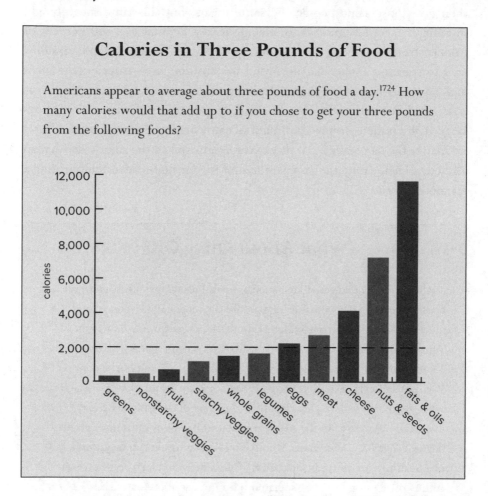

Calories in Three Pounds of Food

Americans appear to average about three pounds of food a day.[1724] How many calories would that add up to if you chose to get your three pounds from the following foods?

Chewing the Fat

If you lower the calorie density of your diet, you could keep eating the same amount of food yet lose weight. If you lower it enough, you could eat even more food than usual and still shed pounds. So how can you decrease the density? A quick look at the two extremes of the Calories in Three Pounds of Food graph should make apparent two methods: abandon added fats and add abandoned vegetables.

As we saw in the Low in Added Fat section, covertly put people on a relatively low-fat diet (20 percent calories from fat), and they tend to lose body fat every day even though they can eat as much as they want. If you then give those same people the same meals, but this time sneakily add in enough extra fats and oils to change it to a high-fat diet (60 percent of calories from fat), they gain body fat every day.[1725] Because people randomized to consume higher-fat diets tend to consume more calories, the term *high-fat hyperphagia* was coined, implying that fat somehow made people eat more, but that wasn't the case. Instead, those secretly switched from low-fat to high-fat diets simply continued to eat nearly the same amount of food no matter the fat content. All that extra fat just spiked the calorie density, so all of a sudden, eating the same amount of food meant inadvertently eating a lot more calories.

What About Olive Oil?

Second only to animal fats, such as lard, tallow, fish oil, bacon grease, and chicken fat, vegetable oil tends to be the most calorie-dense food,[1726] more so even than butter, which is about 16 percent water by weight.[1727] What about olive oil? In many cases, Mediterranean dietary patterns have been found to beat out other diets for weight loss,[1728] and in the context of a truly Mediterranean diet, olive oil has not been found to be associated with significant weight gain. But how the olive oil is being used may make the difference. In the Mediterranean, olive oil is often used to dress beans, vegetables, and salads, so olive oil consumption can be an indicator of a healthier, more traditional diet.[1729] In a more modern context, just adding olive oil to food is associated with increased obesity risk,[1730] so weight loss on a Mediterranean diet may be in spite of, not because of, the olive oil.[1731]

The study subjects were men with big appetites who were already eating about four pounds of food a day. The high-fat diet was so calorie dense that they would have had to have eaten around six pounds a day of the lower-fat meals to cause the same kind of weight gain. Since the subjects didn't even notice the difference between the two diet phases, those who were started on the high-fat diet ate the same four pounds of the lower-fat meals after being switched, so they went from gaining weight to losing weight without even realizing it.[1732] That's why manipulating added fat content can be so powerful.

But if you feed people higher- or lower-fat diets with the same calorie density (by diluting the high-fat meals with water, for example), the high-fat hyperphagia effect disappears. So it isn't the fat per se. With more than twice the calories as carbs or protein, fat is just so calorie dense that it can slip in more calories per bite. So the phenomenon was renamed *passive overconsumption,* which you may remember from the Causes section. Fat doesn't drive us to overeat. Unintentionally, we just may eat more calories without even knowing it.[1733]

A paper in the journal *Public Health Nutrition* entitled "Two Important Exceptions to the Relationship Between Energy Density and Fat Content" added important caveats.[1734] Processed foods with reduced fat claims on the front of their packaging are often so packed with sugar that they may have the same number of calories per serving as a higher fat product. SnackWell's fat-free cookies, for example, at 1,700 calories per pound[1735] are as calorie dense as a cheese danish.[1736]

The other exception noted was that vegetables are so calorie dilute that even high-fat veggie dishes like buttered broccoli tend to be less calorically dense overall than most of what people are eating.[1737]

This brings up the second strategy for lowering dietary calorie density: instead of sneaking out fat, sneak in vegetables.

Souped-Up Weight Loss

If the water content of vegetables is their secret to low-calorie density, what about taking that to its logical conclusion and feeding people liquids, as in soup? Soup consumers tend to have slimmer waists and lower body weight, perhaps as a consequence of the lower average calorie density of their diets, but they also tend to exhibit other healthy eating behaviors, such as eating more greens and beans.[1738] You don't know if it's the soup itself unless you put it to the test.

In a study funded by Campbell's—who else?—people on calorie-restricted diets were randomized to eat either two servings of soup a

(continued)

day or two dry snacks like crackers or pretzels with the same number of calories as the soup servings. After one year, the soup group lost 50 percent more weight, about fifteen pounds compared to around ten pounds.[1739] Of course, their sodium intakes went up—even "low sodium" Campbell's soup may exceed by more than 250 percent my one-to-one sodium-per-calorie ratio recommendation I detailed in *How Not to Die*.[1740] So I encourage everyone to look for no-salt-added soup varieties or make your own. For more on soup, check out the Wall Off Your Calories section.

Dangling a Carrot

The biggest influence on calorie density is not fat but water content.[1741] Since water adds weight and bulk without adding calories, the most calorie-dense foods and the most calorie-dense diets tend to be those that are dry.[1742] Some vegetables, on the other hand, are more than 95 percent water, and, as we saw in the High in Water-Rich Foods section, it's not just iceberg lettuce. Bamboo shoots, bean sprouts, cucumbers, celery, turnips, cooked napa cabbage, bok choy, summer squash, and zucchini may top out at 95 percent water.[1743] They're basically water in vegetable form. A big bowl of water-rich vegetables is practically just a big bowl of trapped water.

The effect on calorie density is so dramatic, the food industry wants in on the action. In a research paper entitled "Food Nanotechnology: Water Is the Key to Lowering the Energy Density of Processed Foods," one researcher proposed "structuring a solid processed food similar to a celery stalk using self-assembled, water-filled, edible nanocells or nanotubes."[1744] No need, as Mother Nature has already done it for us.

If piling on vegetables causes protests at the dinner table, *hidden* vegetables can be used to covertly decrease calorie density, just as hidden fat can be used to covertly increase it. In a famous Penn State study, broccoli, cauliflower, tomatoes, squash, and zucchini were added secretly to familiar entrées, while the dishes' appearance, flavor, and texture were maintained (by puréeing vegetables into pasta sauce, for example).[1745] The kids in the study were none the wiser and ate the same amount of food, thereby taking in significantly fewer calories and significantly more vegetables. Win-win!

Surreptitiously slipping veggies to unsuspecting kids shouldn't be the only way to get them to eat them, though. The researchers stress the importance of using several approaches, including repeated exposure to originally disliked whole vegetables, which has been shown to improve acceptance over time.[1746] Taste familiarity is an important determinant of children's food preferences. The more they are exposed to the taste, the more likely it is they'll eat them.[1747] So the best way to get kids to eat their vegetables is to have them actually eat their vegetables so they can develop a lifelong appreciation.[1748] Covertly incorporating vegetables can be one strategy, but they're not going be living at home forever, and we want to leave them with a legacy of overtly healthy habits too.

The same vegetable sneak-attack strategy has been used successfully in adults.[1749] In fact, study subjects actually preferred some of the "vegetable-enhanced" meals to their non-veggie-fortified options. What's more, even though they ate bigger portions of the meals with added vegetables, they still took in fewer calories.

Again, that's the beauty of calorie density. The subjects were awarded the twin benefit of eating a pound of vegetables a day and consuming 350 fewer calories. More food, fewer calories. Keep that up and over time, you could lose thirty-five pounds just like that.[1750]

What may be an even more effective weight-loss strategy than just adding calorie-dilute veggies is a combination approach. Those randomized to receive advice about reducing fat intake lost more weight than those just told to eat more fruits and vegetables, but those instructed to do both—lower their fat consumption while increasing their fruit and veggie intakes—did the best, losing seventeen pounds and maintaining that reduction for the whole year.[1751] Yes, simply adding vegetables—whether covertly or overtly, like adding chopped greens to rice—can decrease calorie density, caloric intake, and hunger,[1752] but simultaneously adding vegetables while removing fat can attack the problem from both sides. For example, adding puréed broccoli and cauliflower in place of some of the cheese in a pasta sauce successfully decreased calorie density by 25 percent, leading to a full 25 percent reduction in caloric intake in children, 79 percent of whom rated the less cheesy, vegetable-heavier version as tasting the same or better.[1753]

Mushrooming Weight Loss

Mushrooms are a great way to swap out calories and swap in flavor. They only have about one hundred calories per pound,[1754] so incorporating them into our meals can certainly lower calorie density, but it's their savory umami flavor that develops particularly well during cooking that makes them an ideal meat replacer. Studies show substituting mushrooms for meat can cut meal calories in half without compromising palatability or satiety. This led researchers to suggest that even just making one such swap a week could result in more than five pounds of weight loss in a year.[1755]

In another study, Johns Hopkins researchers randomized overweight individuals into one of two groups: those instructed to follow the USDA Food Guide Pyramid–based diet prescription, or another told to adhere to the same diet prescription but to also incorporate mushrooms instead of meat into meals three times a week. A year later, not only did the mushroom group have better metabolic markers and less inflammation (which you would expect from any sort of meat reduction), but they also achieved a significant loss in weight of seven pounds at six months and kept it off for the rest of the year.[1756] Pass the portobello burgers!

Out of Thin Air

Pop Quiz: Aside from fiber and water, what other food component has zero calories? Hint: Maybe I should have called this a Pop*corn* Quiz. Air. Air has zero calories. A cup of corn kernels has four times more calories than a cup of popped corn kernels,[1757,1758] despite having more water. That may be one reason popcorn is more filling than potato chips. Six cups of popcorn was found to be more satiating than about the same weight of potato chips (one cup), though in this case the difference in fat content also affected the calorie density.[1759] To control for both water and fat content, researchers decided to study cheese puffs.

Researchers compared Crunchy Cheetos to Cheetos Puffs. Though both have the same number of calories per pound, the Puffs have fewer calories per volume because they've been puffed up with air. Study subjects were offered a big bowl of each, and, although they consumed nearly 75 percent greater volume of the Puffs, they still ended up taking in about 20 percent fewer calories, presumably because the Puffs had so many fewer calories per cup due to the added air.[1760] Of course, neither cheesy snack food is a good choice, as they both exceed 2,500 calories per pound, worse even than straight-up cheese.[1761,1762]

The Cheetos study wasn't perfect. The two types of Cheetos differed in their ingredients, which could have affected the results. To see if food volume independently affects intake, an ingeniously simple experiment was devised: Researchers crushed up some Wheaties. Reducing the flake size reduced the volume, so they could feed people the identical food, differing not by calories per pound but by calories per cup. The study subjects poured themselves less of the crushed Wheaties, sensing it was denser, but not enough to avoid pouring themselves 34 percent more calories.[1763] So it seems volume really does appear to make a difference.

Since we tend to consistently eat both a certain weight and volume of food,[1764] eating foods higher in both water and air (and therefore lower in calorie density) may facilitate weight loss—which brings us to fruit.

Bearing Fruit

One of the reasons bananas are so light is that 20 percent of their volume is straight-up air.[1765] Because most of the rest of a banana is water, 85 percent of a banana is calorie-free. Fruits even higher in water content—like apples and pears—are more than 90 percent calorie-free. So what would happen if you had people add fresh fruit to their regular diets?

In a study out of Brazil, people were randomized to eat three apples or three pears a day as snacks between meals on top of whatever else they were eating. Fruit is low in calories, but not calorie-free, so if they're adding foods to their diets, won't they gain weight? No, they actually *lost* a couple of pounds. Could that weight loss simply be due to all the additional fiber they were getting from the apples and pears? Enter the cookie group. The study subjects were randomized to three apples, three pears, *or* three oatmeal cookies with enough oats in them to have about the same amount of fiber as the fruit. So all three groups added about the same number of calories and same amount of fiber. Unlike the fruit, however, adding oatmeal cookies to the diet did *not* lead to weight loss, despite the added fiber. No shocker there. Because of its water content, the fruit was five times heavier, so it offered five times as much food as the cookies. Cookies are so calorie dense that you can add hundreds of calories without feeling much of a difference, whereas people appeared to unconsciously compensate for all the extra bulk from the fruit by eating less of everything else and lost weight as a result.[1766]

When three methods of lowering calorie density were compared—covertly manipulating fat levels by removing butter and oil, adding diced or puréed fruits and vegetables, or adding water—decreasing fat seemed to work best in terms of decreasing overall daily calorie consumption. However, this may have been complicated by the fact that the entrées with the added fruits, vegetables, and water were rated moister and were associated with faster eating rates compared to the reduced-fat entrées. The bottom line is that a combination of approaches might work best, like replacing oil with applesauce when baking, achieving both a fat reduction and a fruit enhancement.[1767]

If researchers with no culinary training can covertly reduce calorie counts without anyone noticing, why can't chefs? Nearly all chefs surveyed, 93 percent, thought the calories in menu items could indeed be reduced by up to 25 percent without customers noticing. So why don't they? The greatest barrier they identified was "low consumer demand."[1768]

Are Nuts the Exception?

Nuts have a high calorie density. At the same time, nuts are one of the few foods that, on their own, may literally add years to your life.[1769] Not only may they slow the aging process itself,[1770] but an ounce a day, which is just about a handful or a quarter cup, may also reduce the risk of dying from heart disease, stroke, cancer, respiratory disease, diabetes, and infections[1771]—more than half of our top ten killers. So it comes as no surprise that nut consumption is associated with lower risk of dying prematurely across the board. As the title of a recent editorial in the *Journal of the American College of Cardiology* put it: "Eat Nuts, Live Longer."[1772]

On a global scale, inadequate nut consumption (under twenty grams a day) may be responsible for millions of deaths,[1773] but what does that mean on a personal level? Studies have found, for example, that those eating nuts just twice a week or more appear to cut their mortality risk in half compared to those who almost never eat nuts.[1774] You could flip that around and suggest that not eating nuts doubles your chances of dying prematurely. Is that really true, though? Yes and no.

There are many potentially confounding factors, such as those who consume nuts tend to smoke less, exercise more, and eat less meat and more fruits and vegetables, but the mortality benefits appear to persist even after controlling for these factors.[1775] Even if we knew for certain it was cause and effect, it's important to understand what halving our mortality risk really means.

As a healthy, middle-aged person, our risk of dying over the next ten years may only be about 2 percent, a one-in-fifty chance of dying over the next decade, but that's if we don't eat nuts.[1776] If we do eat them, our risk of dying may drop to 1 percent. So, yes, technically, we just cut our risk in half by going from 2 percent to 1 percent, but, at the same time, we really only cut our *absolute* risk of dying by a single percentage point. That may not sound as impressive, but to me, dying at such a relatively young age seems such a tragedy that it would be worth making lifestyle changes to drive down that risk as low as possible, especially when one such strategy is a simple, delicious dietary tweak.

Given the purported mortality benefits of eating nuts and despite their high calorie density, it would seem worthwhile to include them in our regular diets by consciously substituting them in place of the same number of calories from other foods. Thankfully, our bodies appear to do it for us automatically.[1777] Nuts appear to be so satiating that if you give people a midmorning snack of almonds, not only do they subsequently eat less at lunch, they eat less at dinner, too, spontaneously accounting for the extra almond calories.

This explains how you can make thirty thousand calories "vanish" into thin air. Those randomized to add servings of almonds,[1778] pistachios,[1779] hazelnuts,[1780] or walnuts[1781] to their daily diets for months didn't gain a single pound on average. In the Nuts and Seeds chapter

(continued)

in *How Not to Die,* I cataloged the factors beyond appetite suppression thought responsible for this vanishing act. A new one to add to the list arose from a randomized, double-blind, placebo-controlled brain scan study out of Harvard. The researcher's "fruit smoothie delivery system" involved identically tasting, fat- and calorie-matched smoothies made either with walnuts or with oil and walnut flavoring.[1782] The brain scans showed that those unknowingly consuming the real walnuts exhibited increased activation of a part of their brains thought to involve the ability to control cravings. There's just something in nuts that appears to be especially satisfying.

A significant proportion of the calories in nuts also quite literally gets flushed away. The actual number of calories that our systems absorb from nuts may be as much as 20 percent lower than it says on the nutrition label because the calories are encapsulated inside cell walls.[1783] No matter how well we chew, some of the calories remain trapped inside unbroken cells, each of which is surrounded by an indigestible wall of fiber.[1784] The calories in whole plant foods are effectively walled off, which may help explain why other higher-calorie-density foods like meat and processed foods are associated with weight gain, whereas nuts are not.[1785]

As a high-calorie-density food, the admonition to "eat sparingly" still applies, but that's all one may need. While the optimum benefits of fruits and vegetables may require cups a day, nuts appear so potent that the mortality benefits may be had for mere ounces a week.

FOOD FOR THOUGHT

So how low should we go when it comes to calorie density? The American Institute for Cancer Research has taken the lead on setting calorie-density targets to help lower the rate of obesity-related cancers. The institute recommends that calorie-dense foods, defined as having more than around 70 calories per ounce, only be eaten "sparingly" and set an ambitious public health goal of trying to get the average calorie density of our diets below 35 calories per ounce, or 560 per pound of food.[1786]

It's hard to imagine units of weight, though. Volume is easier to visualize. How many calories is that per measuring cup? Thirty-five calories per ounce translates to about 300 calories per cup.[1787] Which foods have fewer than 300 per cup, and which foods have more? I made a simple chart for you to stick on your fridge to see at a glance which foods you may want to eat more—or less—of:

Calories per Cup

Eat More	On Target	Eat Less	Eat Sparingly
< 100 calories/cup	< 300 calories/cup	300–600 calories/cup	> 600 calories/cup
most fresh fruit	avocados & bananas	dried fruit	nuts & nut butters
most vegetables	starchy vegetables	french fries & onion rings	oil
	pasta & whole grains	bread	chocolate
	beans, lentils & chickpeas	fried tofu	soy nuts
	yogurt	eggs	cheese
	seafood & wild game	beef, pork & poultry	bacon

Note: Calorie-density calculations typically exclude beverages since all drinks quickly drain out of the stomach at about the same rate.

This volumetrics wisdom of choosing foods heavy on bulk and light in calories goes back centuries. The president of the Royal College of Physicians of Edinburgh seemed to be channeling the calorie-density concept in his dietary treatment recommendations for "corpulence" back in the 1700s: "Animal food only once a day and then very moderately. Cheat appetite by eating light things—especially vegetables."[1788]

LOW IN MEAT

Should We Stop Meating Like This?

Rather than promoting produce, most of our U.S. taxpayer-dollar subsidies support the production of meat, dairy, oils, and sugar.[1789] So while I was excited to discover that there is a National Watermelon Promotion Board, its budget is dwarfed by the combined quarter-billion-dollar might of the federal government–administered American Egg,[1790] Cattlemen's Beef,[1791] National Dairy,[1792] and National Pork boards.[1793] Don't expect Dollar Menu melons anytime soon.

So given the cheapness of meat, what role might it be playing in the obesity epidemic? The largest study of those eating plant-based diets found that American vegetarians tend to weigh about twenty-five pounds less than those who eat meat.[1794] Compared to those chewing meat, those eschewing it also appear to gain less weight as they age.[1795] Kids[1796] and teens[1797] eating more vegetarian meals also tend to be leaner than their nonvegetarian peers. They aren't smaller in general, though: Vegetarian boys and girls measure up to be about an inch taller than their "omnivorous classmates."[1798] They just aren't as wide.

It's certainly not all or nothing, though. Quantity matters. A research team sifted through more than a thousand studies published just since the year 2000 to perform a systematic review on which foods were "determinants of long-term weight change." Not surprisingly, they found that white bread, sweets, and desserts all seem to promote weight gain. Their main finding, however, was that evidence is strongest for high meat intake predicting more weight gain.[1799] Those who eat a lot of meat also tend to eat less fruit, whole grains, and nuts,[1800] though, all of which may be protective against gaining weight.[1801] So is the weight gain because they're eating more animal products or because they're eating fewer plants? Or might it be something else entirely? Those who eat more meat also tend to exercise less, for example,[1802] or maybe they're just drinking soda with their burgers.

In the same vein, vegans are forty pounds lighter on average than those who eat conventional diets,[1803] but that doesn't mean that cutting out meat, dairy, and eggs will necessarily make you lose forty pounds. Those who eat healthier also tend to live healthier, so it's not necessarily the diet per se. Maybe vegans eat out less and work out more. To see if meat has an independent effect on obesity, we need to control for both dietary and nondietary factors.

When researchers have tried to account for these differences, controlling for other nutritional and lifestyle considerations like fiber intake and exercise, the link between meat consumption and weight gain remained solid.[1804] Over a twenty-month period, for example, those eating about three more ounces of meat a day had about three times the risk of gaining five or more pounds.[1805] Another study found that those who ate about five ounces of meat a day had eight times the incidence of abdominal obesity over a year compared to those who ate around one ounce of meat daily.[1806] (An ounce of meat is about the size of a golf ball.) Meat intake seems to be more closely associated with abdominal weight gain than peripheral gain—that is, bigger bellies rather than bigger thighs.[1807] Over a ten-year period, the amount of weight gain associated with eating more than seven servings of meat a week (compared to those averaging less than about one serving of meat every other day) was the same as the amount of weight lost by women who walked or men who jogged or ran four or more hours a week.[1808]

Even a Paltry Amount of Poultry?

Could it be as simple as people who eat more meat tend to take in more calories?[1809] Most of those studies linking meat consumption with weight gain controlled for total caloric intake. This implies that if you have two people eating about the same number of calories, the person eating more meat might gain more weight. To find out which meat may be the most fattening, an epic study was performed. EPIC is actually the name of the study, and it lives up to its moniker, having enrolled hundreds of thousands of men and women, assessing their intake diets, and following them out for years.

The EPIC researchers also found total meat consumption linked to increased weight gain, even at similar caloric intakes. They concluded: "Our results are therefore in favor of the public health recommendation to decrease meat consumption for health improvement." The surprise, though, was that poultry appeared to be the most fattening. Consumption of poultry—mostly chicken—was associated with three times the weight gain compared to red meat like beef,[1810,1811] and this was after taking into account age, gender, physical activity level, smoking status, overall dietary quality, and calorie counts.

How did the meat industry respond to the EPIC findings? By suggesting that perhaps the extra weight gain was muscle mass and not body fat.[1812] Could the meat have made the subjects beefier rather than fatter? The researchers responded to the industry's challenge by going back and specifically assessing changes in the subjects' waistlines and found the same thing.[1813] Even when eating around the same number of calories, the more meat we eat, the more our bellies may grow. The researchers even calculated how much our waistlines might be predicted to expand, based on our daily meat consumption. It only came out to be one extra inch around the waist over the five-year follow-up for a daily chicken breast's worth,[1814] but that appears to be *independent* of the calories.

No other such study comes close to EPIC in size, but another one followed thousands of individuals for even longer and confirmed the connection between poultry consumption and increased risk of weight gain over a period of fourteen years. Using statistical methods to adjust for other factors, researchers effectively tried to study men and women who ate about the same number of calories a day, consumed the same amount of vegetables, fruits, and grains, and did about the same amount of exercise—but ate different amounts of meat. On average, at baseline, those who ate less than a small serving of meat a day were not overweight, but the more meat they ate, the heavier they were.[1815] By one and a half servings a day, they crossed the threshold of a BMI of 25 to become officially classified as overweight.

Over the following fourteen years, chicken consumption was associated most with weight gain in both men and women, and it didn't appear to take much. Compared to those who didn't eat any chicken at all, those eating more than 22.8 grams of chicken a day had a significantly greater increase in their body mass indexes.[1816] To put that into context, 22.8 grams is less than an ounce, which is about one single chicken nugget a day[1817] or just one chicken breast once every ten days.[1818]

Chicken Out

The odds of obesity may increase by 18 percent for every 1 percent increase in calories from red meat, poultry, fish, or shellfish.[1819] As we saw in the previous section, animal protein intake in general has been associated with both increased abdominal obesity and general obesity, even after taking into account other dietary and lifestyle factors.[1820] We know you can't control for everything, though. In the population studies above, poultry appeared to be the worst offender, but interventional trials are required to prove cause and effect.

In a head-to-head test of beef, pork, and chicken, no differences were noted in terms of short-term satiety.[1821] What about weight changes over time? No differences there either. People were told to eat mostly beef, pork, or chicken in three-month blocks, and no differences were noted in body composition in any of the three periods.[1822] Might this be like the cholesterol story? There's a common misperception that switching from red meat to white meat lowers cholesterol, but when it was actually put to the test, no significant improvements were noted when people swapped beef, veal, and pork for chicken and fish.[1823] So are we seeing the same when it comes to weight loss? The only meat shown to be less fattening than chicken in a randomized controlled trial was chicken-free chicken, a plant-based meat made from the mushroom kingdom first popularized in Europe called *Quorn*.

When the meat industry funded an obesity study on chicken, they pitted it against "cookies and sugar-coated chocolates."[1824] This is a classic drug industry tactic: Make your product look better by comparing it to something known to be substandard.[1825] (Apparently, regular chocolate wasn't enough to make chicken look better.) But what happens when chicken is pitted head-to-head against a real control like meatless chicken? Chicken chickens out.

Quorn-brand chickenless chicken was found to be more satiating among both lean[1826] and overweight[1827] individuals, cutting down on subsequent meal intake hours later. Feed people a chicken-and-rice lunch, and four and a half hours later, they eat 18 percent more of a dinner buffet than those who had been given a lunch of chicken-free chicken and rice. In terms of calories, the chicken-and-rice lunch diners ate about 1,200 calories for dinner, compared to the 1,000 dinner calories eaten by subjects after the Quorn meal. Tofu also beat out chicken in a similar manner.[1828] These findings are consistent with childhood obesity research that found meat consumption seemed to double the odds of schoolchildren becoming overweight, whereas the consumption of plant-based meat products appeared to have no effect. Whole-food sources of plant protein, such as beans, did even better, though, associated with cutting the odds of kids becoming overweight in half.[1829]

TMAObesity?

Ancient doctors evidently used to use ants to diagnose people with diabetes.[1830] They (the ants, not the doctors) were attracted to the sugary urine. This is an archaic example of the modern science of metabolomics, which tries to uncover the molecular signatures of disease. For example, with each breath, we exhale hundreds of different compounds.[1831] Imagine how, with enough people and enough computing power, we might be able to diagnose a disease like lung cancer with some sort of Breathalyzer test. We just have to figure out the specific patterns of chemicals in the body fluids of those with and without disease. This is how Cleveland Clinic researchers discovered the role of TMAO.

The blood of patients who had experienced a heart attack or stroke was compared to the blood of those who hadn't, and that's how TMAO, short for *trimethylamine oxide,* was identified.[1832] The more TMAO people had in their blood, the more likely they were to go on to suffer a heart attack, stroke, or otherwise die prematurely.[1833] Where does TMAO come from? Just as short-chain fatty acids are produced by good bacteria in our gut when we eat fiber, TMAO originates from bad bacteria in our gut when we eat lots of choline (concentrated in eggs, but also lecithin supplements) or carnitine (concentrated in meat, but also some energy drinks).

If you eat eggs[1834] or meat,[1835] you get a bump in TMAO levels within hours, unless you recently took antibiotics that wipe out your gut flora. In that case, it can be weeks before your bad bacteria grow back. Alternately, you can prevent the growth of these bad bacteria by not feeding them in the first place. Feed a vegan a steak, and they make virtually no TMAO, presumably because they hadn't been fostering the growth of steak-eating bacteria.[1836]

The egg and beef industries combined forces to fund a study showing that eating fish was even worse than their products, but TMAO levels rose within fifteen minutes after eating fish, suggesting the TMAO is preformed in the fish and may be handled differently by the body. Regardless, their own study showed TMAO levels were *lowest* after eating the non-fish, non-egg, non-beef control food: fruit.[1837] Even relatively choline-rich plant foods don't seem to cause a problem. For example, two ounces of pistachios every day actually seemed to cause a reduction in TMAO levels.[1838]

TMAO may help explain why those who eat more plant-based diets are more protected from heart disease,[1839] but what about obesity? Well, obese individuals do seem to churn out more TMAO,[1840] and blocking TMAO in mice protects them from weight gain, but what we care about is whether avoiding carnitine and choline-rich foods helps with weight loss in people.[1841] We finally got an answer in 2018 from the POUNDS Lost Trial. (*POUNDS* stands for *Preventing Overweight Using Novel Dietary Strategies*.) Those with greater reductions in carnitine and choline were significantly more likely to experience weight loss and waist slimming, while those with increases in carnitine or choline were about twice as likely to fail to lose weight over a two-year period.[1842] But it's not all or nothing.

True, you can feed a vegan an eight-ounce sirloin and not get a TMAO spike,[1843] but even those who eat meat on a regular basis appear to be able to modulate the populations of meat-eating bacteria in their gut. Feed people sausage, egg, and cheese biscuits before and after being on a five-day high-fat diet (55 percent calories from fat), and they end up producing more TMAO after the five-day binge.[1844] This shows we may be able to shift our gut bacteria on a week-to-week basis—for better or for worse.

You (and Your Grandkids?) Are What You Eat

If you expose a pregnant cricket to a predatory wolf spider, her babies hatch exhibiting increased antipredator behavior and, as a consequence, have improved survival from wolf spider attack.[1845] The mother cricket appears to be able to forewarn her babies while they are still inside her about the threat so they come out preadapted to their external environments. How is that possible? Isn't their DNA already set in stone?

This same phenomenon happens in plants too.[1846] If you take two genetically identical plants and grow one in the sun and the other in the shade, the sun-grown plant will produce seeds that grow better in the sun, while the shaded plant will produce seeds that grow better in the shade—even though the two plants are genetically identical. Same DNA, different behavior. This is the epigenetics I talked about in the Causes section, changes in how the genes we have end up expressing themselves.

Another example can be seen with vole pups birthed in the winter, who are born growing thicker coats.[1847] Vole mothers are able to

(continued)

communicate the season to their babies in the womb and tell them to put on a heavier coat even before they're born! And people are no different. You know how some people have different temperature tolerances, resulting in battles over the thermostat in the bedroom or the office? Whether you're born in the tropics or in a cold environment determines how many active sweat glands you have in your skin.[1848]

What does this have to do with diet? Can what a pregnant woman eats permanently alter the biology of her children in terms of what genes are turned on or off throughout life? Children born during the 1944–45 Dutch famine imposed by the Nazis ended up with higher rates of obesity fifty years later.[1849] It seems that the babies' gene expression was reprogrammed before birth to expect to be born into a world of famine and to conserve calories at all cost. But when the war ended, this propensity to store fat became a disadvantage.

What pregnant women eat and don't eat doesn't just help determine the child's birth weight but their future adult weights. For example, maternal animal protein intake during pregnancy (primarily from meat) appears to increase the risk their children will grow up overweight.[1850] Every daily portion of meat intake during the third trimester was correlated with about an extra percent of body fat mass in their children by their sixteenth birthday, potentially increasing their risk of becoming obese later in life, and this appeared to be independent of how many calories they ate or how much they exercised.[1851]

Epigenetics, the science of altering the expression of our genes, is good news. That means your DNA is not your destiny. No matter your family history, some genes can be effectively turned on and off by the lifestyle choices you make, affecting you, your children, and maybe even your grandchildren. Being pregnant during the Dutch famine didn't just lead to an increase in diseases among their kids but even, apparently, their grandkids.[1852] So what a pregnant woman eats now may affect future generations. The possibility of generation-spanning effects of poor dietary conditions during pregnancy may help shine some light on our explosive epidemics of diabetes, obesity, and cardiovascular disease.

Food for Thought

Cutting down on meat is just one of the many ingredients of what could be considered an optimal weight-loss diet. If you continue to eat meat, your best choice would likely be wild game[1853] (critically, felled with lead-free ammunition only).[1854] Today, even our meat could be considered junk food. For more than a century, one of the major goals of animal agriculture has been to increase the carcass fat content of farm animals. Those with the highest fat-to-lean content are branded "prime" and command the highest prices,[1855] but can end up as prime contributors to America's caloric intake.[1856] It's not your grandma's meat.

Take chicken, for example. In 1896, the USDA determined chicken was about 23 percent protein and less than 2 percent fat by weight,[1857] which is even leaner than some wild game like venison.[1858] Today, with ten times the fat, chicken has 1,000 percent more fat than it did just over a century ago.[1859] These days, more than 70 percent of the calories in chicken may come from fat. The birds have been genetically manipulated through selective breeding to contain more fat than protein.[1860] Chicken Little has become Chicken Big and may be making us bigger too.

LOW IN REFINED GRAINS

Going Against the Grain

Most of what we eat in America is processed junk. *Ultraprocessed* foods are defined as "industrial formulations which, besides salt, sugar, oils and fats, include substances not used in culinary preparations, in particular additives used to imitate sensorial qualities" of real food.[1861] Think Frosted Strawberry Pop-Tarts. Ultraprocessed foods comprise an unbelievable 58 percent of the daily caloric intake in the United States.

The number one source of calories in the U.S. diet is refined grains like white flour, followed by added fats like oils. Then come meat and added sugars. Refined carbs and refined fats make up more than half the American diet.[1862] Food-wise, grain-based desserts like cakes, cookies, pastries, and pies are our single largest calorie contributor. Second is white bread, followed by soda.[1863] For our children and adolescents, it's the same top three, but with pizza replacing the bread.[1864]

When proponents of low-carb diets demonize carbohydrates, public health advocates are quick to point out that it's the source that matters—carbohydrates can mean everything from lentils to lollipops.[1865] Though that's true, the Standard American Diet sadly tends to lean more toward the lollipop end of the spectrum. We eat about three times as many calories from refined grains and added sugars as we do from all whole plant foods combined.[1866] So the problem identified by the low-carb proponents is real. We are awash in refined grain garbage, but the answer isn't to switch to high-fad, high-fat diets but rather to low-crap ones.

The consumption of refined grain products appears linked to increased weight gain, but is that just because refined grains are components of fatty foods like pizza, sugary foods like SnackWell's, or the twin menace of fatty sugar bombs like donuts? The Harvard cohort studies involving more than one hundred thousand male and female health professionals found that refined grains like white rice and white bread were associated with weight gain *independent* of all the other dietary and lifestyle factors they measured.[1867] This suggests that it's not just that people who eat lots of Wonder Bread are eating more salami sandwiches or otherwise eating or living unhealthfully. The researchers estimated that every daily serving of refined grains may translate into about a four-tenths of a pound increase in weight over a four-year period. (To put that into perspective, a single large bagel may equal four servings of refined grains.[1868])

Are grains in general the problem, or only refined grains? Observational studies in which people and their diets are followed over time have consistently shown whole-grain consumption not only to be neutral but even associated with *better* weight control.[1869] Children who consumed more than one and a half servings of whole grains per day were found to have 40 percent lower odds of being obese compared with those who consumed less than one daily serving.[1870] In adults, weight gain might be reduced over the long term as much as two pounds for each extra one-ounce increment in daily whole-grain consumption.[1871] But is seeking out foods like brown rice and whole wheat simply a marker for a healthier lifestyle?

Only 6–8 percent of American adults follow my recommendation to eat at least three servings of whole grains a day,[1872] and those who choose oatmeal for breakfast instead of bacon and eggs may also be making other healthy life choices. Indeed, high whole-grain consumers tend to be more physically active, smoke less, and consume more fruits and vegetables.[1873] Statistically, one can try to control these factors like the Harvard studies did, effectively comparing nonsmoking whole-grain eaters to nonsmoking non-whole-grain eaters, all with similar exercise and diet. The result? Whole grains were still found to be associated with better weight control.[1874]

You can't control for everything, though. Could it be that people who make the choice to eat whole grains also choose to wear seat belts and bike helmets, install smoke detectors, and forgo sky diving? There are lots of potential mechanisms by which whole grains might facilitate weight loss—higher fiber, lower calorie density, lower glycemic response, a slower eating rate due to more chewing[1875]—but you don't know, of course, until you put it to the test.

Separating the Wheat from the Chaff

If you feed people a whole-grain rye porridge for breakfast (like oatmeal, but with rolled rye instead of rolled oats), they report significantly prolonged satiety and lowered hunger and desire to eat for up to eight hours after consumption compared to having eaten the same number of calories of white bread.[1876] Because of the high water content of the porridge, a larger portion had to be given to match the calories in the bread. A fairer test would be to compare foods in the same form, like whole-wheat rolls compared to white-flour rolls, which is exactly what a group of British researchers did. A beneficial effect on blood pressures was noted in the whole-wheat group, but no effect was found for appetite or food intake.[1877] Even in the porridge study, the whole-grain group said they felt fuller, but that didn't translate into them actually eating any less at lunch later on.[1878]

Longer-term studies proved similarly disappointing, both for dropping daily caloric intake[1879] or body weight in children[1880] or adults.[1881] Though there were other benefits noted when people were randomized to add whole grains to their diets, like improved artery function,[1882] decreased inflammation[1883] and blood pressure,[1884] why not weight loss?

The WHOLEheart study was one such trial that randomized hundreds of overweight individuals to either continue their usual diets or be provided with a free variety of whole-grain products like granola bars and other snack foods.[1885] The subjects in the freebie group were instructed to substitute the foods "like for like" with refined-grain foods in their diets, but you can imagine what actually happened. Dietary reports suggested participants ate the free products as additions, rather than substitutions, to their regular diets.[1886] No wonder they didn't lose any weight! Some of the participants apparently also replaced the wrong foods. For example, those who added the most whole grains apparently cut down on their fruit consumption.[1887]

In the Framingham Heart Study, thousands of individuals underwent CT body scanning to determine precisely how much fat they carried in their abdomens. Those who met my minimum of three daily servings recommendation for whole grains harbored about twenty cubic inches less fat around their abdominal organs and an additional twenty cubic inches less superficial belly flab. That's pretty impressive. The researchers' unique insight, though, was that the whole-grain benefit appeared to vanish among those who were also eating four or more daily servings of refined grains.[1888] So it may not be enough to just add whole grains to our diets—we also need to cut the crap.

Compliance is also an issue. Another large study that failed to show a weight-loss advantage to the provision of free whole-grain products sought to understand why by analyzing people's blood. There's a compound in the bran layer of certain whole grains (called alkylresorcinol) that's stripped away when grains are refined. So, by measuring the levels in people's blood, you can get an objective measure of roughly how much whole grain they're eating. After all the time, money, and effort that went into the study, it turns out more than 60 percent of the participants who were ostensibly in the "whole-grain" group had such low blood levels of the compound that it's likely they ate little or none of the whole-grain products that were provided, basically rendering the results meaningless.[1889]

Other studies didn't provide food at all and instead simply instructed people to choose whole-grain products when they shopped. Now that "Made with WHOLE GRAIN" is plastered on the front of Froot Loops cereal boxes and even cheesecake manufacturers are trying to get in on the trend,[1890] it's no wonder such studies may fail to show a benefit. Even in tightly controlled trials, some of the intervention choices were questionable, randomizing people to meat loaf made with whole-wheat bread crumbs versus white bread crumbs,[1891] or snacks made from whole-wheat flakes, sugar, and M&M's versus refined-grain flakes, sugar, and M&M's.[1892] (I couldn't make this stuff up.) What's more, some of the whole-grain doses used were so small they resulted in less than a half-ounce difference in fiber intake—insufficient, perhaps, to show a difference in body weight regulation.[1893]

Grain of Truth

There have been successful whole-grain weight-loss interventions that involved, for example, switching people from white rice to brown rice[1894] or incorporating two packets of oatmeal every day versus a placebo-control hot cereal.[1895] In both cases, waistlines significantly slimmed, suggesting a change in body fat. A Japanese study that measured body composition changes directly with CT scans found a significant decrease in visceral belly fat in those given whole-wheat versus white bread.[1896] Indeed, if you go back and perform a meta-analysis of all the randomized controlled studies, even though an overall weight change didn't materialize, there was a small but significant drop in body fat in the whole-grain groups.[1897] Why?

Two main mechanisms have been suggested to explain the apparent benefit. Substituting whole grains for refined grains in a tightly controlled setting leads to (1) an increase in resting metabolic rate and (2) increased calorie loss through the stool.[1898] The metabolic boost is attributed to the waste heat produced by the fermentation of fiber in the bowel,[1899] and the extra calories flushed are due to the diminished ability of your body to extract energy from a high-fiber diet.[1900] The combined effect may add up to a loss of about ninety calories a day, which almost exactly predicts the weight loss found in the Harvard cohorts over a four-year period.[1901] So whole grains may indeed help with fat loss but only, perhaps, when there's a parallel drop in refined grain junk.

FOOD FOR THOUGHT

To remove refined grains from your diet is to remove America's number one source of calories. Switching to whole grains may help reduce body fat, but there's an even better swap. See the Wall Off Your Calories section for taking your grain game up a notch and graduate from mere whole grains to *intact* whole grains, such as oat groats (also known as *hull-less* or *hulled oats*).

LOW IN SALT

Don't Shake on It

One of the most dramatic changes in our diets has been the skyrocketing intake of salt. For most of human existence, we were only getting the pinch of salt a day naturally found in whole foods.[1902] Now, thanks mostly to processed foods, we're exposed to ten times more than our bodies were meant to handle.[1903] What role might this play in our obesity epidemic?

For nearly forty years, studies have linked salt intake to excess body fat.[1904] A 2017 meta-analysis of more than a dozen such studies found that higher sodium consumption was associated with nearly a two-inch-larger waist.[1905] A subsequent study found an extra pound of body fat for each quarter-teaspoon-higher salt intake a day.[1906] Children with the saltiest diets may have double the odds for abdominal obesity,[1907] but how do we know it's the salt itself? Think of some childhood favorites: pizza, potato chips, mac 'n cheese. They are packed with sodium, but they're also packed with calories. Perhaps the only reason sodium intake is correlated with obesity is because high salt and calories tend to travel together in the same foods.[1908]

Why does the food industry add salt to so many products? It's simple: to make processed food more palatable so you'll eat more of it. Which are you more likely to overeat? Unsalted nuts or salted nuts? Unsalted pretzels or salted pretzels? Salty foods can have an addictive quality. The overlap in pleasure circuitry within the brain between our appetites for salt and the effects of opioids and cocaine has led some to speculate that drug addiction is a hijacking of our inborn salt cravings that kept us alive through the long millennia before the advent of saltshakers.[1909] Now, those same salt cravings are killing us (by contributing to cardiovascular disease[1910] and stomach cancer[1911] risk), but are they also making us fat?

Salt doesn't just make us want to eat more but drink more as well. And what do most Americans over age two drink on a given day? Sugar-sweetened beverages like soda.[1912,1913] Based on studies measuring fluid intake after manipulating the salt content of people's diets, Americans might end up drinking an estimated forty billion fewer soft drinks per year if we cut our sodium intake in half.[1914] That's a lot of calories.

Pinch an Inch

Until recently, that was all we thought was going on: Salt increases body fat by causing us to eat and drink more calories. But now, there is growing evidence that there may be a more direct link between sodium intake and obesity.[1915] Studies controlling for total caloric intake including sweetened beverages *still* found a link between salt intake and body fat or obesity in adults, children, and adolescents,[1916,1917,1918,1919] but these studies are fraught with difficulties.

Salt can make you retain water, which can affect bioimpedance measurements of body composition.[1920] But studies that have used more rigorous measures like x-ray or MRI scanning have also found a link between salt and body fat.[1921] It's also hard to accurately estimate how much salt people are eating without having them carry a jug to collect their urine all day, or how many calories they're consuming without carrying out expensive "doubly labeled" water experiments. But again, even studies that have used these kinds of gold-standard techniques still found a link between salt intake and body fat, independent of how many calories people were eating.[1922] Most of these studies were cross-sectional in nature, only a snapshot in time. When researchers followed hundreds of individuals over time, their salt consumption didn't predict changes in overall body weight in terms of the numbers on a scale, but all the while, body fat appeared to be increasing while their fat-free mass shrank. After controlling for a number of potential confounding factors, those who ate the most salt appeared to shift their body compositions to more fat and less lean tissue.[1923]

Nearly all of these are observational studies and so can't prove cause and effect. Maybe high-salt consumers practice other bad health behaviors like sedentary living. Studies have controlled for physical activity,[1924] but you can't control for everything. The only interventional studies have been performed on rodents. Yes, you can fatten rats just by boosting their salt intakes,[1925] but the opposite effect has been described in mice.[1926] So are we more like rats or mice? Clinical researchers use animals to run tightly controlled experiments, but no matter how good the data, they always end up on the wrong species.

There is one recent human experiment that could provide a mechanism by which salt may contribute to obesity. When people were switched to a low-salt diet, the levels in their blood of the gut hormone ghrelin dropped, and when shifted to a high-salt diet, their ghrelin levels shot up.[1927] Ghrelin, the so-called hunger hormone I discussed in the High in Fiber-Rich Foods section, is the target of attempts by drug companies to create an anti-obesity vaccine,[1928] but we may be able to help block its action naturally by lowering our sodium intake.

Some are so convinced that salt is such a key player in our obesity epidemic they have suggested "partial resection of the nerve branches innervating the lingual mesolimbic receptor system"—in other words, cutting the nerves going to the salt-sensing taste buds of morbidly obese individuals.[1929] The link between salt and weight remains much too speculative for such a drastic approach, but given that sodium consumption is already considered the leading dietary risk factor for death on the planet,[1930] there's reason enough to cut down, and it may just have the happy side benefit of facilitating fat loss—no scalpel needed.

FOOD FOR THOUGHT

A *New England Journal of Medicine* editorial entitled "Compelling Evidence for Public Health Action to Reduce Salt Intake" argued that since about 75 percent of salt exposure comes from manufactured foods, "the individual approach is probably impractical"[1931]—as if the consumption of processed foods is somehow preordained. But we not only have control over how much salt we add at home, we also have control over which foods we buy.

In the very least, we can try to steer away from the worst offenders. For adults over fifty, the number one source of sodium intake is bread. For younger adults, the greatest contribution of sodium to the diet is not canned soups, pretzels, or potato chips but a seemingly unprocessed food—chicken.[1932] Salt is actually injected into the chicken meat, in part to solubilize the muscle proteins to a gel for optimum texture.[1933] The commentary notes that although sodium levels are going down in some sectors of the food industry, the opposite seems to be happening in the meat industry, where "the addition of salt to poultry, meats, and fish appears to be occurring on a massive scale."[1934] Impractical or not, we can shop for low-sodium options, eat out less, and stop adding salt in the kitchen and dining room.[1935]

LOW INSULIN INDEX

The Hormone of Plenty

Insulin can be thought of as the "hormone of calorie prosperity."[1936] After a meal, our blood is awash with calories. The starches we eat are broken down into simple sugars, the proteins into amino acids, and the fats into fatty acids, all of which are absorbed into our bloodstreams. Insulin then goes to work to distribute and store this bounty. It moves the blood sugars into our muscles to fuel our movement, gets our cells to take up the amino acids to build new proteins, and stockpiles circulating fatty acids into our fat stores. Insulin drives fat storage both by directing fat from our bloodstreams into our fat cells and by telling our fat cells to stop burning calories. Insulin is, after all, the signal of abundance.

Should we become obese, fat can spill out from our overbloated fat cells back into our bloodstreams and get lodged in our muscles. When this happens, it can interfere with insulin signaling, causing our muscles to become less responsive to insulin, a phenomenon known as *insulin resistance*. Normally, our muscles take up blood sugar in response to insulin, but if they become resistant to the effects of insulin, the sugar remains in the blood and can build up to dangerous levels. To prevent this, our bodies produce even more insulin to force more blood sugar into our muscles. But all that extra insulin in our system can cause additional fat storage and result in a vicious cycle: obesity leading to insulin resistance, which leads to higher insulin levels that then lead to more obesity and even more insulin resistance.

When insulin resistance gets so bad that our insulin production can no longer keep up and overcome it, our blood sugars start creeping up and we become prediabetic and then progress to full-blown diabetes. Instead of treating the cause—insulin resistance—with lifestyle medicine to try to reverse the diabetes, what do most doctors do? Prescribe even *more* insulin, which can perpetuate the cycle. With injections, insulin levels can be forced so high that even resistant muscles will concede, but what effect will all that extra insulin have on our fat stores? Within the first year of starting insulin, type 2 diabetics typically gain between seven and twenty pounds of "insulin-associated weight gain."[1937]

The Insulin-Obesity Cycle

Obesity can kick-start the vicious cycle leading to the insulin resistance, which leads to elevated insulin levels, which leads to more obesity, as illustrated in the figure below.

You can also become insulin resistant without being obese. The fat that ends up clogging our muscles and causing insulin resistance can come from the fat we wear *or* the fat we eat. Normally, we may have as little as 100 µmol/l of free fat floating around in our bloodstreams at any one time, but

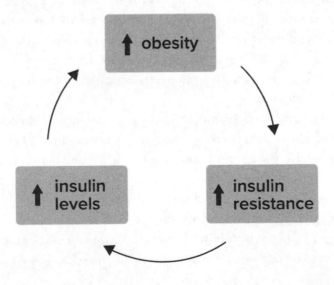

those who are obese may have up to 800 µmol/l. However, skinny people can reach 800 µmol/l just eating a high-fat diet. In other words, a thin person eating a low-carb diet can have the same level of fat in their blood that an obese person does.[1938]

Infuse fat into people's veins through an IV, and, by using a high-tech type of MRI scanner, you can show in real time the buildup of fat in muscle cells within hours, accompanied by an increase in insulin resistance. The same thing happens when you put people on a high-fat diet.[1939] Feed folks even a single high-fat meal, and within six hours, their insulin sensitivity can be cut in half, meaning their insulin resistance shoots up.[1940] Do this day after day, and insulin levels can rise to compensate, which can then lead to weight gain as the vicious cycle starts turning.[1941]

Some people are born with higher-than-normal insulin levels and naturally have a higher propensity to gain weight, suggesting that the cycle can also start with an elevated insulin level, leading to elevated obesity and, subsequently, elevated insulin resistance.[1942]

The causal role of high insulin levels in obesity was established in a study published in 2018 entitled "Reducing Insulin . . . in Adults Reverses Diet-Induced Weight Gain," but the adults they were talking about were adult mice.[1943] You can prove insulin drives obesity by genetically engineering a low-insulin mouse that is essentially immune to obesity, but how can you prove it in people?[1944] The closest we've come is the demonstration that drugs that lower insulin levels do cause weight loss in obese adult humans,[1945,1946] but the drugs also may have direct effects on body fat that could account for the benefit.[1947] So while we don't know for certain, I think there's enough evidence to try to keep our insulin levels within the normal range.[1948]

Break the Cycle by Improving Insulin Sensitivity

One way to lower our insulin levels is to make our insulin work better. The reason our bodies pump out so much insulin is to overcome any resistance, so by improving the insulin sensitivity of our muscles, we can make a little insulin go a long way. How? You can do it with exercise (both endurance and resistance training), weight loss, or reducing your intake of fat—but not necessarily all types of fat.[1949] While the monounsaturated fats concentrated in nuts, olives, and avocados appear more likely to be detoxified or safely stored away, the saturated fats concentrated in meat, dairy, and junk can create the toxic breakdown products in our muscle cells thought responsible for the development of insulin resistance.[1950]

Experimentally shifting people from animal fats to plant fats can improve insulin sensitivity even without changing the overall quantity of fat eaten.[1951] Thinking this may help explain why those eating more plant-based diets have less insulin resistance, researchers at Imperial College London set out to compare the amount of fat clogging the muscle cells of vegans versus omnivores.[1952] So as not to give the vegan group an unfair advantage, the researchers recruited omnivores who were as slim as the vegans. The researchers wanted to know if plant-based eating had a direct benefit beyond simply indirectly pulling fat out of the muscles by helping people lose weight in general. The vegans were found to have significantly less fat trapped in their muscle cells, which can translate into less insulin resistance and lower insulin levels.[1953]

So can switching fats help with weight loss? Amazingly, Australian researchers found that even if you feed people about the same number of calories and the same amount of fat, but switch out meat and butterfat for olive oil, nuts, and avocados, you lose nearly six more pounds of fat in a single month.[1954] You can certainly overdo plant fats, though. On high-fat diets, the type of fat appears to matter less.[1955] Have people drink nearly a half cup of oil, and you can temporarily triple their insulin resistance in a matter of hours.[1956]

Break the Cycle by Lowering Insulin Spikes

In addition to making our insulin work better by improving our sensitivity to it, we can lower our insulin exposure by choosing foods that cause less of an insulin surge. Although those who are born with[1957] or develop higher-than-normal insulin spikes after meals are at elevated risk of weight gain[1958] and obesity,[1959] anyone can get an exaggerated insulin response to Wonder Bread.

High glycemic loads are the primary stimulus for insulin release as our bodies desperately try to sock away blood sugar from the rapidly digested sugars and starches, as I described in the Low Glycemic Load section. Randomized controlled trials clearly show that swapping out refined grains in favor of whole grains reduces insulin spikes[1960] (likely due to the fiber content).[1961] Remember, though, insulin doesn't just deal with carbohydrates after a meal but protein and fat as well.

To their credit, low-carb and paleo diet advocates identify insulin as playing a role in the obesity epidemic, but they often don't appear to recognize the broader scope of insulin triggers. Since carbs increase insulin, the argument goes, we should eat lots of meat, which is just fat and protein with zero carbs. That wouldn't cause an increase in insulin, right? Wrong. We've known for more than a half century that if you feed people a steak, their insulin levels go up.[1962] Pretty much pure protein (like whey powder) and pure fat can have a similar effect.[1963] Have people eat some lentils with butter, and you get a 60 percent higher insulin reaction to pure sugar compared to lentils alone.[1964] That's why we need more than a glycemic index. We need an insulin index. We need to feed people dozens of different foods and just measure what kind of insulin reactions they get. And that's exactly what researchers did.

What do you think causes the biggest insulin reaction: a large apple, an orange, a cup of oatmeal, a cup and a half of white-flour pasta, four Chips Ahoy! chocolate chip cookies, a bunless burger, or a fish fillet?

Is that your final answer?

Well, surprisingly, beef and fish cause more insulin to be released.[1965,1966] In terms of meat, the original study looked only at beef and fish, but subsequent studies found the insulin response to chicken and pork was just as high.[1967] It turns out meat protein causes almost exactly as much insulin release as pure sugar.[1968] So, based on their own logic, low carbers and paleo folks should be reaching for big bowls of pasta rather than meat.

Those eating plant-based diets average significantly lower insulin levels and have less insulin resistance, even compared to nonvegetarians at the same body weight.[1969,1970] In fact, those who eat meat have up to 50 percent higher insulin levels in their bloodstreams.[1971,1972] Might that just be because they're more sedentary or something? Researchers from the University of Memphis decided to put it to the test by placing men and women on a plant-based diet and got significant drops in insulin within just three weeks.[1973] But add some egg whites to the plant-based diet, and you can cause a "dramatic"[1974] rise in insulin output—as much as 60 percent within just four days.[1975]

Fish and poultry may be even worse than the egg whites.[1976] Add about half a can of tuna to some spaghetti, and induce about a 70 percent higher insulin spike in diabetics.[1977] Skinless chicken breast and white rice cause an insulin reaction closer to straight sugar than rice alone.[1978] Compared to chicken, the meat-free tastes-like-chicken Quorn causes up to 41 percent *less* of an insulin reaction within fifteen minutes.[1979]

Low-Carb and Paleo Diets Put to the Test

In a study out of MIT, researchers increased the carbohydrate intake of subjects by up to hundreds of grams a day, yet their insulin levels went down.[1980] How is that possible? The researchers weren't feeding people jelly beans and sugar cookies; they fed them whole plant foods—lots of whole grains, beans, fruits, and vegetables.

What if you instead put someone on a very-low-carb diet like an Atkins diet? Low-carb advocates such as Dr. Eric Westman, author of the *New Atkins Diet* books and the person who took over after the old Dr. Atkins died, assumed doing so would lower insulin levels.[1981] But what they found was that there is no significant drop in insulin levels on very-low-carb diets. Instead, there is a significant rise in bad LDL cholesterol levels[1982] and a significant crippling of artery function,[1983] which helps explain why those eating more low-carb diets tend to live significantly shorter lives.[1984]

Atkins is an easy target, though. No matter how many newer-than-new Atkins diets come out, it's still old news. What about the paleo diet? The paleo movement gets a lot of things right. It tells people to ditch dairy and donuts, eat lots of fruits, nuts, and vegetables, and cut out a lot of processed junk. But a study published in the *International Journal of Exercise Science* has raised concerns.

Researchers took young healthy people and put them on a paleo diet along with a CrossFit-based, high-intensity circuit training exercise program. If you lose enough weight by any means, whether by exercise, stomach stapling, chemotherapy, or a hearty cocaine habit, you can temporarily drop your cholesterol levels no matter what you eat. After ten weeks of hard-core workouts and weight loss on the paleo diet, however, the study participants' LDL cholesterol *still* went up—and it was even worse for those who started out the healthiest. Those who started the study with optimal levels (under 70) had a 20 percent elevation in this leading risk factor for heart disease, our number one killer.[1985] The researchers concluded that "the Paleo diet's deleterious impact on blood lipids [fats] was not only significant, but substantial enough to counteract the . . . improvements commonly seen with improved fitness and body composition."

Exercise is supposed to make things better.

On the other hand, put people on a plant-based diet and a modest, mostly walking-based exercise program, and within three weeks, their bad cholesterol can drop 20 percent and their insulin levels can plummet 30 percent, despite a 75–80 percent carbohydrate diet.[1986] In contrast, the paleo diet appeared to have "negated the positive effects of exercise."[1987]

Animal Protein vs. Plant Protein

What about plant proteins? Although isolated soy protein causes an insulin surge similar to meat, dairy, and eggs, comparing foods to foods,[1988] adding fish or egg whites to rice amplifies the insulin reaction, but adding tofu does not.[1989] Similarly, a whole soy food significantly lowers insulin levels, but soy protein supplements do not.[1990]

Add tuna to mashed potatoes, and the insulin reaction is about 50 percent higher than eating the mashed potatoes alone.[1991] Adding broccoli instead, however, results in the insulin response being cut about 40 percent within the first thirty minutes.[1992] This didn't appear to be a fiber effect, since giving the equivalent amount of isolated broccoli fiber provided no significant benefit. The differential effect of plant versus animal protein has been attributed to their contrasting amino acid profiles.[1993]

Plant proteins tend to be lower in the branched-chain amino acids (BCAAs) and the sulfur-containing amino acid methionine, which both have been associated with insulin resistance.[1994] To date, most of the research on restricting methionine intake has been about preventing cancer growth and slowing aging,[1995] but more recently, it has been presented as a "useful nutritional strategy" to combat insulin resistance.[1996] Sticking to plant-based sources of protein would cut methionine intake about in half, resulting in significantly lower blood levels.[1997] As such, following purely plant-based diets has been put forth as a feasible "life extension strategy,"[1998] but there are myriad reasons why plant-based diets have been shown to improve insulin resistance.[1999] You can't prove methionine is playing a specific role until you isolate it out. To date, the trials demonstrating better insulin sensitivity on diets that just specifically restrict methionine have all been done on rodents,[2000] but that's not the case for branched-chain amino acids.

What Are Amino Acids?

Amino acids are the building blocks of proteins. There are about twenty different kinds,[2001] similar to the number of letters in the alphabet. Just as different sentences can be made from different combinations of letters, different proteins are made from stringing together different sequences of the various amino acids. Three of the amino acids—leucine, isoleucine, and valine—have fatty side-chains that branch off from their central structure and are thereby referred to as *branched-chain amino acids*.

Branch Out Your Proteins

When researchers analyzed differences in the blood among people with different insulin levels,[2002] in addition to finding the saturated fat connection, they uncovered that the levels of branched-chain amino acids in the blood were correlated with insulin resistance.[2003] A number of potential mechanisms were identified, from toxic metabolites[2004] to the stimulation of a fat-generating enzyme complex.[2005] Since that initial publication, an "overwhelming" number of studies[2006] have consistently shown that blood and urine levels of branched-chain amino acids are tied to insulin resistance. This doesn't necessarily mean that decreasing intake of BCAAs will help, though, since there are other factors that influence BCAA levels in the blood.[2007]

Short-term dietary tweaks like swapping out meat lasagna for vegan lasagna can lower levels a bit,[2008] but even those sticking entirely to plant proteins only have about 5 percent lower BCAA levels in their bloodstreams.[2009] Is that enough to make a difference? Well, meat consumption is associated with increased insulin levels,[2010] weight gain,[2011] and higher diabetes risk,[2012] and substituting in even just 5 percent of plant protein for animal protein may decrease diabetes risk by 23 percent.[2013] These data circumstantially support the contention that insulin resistance could help explain the meat-obesity connection,[2014] but you don't know if amino acids are playing a starring role until you run the experiment and put it to the test.

Indeed, just like you can make someone insulin resistant by infusing fat into their bloodstreams, you can do the same thing by infusing amino acids.[2015] Down a protein drink of just straight whey and water, and it can cause insulin resistance within hours.[2016] Give some vegans BCAAs, and you can make them as insulin resistant as omnivores.[2017] Or you can do it the other way: Take some omnivores and put them through even just a "48-hour vegan diet challenge," and you can produce significant improvements in metabolic health. After two days on a healthy plant-based diet, not only did cholesterol and triglycerides drop but so did insulin and insulin resistance, presumed to be due in part to the "strong modulatory effect" on circulating BCAA levels. Because the benefits appeared so rapidly, the researchers suggested metabolic benefits could be gotten from an "intermittent vegan diet" or even the "flexitarian approach" of alternating between animal and plant protein choices.[2018]

In that case, does protein manipulation then translate to weight loss? To see if lowering amino acids would improve insulin resistance—and, ultimately, accelerate weight loss—researchers put a group of overweight men on a "protein-restricted diet," which is to say a *normal* protein diet. The recommended dietary allowance for protein is about 50 grams a day (46 for women, 56 for men).[2019] The researchers took men who were averaging twice that—112 grams, which is about the average of what many American men get[2020]—and randomized them down to 64 grams of protein a day. They were still getting more protein than they needed.

The levels of branched-chain amino acids circulating in the lower-protein group dropped as suspected, but did they lose weight? Both diets were designed to have the same number of calories, so six weeks later, both groups should weigh the same, right? The body weight and fat mass of the regular protein group didn't change, but the lower protein group lost about six pounds.[2021] BCAAs may explain why those randomized to a plant-based diet eliminate significantly more of the deeper, more dangerous fat, even when taking in the *same* number of calories.[2022]

FOOD FOR THOUGHT

Given the metabolic harms of excess BCAA exposure, leaders in the field have suggested the invention of drugs to block BCAA absorption, which "may represent a translatable and sustainable approach to promote metabolic health and treat diabetes and obesity without reducing caloric intake."[2023] Or we can just not eat so many branched-chain amino acids in the first place. BCAAs are found mostly in meat, including chicken and fish, dairy products, and eggs.[2024] This is one postulated explanation of why animal protein has been associated with higher diabetes risk, whereas plant protein appears protective.[2025]

Figuring out the "appropriate upper limits" of animal protein intake "may offer a great chance for the prevention of T2D [type 2 diabetes] and obesity,"[2026] but it need not be all or nothing. Cutting down on dairy consumption may not be enough,[2027] but even "intermittently substituting vegan meals in otherwise animal-based diets" may be beneficial in this regard.[2028]

From an insulin standpoint, the worst of both worlds would presumably be the combination of animal protein and a high glycemic load—think burger on a bun, meat and potatoes, or a deli meat sandwich. The joint induction of insulin resistance and spiking blood sugars is a bad combo.[2029]

The advice to avoid eating animal protein and refined carbs together was one of the tenets of the "food combining" dogma popularized in books like *Fit for Life*. Though the rationale given at the time was "frankly laughable"[2030] from a scientific standpoint, they may have stumbled onto something. When people were randomized to a "low-insulin-response" diet that included advice to separate out the consumption of foods rich in carbohydrate or protein at different meals, their insulin levels dropped and they lost an extra six pounds over twelve weeks compared to people on a diet designed with the same number of calories but no special insulin-reducing aspects.[2031]

Thankfully, the combo effect doesn't appear to extend to legumes. Despite being rich in protein and starch, the insulin index of legumes, such as beans, split peas, chickpeas, and lentils, appears to parallel their very low glycemic index.[2032] So to reduce insulin levels to potentially facilitate weight loss: Rule #1: Avoid high-glycemic foods; Rule #2: Make plant protein your preference; and Rule #3: When you do eat animal protein, try to pay particular attention to Rule #1.

MICROBIOME-FRIENDLY

Tenant Building

Surrounded on all sides by fattening temptations, our obesogenic—obesity-generating—environment is hard to escape,[2033] though some people do manage to navigate their svelte selves through. If the epidemic were purely due to external factors, wouldn't everyone be obese? Some individuals seem to be more susceptible than others, which suggests a genetic component. Partial heritability is supported by studies of twins and adopted kids, but the genes we've identified only account for a small amount of the variation in body size between individuals.[2034] Might a role be played by the variation in our "other genome"? That is, the DNA contained in all the different microbes that inhabit our bodies? We have one hundred times more bacterial genes inside us than human genes.[2035]

We have trillions of bacteria living inside each of us. One professor emeritus went as far as to say, *"Nous sommes toutes les bacteries,"* which translates to "We are all bacteria,"[2036] a provocative way of acknowledging there are more bacterial cells and genes in our own bodies than there are human cells and genes. And most of those bacteria live in our gut.

The colon used to be viewed as merely a retention tank for waste and that water absorption was its big biological function.[2037] Our ignorance arose from "difficult access to the large intestine"[2038] and the fact that we weren't able to culture most of the gut flora outside of the body. About three-quarters of gut microbes fail to grow under standard laboratory conditions,[2039] and so remained the "dark matter" of fecal matter.

How do you study something you can't study?

Today, we have advanced DNA fingerprinting techniques to unravel the mystery. The first time scientists attempted to sequence all the genes of a bacterium, it took thirteen years.[2040] These days, the same feat might take only a few hours.[2041] With all this new knowledge, what we learned is that each one of us can be thought of as a superorganism, a kind of human-microbe hybrid.[2042]

The human colon has been considered the most biodense ecosystem in the world, meaning there's more life concentrated in our colons than anywhere else on Earth.[2043] Many probably think that stool is composed primarily of undigested food, but most of it—about 75 percent—is pure bacteria.[2044] Trillions and trillions of them—about half a trillion per teaspoon, in fact.[2045] We are bacteria factories. As Neil deGrasse Tyson put it, "More bacteria live and work in one linear centimeter of your lower colon than all the humans who have ever lived."[2046]

What's in it for us? What do we get for housing these trillions of tenants? Rent is paid in the form of boosting our immune systems, balancing our hormones, improving digestion, and making vitamins for us. We feed them, and they feed us right back. Our gut bacteria have been referred to as a "forgotten organ."[2047] They weigh as much as one of our kidneys and are as metabolically active as our livers.[2048] They may have control over as many as one in ten metabolites measured in the bloodstream.[2049] We have about twenty-three thousand genes,[2050] but, collectively, our gut bacteria have about three *million* genes. Our gut flora don't just constitute any organ but perhaps the "main organ" involved in the cause of obesity.[2051]

A Bitter Pill

How do we know gut bacteria have anything to do with gaining weight? More than seventy years ago, we learned that low doses of antibiotics fattened farm animals,[2052] but, when penicillin is fed to "bubble boy" chicks hatched without any gut bacteria into a sterile environment, the antibiotics have no effect on their weights.[2053] That was how it was first discovered microbes could affect body weight.

According to the FDA, animal agriculture now feeds about thirty million pounds of antibiotics to livestock every year,[2054] four times the amount sold to treat human infections.[2055] This has raised concerns about the fostering of antibiotic resistance,[2056] but if these drugs can cause weight gain in farm animals, might exposure to antibiotic residues left in meat contribute to the human obesity epidemic? Public health scientists have raised this as a theoretical possibility,[2057] especially given the rise in fish farming.[2058] It can take as much as a half pound of antibiotics to produce just one pound of salmon,[2059] for example, which helps explain why the researchers found most of the samples from common seafood in the United States tested positive for trace amounts of antibiotics.[2060] The dose consumed would be minuscule compared to that which doctors too often overprescribe, though.

The average American child may receive three courses of antibiotics by age two, about ten courses by the age of ten, and around seventeen antibiotics courses by age twenty. This is more than twice that of countries like Sweden, suggesting much of the prescribed antibiotic use in the United States is unnecessary.[2061] The American Academy of Pediatrics estimates that as many as ten million antibiotic prescriptions are given out unnecessarily every year.[2062] Undoubtedly, antibiotics can be lifesaving wonder drugs, but they should be used judiciously—not only to prevent the development of resistant strains but because even a common seven-day regimen can alter your gut flora for years.[2063] What role might this be playing in the obesity epidemic?

A compilation of more than a dozen studies involving about a half million children found that exposure to antibiotics during infancy was associated with an increased risk of becoming overweight during childhood.[2064] And the greater the exposure, the greater the risk.[2065] Each additional course of antibiotics in early life was found to be associated with a 7 percent increased risk of our kids becoming overweight.[2066] How do we know it's cause and effect, though? Maybe parents who overfeed their kids are more likely to pester doctors for prescriptions?[2067]

Studies have shown that, compared to control subjects, those treated with antibiotics gain more weight—and in some cases, much more weight, like an average of nine pounds over a control group.[2068] The controls didn't need antibiotics, though, because they weren't sick. Perhaps simply having an infection may lead to weight gain,[2069] or even having an infection cleared up. For example, a group of patients with a stomach infection called *Helicobacter pylori* were randomized to either antibiotics or placebo. The antibiotic group gained more weight, but maybe it was due to their appetites being restored because their infections were cleared.[2070] How can we know for certain?

To truly put it to the test, you'd have to randomize healthy people to either antibiotics or sugar pills. Just such a study was published on U.S. Navy recruits in 1955.[2071] Those on the antibiotics gained about a pound a month more than the placebo group, suggesting that our gut flora do indeed play a role in controlling our weight.

Eating for Trillions

When antibiotics are necessary, doctors can try to limit their collateral damage by using a more laser-like approach in their prescribing, rather than carpet-bombing germs with broad-spectrum antibiotics. There's even been a proposal to "bank every healthy child's fecal specimen" so we can chase each antibiotic course with a dose of their pretreatment microbes.[2072] Another controversial suggestion involves how to best start our children's gut flora out on the right foot.

Most of the microbes populating our colons first originate from our mothers' vaginal flora, which we acquire during birth. What about those born via cesarean section? Instead of getting their mothers' vaginal flora, infants born by cesarean delivery start out with microbiomes more closely representing that of the operating room.[2073] This may help explain why children born by C-section have a 33 percent greater risk of childhood obesity.[2074] With so much at stake, "vaginal seeding" has been proposed, in which maternal vaginal fluids are transferred into the mouths of cesarean babies. The American College of Obstetricians and Gynecologists opposes the practice for fear of transmitting any STDs,[2075] but a study in which women were first screened for such infections found that vaginal seeding was successful in establishing a more natural gut flora in their infants.[2076]

Breast milk naturally contains special compounds that can nourish the infant's microbiome, which may help explain why breastfed infants are less likely to become obese as children.[2077] This benefit appears to be limited to those who didn't receive antibiotics during the breastfeeding period, however, underscoring the importance of our gut flora for weight control.[2078] Breast is best, but after weaning, what should we eat, and what should we avoid to promote a healthy, slimming microbiome?

They Are What We Eat

Every food choice we make may affect the growth of trillions of bacteria.

I've already explored some of the effects of what we feed our flora, from the benefits of the short-chain fatty acids produced when we feed them fiber to the risks from the TMAO when we feed them meat or eggs. What we eat affects not only what our gut microbes make but also which microbes exist. Remember the steak-munching vegan from page 204? Just as they didn't harbor the bad bugs that make TMAO, those who've been living off cheeseburgers and milkshakes their whole lives may take months to realize the full potential of increased fiber consumption as they slowly build up the communities of fiber-eating organisms.[2079]

No known single microbial signature exists for obesity,[2080] but when the microbiomes of obese and nonobese individuals are compared, there are some specific bugs associated with more, or less, weight gain over time. One influential study found eight species of bacteria that appeared protective against weight gain, and they all ate fiber.[2081]

There's a hormone called *FIAF,* which stands for *fasting-induced adipose factor.* When you fast, your body stops storing fat and instead starts burning it off. FIAF is one of the hormones that signal our bodies to make this switch. This may be one way our gut flora manage our weight. Some bacteria repress this hormone, thereby increasing the tendency to store fat, whereas the short-chain fatty acids made by our fiber-eating bacteria can boost FIAF production.[2082]

Eating fiber-rich foods has the double benefit of directly resulting in the formation of short-chain fatty acids and selectively cultivating the bugs that make it. Ounce for ounce, the colon contents of those eating more plant-based diets have nearly three times the capacity to form short-chain fatty acids.[2083] In this way, eating healthfully not only provides more raw materials for short-chain fatty acid production but improved microbial machinery to churn out more of it. In contrast, putting people on a low-carb diet can slash short-chain fatty acid production by up to 75 percent.[2084]

Another way your gut flora can differentially affect your weight is through enhanced or reduced energy harvest. Some types of bacteria are better than others at extracting calories from our gut contents. Feed a group of people the exact same 2,400 calories, and based on the calorie content of their stools, some retain 2,350 of those calories, while others may only hold on to about 2,200.[2085] Calories that end up in the toilet are calories that can't end up on our hips.

Certain obesity-related bacteria in your colon can take your waste, break it down even further, and release calories that are then absorbed back into your bloodstream. Just when your body is trying to get rid of all your waste, the calories can come bouncing right back. Take, for example, a grouping of bacteria called *Firmicutes.* A 20 percent relative increase in *Firmicutes* was associated with an increase of about 150 calories in daily calorie absorption, whereas a 20 percent increase in a different grouping of bacteria was associated with a *decrease* of about 150 daily calories.[2086] This may help explain some of the edge those eating more plant-based diets have for weight control, as DNA fingerprinting of vegetarian feces has found significantly more of the lean-type bacteria.[2087]

Change Your Diet, Change Your Microbiome

More than two thousand species of bacteria have been characterized in the human gut, yet each of us tends to have a unique collection.[2088] Remarkably, however, all of humanity appears to cluster toward one of two broad categories called *enterotypes*.[2089] Enterotypes are not like blood types, which put us distinctly into specific immutable categories.[2090] Instead, our gut flora exist in more of a continuous gradient with tendencies to drift one way or another. And when it comes to our gut flora, there are apparently two types of people in the world: those who grow mostly *Bacteroides* species and those who grow mostly *Prevotella*.

It's pretty amazing that despite so many different types of gut bacteria, people tend to settle into just one of two groups. Researchers figure our guts are like ecosystems.[2091] There are a lot of different species of animals on the planet, for example, but they aren't randomly distributed. You don't find dolphins in the desert. In the desert, you find desert species, and in the jungle, you find jungle species, because each ecosystem has different selective pressures like rainfall or temperature. The enterotype data suggest there are two types of colon ecosystems, so you can split humanity into people whose guts grow a lot of *Bacteroides*-type bacteria and those whose guts are better homes for *Prevotella* species.

Your enterotype doesn't seem to depend on where you live, whether you are male or female, or how old you are. What matters is what you eat. Researchers looked at more than one hundred different food factors, and it turns out *Bacteroides* and *Prevotella* are kind of opposites. *Bacteroides'* prevalence is correlated to the consumption of components found in animal foods, such as animal fat, cholesterol, and animal protein, whereas *Prevotella* are linked to constituents found almost exclusively in plant foods.[2092] *Prevotella* are fiber-feeders and pump out more short-chain fatty acids.[2093]

Native Africans who eat largely plant-based diets tend to have a *Prevotella* enterotype, while African Americans eating a typical Western diet tend to be in the *Bacteroides* camp. This may help explain why African Americans have fifty times more colon cancer, since short-chain fatty acids don't just protect against obesity but have anticancer properties as well.[2094] The question then becomes: *How long does it take to shift your gut flora from one enterotype to the other?*

Researchers started giving Africans an American-style diet and African

Americans a much more plant-based, African-style diet. Perhaps skeptical that Americans would actually eat real food, the researchers made exchanges like swapping out hot dogs in favor of veggie dogs rather than feeding them more typical African fare (such as phutu, a grain-based porridge).[2095] Still, within only two weeks, remarkable mirror-image changes were found in the gut flora in the respective groups, with the colonic health of the Africans taking a dive and that of the Americans significantly improving.[2096]

What's the absolute fastest you can change your microbiome? Researchers came up with diets from both extremes to find out: a plant-based diet rich in grains, beans, fruits, and vegetables, and an "animal-based" diet composed of meats, eggs, and cheeses. Within twenty-four hours of switching between the two diets, there was a substantial shift. So, to answer the question: basically as soon as food hits our colons. What happened, for example, to the lifelong vegetarian who got placed on the animal-based diet? Predictably, he started out *Prevotella,* but within days, his *Prevotella*-to-*Bacteroides* ratio completely flipped. His entire gut flora got turned on its head.[2097]

The fact that our gut can so rapidly switch between herbivorous and carnivorous functional profiles presumably has evolutionary benefits. If you take down a mammoth and eat meat for a couple of days before reverting to plants, you want your gut to be able to adjust. This flexibility is manifest in the diversity of human diets to this day, but what's the healthier state to be in most of the time? On the plant-based diet, the subjects' guts yielded more protective short-chain fatty acids, fewer carcinogens, and less of the rotten-egg gas hydrogen sulfide. Hydrogen sulfide is made by pathogens such as *Bilophila wadsworthia,* which increased on the animal-based diet. That stinks because . . . well . . . it stinks and because hydrogen sulfide can damage DNA.[2098] (The only pathogens found more of on the plant-based diet were plant viruses such as those that attack spinach.[2099])

The benefits of plant-based eating need not be all or nothing, though. Those highly adherent to a Mediterranean diet filled with fruits, vegetables, and beans, while averaging no meat (including fish), eggs,[2100] or dairy on a day-to-day basis, had comparable short-chain fatty acid levels to vegans, even though the Mediterranean diet adherents weren't completely plant-based all the time.

Garden Variety

Having a greater diversity of gut flora, a greater "bacterial richness," is also associated with less body fat[2101] and less weight gain over time.[2102] The richest microbiomes ever recorded were those of the Yanomami tribe in the Amazon jungle who had no previous contact with the modern world.[2103] Traditional societies tend to have more diverse gut flora in general, and the key is thought to be their extraordinary fiber intakes, which can reach 120 grams a day,[2104] nearly eight times the American average.[2105]

Our modern, low-fiber diet is considered a "key reason of microbiome depletion."[2106] Pregnant women who eat more fiber have heightened microbial richness, which may have long-term effects on the future health of the next generation.[2107] We're slowly losing more and more of our microbes with every generation, placing some of our good bacteria at risk for extinction.[2108] It may be a case of *use it or lose it*. "You just might consider choosing a salad at lunch today or an extra serving of beans at dinner," one microbiologist commented. "Future generations may thank you, too."[2109]

Can't you just take a fiber supplement? Unfortunately, they don't seem to work in terms of improving richness of the microbiome,[2110] whereas whole foods can. Feed folks whole-grain barley, brown rice, or both for a month, and microbiome diversity improves.[2111] Interestingly, the combination of equal portions of barley and brown rice resulted in metabolic benefits superior to the benefits from either grain alone, suggesting a synergistic effect. This may help explain the discrepancy between the apparent benefits of whole grains found in population-based studies, versus the disappointing results found in many interventional studies— namely, the failure to produce weight loss.[2112] Perhaps simply switching to whole-wheat rolls from white bread may be insufficient to diversify the gut.[2113]

Food Additives That May Make Your Gut Leak

Our skin keeps the outside world outside, and so does the lining of our gut. Should our intestinal barrier break down, bacteria can slip into our bloodstreams and trigger inflammation. This may not only spark inflammatory bowel diseases[2114] but also, potentially, obesity.[2115] How can we keep our gut from getting leaky?

Fiber appears to play a vital role in maintaining our gut barrier,[2116] but how? We have specialized cells lining our gut that secrete a mucus layer that forms our first line of barrier defense. When we starve our microbial selves by eating a fiber-depleted diet, our famished flora may turn to munching our mucus as an alternative fuel source and thereby undermine our defenses.[2117] Researchers were able to re-create layers of human intestinal cells in a lab and showed that E. coli bacteria could be prevented from breaching the barrier by dripping fiber onto the cells at dietary doses. (They used plantains and broccoli.)

The researchers also made a second discovery. Bacterial invasion was facilitated by the food additive polysorbate 80,[2118] an emulsifier commonly found in such processed foods as ice cream, whipped toppings, and cottage cheese.[2119] Food additives like polysorbate 80 and carboxymethylcellulose (a thickener sometimes found in foods such as ice cream, salad dressing, and sauces) have in fact been shown to cause weight gain in mice, but they've never been tested directly in people.[2120] Until they've been proven to be safe, you may want to scrutinize ingredient labels, as well as make sure to rinse your dishes. Traces of dishwashing detergent could have similar adverse effects. Apparently, some people wash dishes and then just leave them to dry without rinsing them, which some gastroenterology researchers have suggested is probably not a good idea.[2121]

Eat Lots of Big MACs

If our microbiome is to be considered a separate organ in our body, it's an organ that runs on MAC, or microbiota-accessible carbohydrates. *MAC* is another name for *prebiotics,* primarily the fiber and resistant starch that fuel our gut flora, and is one reason why you can get an increase of nearly two grams of stool for every one gram of fiber: You're boosting bacterial growth.[2122] When we eat a whole plant food like fruit, we're telling our gut flora to be fruitful and multiply.

If you don't eat healthfully enough, you can actually starve your microbial self.[2123] It's like when astronauts return from spaceflights missing most of their good bacteria because they had limited access to real food. Too many of us may be leading astronaut-like lifestyles here on Earth by not getting enough fresh fruits and vegetables. Astronauts have been documented losing nearly 100 percent of their *Lactobacillus plantarum*,[2124] a particularly strong fiber-feeder, but most Americans don't have any to begin with. Common in probiotic preparations, these bacteria were found to be missing from the guts of 76 percent of those eating a Standard American Diet. Close to two-thirds of those eating plant-based diets, however, house this friendly flora.[2125]

What we eat today can affect our microbiomes tomorrow. Stool and saliva samples were collected from study subjects for an entire year while hundreds of diet and lifestyle factors were tracked daily. Flossing was found to benefit the microbiome in their mouths, and fiber was found to benefit the microbiome in the gut within a single day.[2126] But do those benefits translate into weight loss?

Most prebiotic intervention studies to date show improvements in satiety[2127] and a reduction in body fat,[2128] including among overweight children[2129] and adolescents.[2130] Some used prebiotic powders versus matched placebos, and others tried exchanging different foods. For example, swap out meat for the same number of calories of whole grains, and people lose more weight. The noted increase in microbial diversity may be one of the factors contributing to the extra weight loss.[2131]

The Three Ps

The Three Ps for gut health restoration are *prebiotics, polyphenols,* and *probiotics.*[2132] Polyphenols are a class of phytonutrients (health-promoting plant compounds) that have long been investigated as potential candidates to explain some of the benefits of better diets against disease.[2133] Polyphenols are produced by plants to protect themselves,[2134] and we may be able to expropriate and commandeer them for the same purpose.[2135]

Plants live the ultimate sedentary lifestyle. Because they can't move, they've had to evolve a whole other way to respond to threats, and they do so biochemically. They manufacture—from scratch—a dizzying array of compounds to deal with whatever's coming their way.[2136] For example, if we get too hot, we can move into the shade. But if plants get too hot, they're stuck—they *are* the shade!

Plants have had nearly a billion years to create a whole chemistry set of protective substances, some of which can play a similar role in us. When plants get infected, they produce aspirin, which can come in handy when we get infected ourselves. Plants heal wounds, and so do we, using similar signaling systems.[2137] Plants have DNA they need to protect from free radical damage, so they cook up complex antioxidants that we can use for ourselves instead of reinventing the wheel. In a sense, the crispers in our fridges are like nature's medicine cabinet.

Naysayers of the power of polyphenols often point to studies showing their low bioavailability. For example, up to 85 percent of the polyphenol pigments that make blueberries blue don't even get absorbed and end up getting dumped into our colons.[2138]

But that may be exactly where some of the magic happens.

Mix those blueberry polyphenols[2139] with a culture of fecal bacteria, and out pops the growth of beneficial bugs like *Bifidobacteria* and *Lactobacillus*.[2140] Just as plants establish symbiotic relationships with bacteria living inside them (like the nitrogen-fixing bacteria in the roots of legumes that provide built-in fertilizer), they may be able to get along with our gut flora too.

Protein, carbs, and fat are *macronutrients* because we eat them by the gram each day, whereas vitamins and minerals are *micronutrients,* as we may only get thousandths or even millionths of a gram a day. (A gram is about the weight of a raisin.) Even those eating pitifully few plants may take in as much as a full gram of polyphenols a day, though.[2141] What effect might they have on our gut bacteria and body weight?

Boosting *Bifidobacteria*

Given the complexity of the human microbiome and our poor state of knowledge, researchers often restrict their focus to the effects of foods on a few familiar species that serve as a proxy for the overall balance of benefit. The bifidogenic effects of foods, for example, may be a good starting point.[2142] *Bifidogenic* refers to foods that foster the growth of *Bifidobacteria,* generally recognized as beneficial bugs. Several studies have reported a relative depletion of *Bifidobacteria* correlating with the development of obesity[2143] in both children and adults,[2144] and as such, they are commonly found in commercial probiotics.

Certain *prebiotics* like inulin, concentrated in such vegetables as garlic and onions, can have a "huge" bifidogenic effect.[2145] Ironically, inulin is a type of FODMAP, or fermentable oligo-, di-, and monosaccharides and polyols, which are actively avoided by some people with irritable bowel syndrome. Those placed on FODMAP-restricted diets do seem to end up with depleted levels of *Bifidobacteria,* so, in theory, such diets could actually be counterproductive for long-term gut health.[2146]

Polyphenols can boost *Bifidobacteria* growth in a test tube within a matter of hours, but can those results be replicated in the real world with polyphenol-rich foods?[2147] Randomize people to about a cup of wild blueberries,[2148] and you can get a significant bump in *Bifidobacteria* in their stools,[2149] but how do you know it was due to the polyphenols and not just the fiber? Well, apples boost *Bifidobacteria,* too,[2150] but the isolated apple fiber pectin alone does not.[2151] Bananas have a similar fiber content to berries, but fewer polyphenols. Does eating bananas significantly boost *Bifidobacteria?* No,[2152] which again suggests polyphenols may be playing a special role.

Polyphenol-rich beverages probably provide the best proof. Tea leaves and coffee beans have lots of polyphenols that end up in the brew, leaving behind the fiber. Both green tea[2153] and coffee[2154] are bifidogenic. For example, three cups of coffee a day can significantly raise *Bifidobacteria* levels in the gut within three weeks.[2155] Adding milk, though, may block some of the benefits. Proteins from dairy, as well as eggs, bind to the polyphenols in coffee.[2156] Soy protein does, too, but unlike milk proteins, your gut flora apparently can strip away the polyphenols from the plant protein in the gut to release them.[2157]

So does eating polyphenol-rich foods lead to weight loss? The Harvard studies, following more than one hundred thousand professional men and women, and their diets, for decades, found that those who choose high-polyphenol fruits and vegetables, such as apples, pears, berries, and peppers, gained significantly less weight. This association appeared to be independent of other diet and lifestyle factors, such as total daily fiber intake.[2158] Polyphenols could be another reason to help explain why people randomized to eat three apples or pears a day lose more weight.[2159]

Do Probiotic Supplements Work?

If *Bifidobacteria* are so good, why not just take them in a probiotic pill? Probiotic supplements have been shown to be effective in randomized placebo-controlled trials for conditions such as antibiotic-associated diarrhea,[2160] but what about weight loss? Can't hurt, right? Well, a study published out of the Netherlands has raised concerns about probiotic safety.[2161]

Acute pancreatitis is on the rise and can become life-threatening in some cases. This sudden inflammation of the pancreas allows bacteria to break through our gut walls and infect our internal organs.[2162] Antibiotics don't seem to prevent this complication, but how about probiotics? They seem to work on rats. If you cause inflammation by mechanically damaging the pancreas, not only may probiotics show "strong evidence for efficacy," but there were "no indications [of] harmful effects."[2163] But that was with rats—what about us? Clinical researchers decided to put it to the test.

Half of a group of pancreatitis patients were given probiotic pills, while the other half got sugar pills. Within ten days, the mortality rates in the probiotics group shot *up* compared to placebo. More than twice as many people died on the probiotics. Thus, the researchers concluded, probiotics "can no longer be considered to be harmless." The researchers were criticized for not cautioning patients about the risk before they signed up for the study.[2164] (The study subjects were told probiotics had what the researchers described as "a long history of [safe] use" with no known side effects.[2165]) In response to the criticisms, the researchers replied that there were no known side effects—*until* their study.[2166]

Risks for healthy individuals are likely to be rare,[2167] but probiotics still may not work as intended. Animal agribusiness doesn't only fatten farm animals with antibiotics but probiotics as well.[2168] A compilation of studies found that human probiotics like *Lactobacillus acidophilus,* for example, commonly found in fermented dairy products, may cause significant weight gain[2169] in piglets[2170] and persons.[2171]

What about probiotics in general? Probiotic supplements are a multibillion-dollar industry, which raises concerns about conflicts of interest and "publication bias" in the scientific literature.[2172] We know that Big Pharma is infamous for this; industry-funded studies that yield negative results are quietly shelved and buried, so all your doctors get to read are the glowing reports. In making evidence-based decisions for our patients, the peer-reviewed medical literature is the gold standard, but all too often, those with the gold make the standards.[2173]

An investigation into bias in the probiotics literature uncovered that conflicts of interest were commonly not reported, even when the authors were sponsored directly by a yogurt company, for example, and as many as twenty unflattering studies appear to have been hidden from public view.[2174]

Still, put all the studies on treating obesity with probiotics together, and overall, a small loss in body weight was found—though there was no significant loss of body *fat,* which is what we really care about when it comes to weight loss.[2175] That small loss in body weight was on average, though, and there are endless variations of probiotic bacterial combinations and dosing, so it's difficult to make sweeping generalizations. However, even some of the most successful trials appear to show only modest benefit, such as a two-pound weight loss over a three-month period.[2176]

Probiotics Bearing Fruit

Is it better to get probiotics the way nature intended? If you've ever made sauerkraut at home, you know you don't have to add starter bacteria to get the cabbage to ferment. Why? Because the cabbage leaves acquire lactic acid–producing bacteria while growing out in the fields. This suggests raw fruits and vegetables may not only be a source of prebiotics—that is, fiber—but also a source of probiotics.[2177] Some may even help us reap the rewards. There are bacteria on cruciferous vegetables, for example, that express that magical enzyme myrosinase I talked about in *How Not to Die.* So by eating broccoli-family vegetables, for instance, you may be lining your gut with the very microbes necessary to maximize their benefits.[2178]

While working on characterizing these bacterial communities on plants, researchers found that populations on each produce type were significantly distinct from one another. The tree fruits harbored different bacteria from vegetables on the ground, for example, and grapes and mushrooms seemed to be off in their own little worlds. So if indeed these bugs turn out to be good for us, that discovery would underscore the importance of eating not just a greater quantity but also a greater variety of fruits and vegetables every day. The researchers also found that there were significant differences in the microbiomes of conventional versus organic produce, though we don't yet know enough about these bugs to understand any potential health implications.[2179]

Note that it's still important to wash and scrub your fruits and veggies under running water to cut down on food-poisoning bacteria. Don't worry, you're not going to eliminate all the potentially good microbes, since many actually live inside the plant tissues and couldn't be washed off even if you tried.[2180] Because microbes and fresh produce are inseparable, cancer centers used to put patients undergoing chemotherapy on *neutropenic* diets devoid of uncooked fruits and vegetables for fear of foodborne infections in their immunocompromised states. When actually put to the test, though, none of the randomized controlled trials showed a benefit to restricting fresh produce,[2181] and one study even found evidence of a *higher* rate of infections.[2182] The researchers speculated that the produce was protective because the friendly flora from fruits and vegetables may have successfully crowded out any bad bugs in the gut.

The Tao of Poo

Given our limited understanding of which bugs are best, combined with the lack of regulatory oversight and quality control in the supplement industry,[2183] wouldn't it make more sense to reestablish good gut flora with actual gut flora? If our microbiome is an organ, what about an organ transplant?

During World War II, soldiers in Africa were recommended by Bedouins to treat dysentery with "consumption of fresh, warm camel feces," but wouldn't healthy human dung work better?[2184] Remarkably, this concept dates back to the fourth century, when patients with severe diarrhea in China were treated with various preparations of fecal matter, euphemistically presented as "yellow soup" or "golden syrup."[2185] Incidentally, this came from the same medical text that described wormwood as an effective herb against malaria,[2186] a discovery that led to a Nobel Prize in Medicine 1,700 years later in 2015.[2187]

What do we know about fecal transplants? Such research could not only offer the potential to treat disease, it could cement the cause-and-effect relationship between our microbiomes and our health.[2188] The first fecal transplant trials were for a potentially life-threatening overgrowth of a hospital-acquired pathogen called *Clostridium difficile*. Prior to the advent of centralized stool banks, patients would have to seek "donations" from friends or relatives.[2189] (It's like what one fly said to the other: "Is this stool taken?")

Once the "logistical challenges of delivering fresh treatment preparations"[2190] were overcome, the specimens were homogenized using a "dedicated" blender and then infused from the bottom up with an enema or top down through a nasogastric tube (a hose through the nose).[2191] No turkey basters necessary. More recently, capsules have been developed, but a single dose requires swallowing up to forty large capsules. Definitely not the time to suffer from reflux!

For *Clostridium difficile* infection, fecal transplantation can be a lifesaver. After thousands of successful transplants, it has been proven to be the single most effective therapy for recurrent infection,[2192] with symptom resolution seen in 85 percent of cases.[2193] (Want to learn more about how you can "Save Lives. Earn Money. Donate Your Stool" to a nonprofit stool bank? Visit www.givepoop.org.)

Doctors who want to try fecal transplants for other conditions must first acquire a special FDA permit.[2194] This is due largely to theoretical concerns about disease transfer. (No such cases have yet been reported.[2195]) A case report published in 2015 called "Weight Gain After Fecal Microbiota Transplantation" definitely raised the stakes, though, for both the potential risks and benefits of the procedure.

A thirty-two-year-old woman "had always been of normal weight" until she received a fecal transplant from a healthy but overweight donor (her daughter).[2196] This was in the United States, so by "normal," they mean the patient was actually slightly overweight herself with a BMI of 26. After the transplant, however, she gained more than forty pounds, ballooning to obesity at a BMI of 34.5. "She said she felt like there was a switch inside her body," her gastroenterologist reported.[2197] "No matter how much she ate or exercised, she couldn't take the weight off . . . she's very frustrated." The fecal transplant researchers concluded: "We recommend selecting non-overweight donors."[2198]

The same thing happens in mice. Giving mice fecal pellets from an obese mouse resulted in a near doubling in fat mass compared to lean mouse pellets, despite eating the same number of calories.[2199] This proves gut flora can play a pivotal role in obesity . . . in mice. What about in people?

Taking a Crack at Weight Loss

Researchers decided to study pairs of human twins "discordant" for obesity, meaning one twin was fat and the other was skinny. What would happen if you switched their microbiomes? The siblings may have been squeamish, so the researchers reverted again to mice. Mice fed stool from the obese twin rapidly swelled in size, but not those fed from the lean twin, despite comparable caloric intakes. Cohousing the mice together prevented the weight gain, however. The lean-type bacteria jumped over to rescue the mouse fed stool from the obese twin, but only in the context of a healthier diet—that is, the microbial cure only worked when the mice were fed diets low in saturated fat and high in fiber, which makes sense since the lean-type bacteria appeared to be fiber-munching, short-chain fatty-acid producers. "Together," the researchers concluded, "these results . . . illustrate how a diet high in saturated fats and low in fruits and vegetables can select against human gut bacteria . . . associated with leanness."[2200]

The results of the twin study suggest that the role of our gut flora in obesity is simply to help take fuller advantage of a more healthful diet. So if the twins had actually swapped their stools, the obese twins might have only lost weight if they had combined the microbial makeover with healthier eating to aid the colonization of the better bugs.[2201] With the new bacteria on board, though, the healthier diet could have resulted in more weight loss, even while eating the same number of calories. But you don't really know until you put it to the test.

If you were surprised by the case report of the mother–daughter fecal transplant, there are even stranger accounts coming out of that world. One gastroenterologist, for example, described a man with alopecia (baldness) who started growing hair after getting a stool transplant.[2202] You can't know if these anecdotes are just one-offs without subjecting them to rigorous randomized controlled trials. Currently, just such a study is under way at Harvard: Stools from lean individuals are being transplanted into obese individuals to see if they suddenly start to lose more weight.[2203] Stay tuned.

There was one study in which gut flora were transferred from lean to obese folks to see if their metabolic states would improve.[2204] The researchers wanted it to be a placebo-controlled study. For drug trials, that's easy: Just give a sugar pill. When you're sticking a tube down someone's throat and transplanting feces, though, what do you use as a "poo-cebo"? Both the lean donors and the obese subjects brought in fresh stools, and the obese subjects were randomized to get transplanted with either the donor stool or their own collected feces. That was the placebo—you get your own back! Isn't that brilliant?

The insulin sensitivity of the skinny donors was up around 50 μmol/kg/ min. That's a good thing, because high insulin sensitivity means their insulin resistance, the cause of type 2 diabetes and a potential risk factor for worsening obesity, is low. The obese subjects started out down around 20 μmol/kg/ min. After an infusion of their own feces, they stayed at around 20 as you'd expect. However, the insulin sensitivity of the group of obese subjects who got the skinny transplant shot up to near where the slimmer folks were.[2205] Eureka! Finally, proof in the power of poop.

Some lean-donor stools delivered more benefit than others. It turns out this "super-donor effect" is most likely conveyed, once again, by the numbers of short-chain fatty acid–producing fiber-feeders.[2206] Within a few months, however, the bacterial composition returned back to baseline, so the effects on the obese subjects were only temporary.[2207] You can get similar benefits by just feeding what few good gut bacteria you may already have. In my NutritionFacts.org video on the subject, we have an animation to illustrate this concept using a bunny analogy:

Imagine you have a shed full of rabbits. If you just fed them pork rinds, they would all die. Of course, you can always repopulate the hutch by infusing new bunnies, but if you keep feeding them pork rinds, they'll eventually die off too. That's like taking probiotics or getting a fecal transplant without changing your diet. On the other hand, even if you start off with just a few bunnies, if you feed them what they're meant to eat, they'll grow and multiply on their own.

Stool transplants and probiotics may only be temporary fixes if we keep putting the wrong fuel into our gut. If we don't change our diets, it may be a waste of money to go shopping for vegan poop on the black market (brown market?). On the other hand, by eating foods rich in *pre*biotics, in other words, increasing "whole plant food consumption," we may select for *and* foster the growth of our own good bacteria.[2208]

Is Obesity Contagious?

The fat twin / thin twin study proved obesity could be transmissible from human to mouse, but what about human to human? We've known for years that people who live together share a greater similarity in gut bacteria than those who live apart.[2209] Is this just because people living together are eating similar diets, or might they be inadvertently swapping bacteria back and forth? A clue to this mystery came when it was realized that family members don't just share gut microbes with each other but also with the family dog,[2210] who, one would hope, is eating a different diet.

It turns out homes can harbor a distinct microbial fingerprint. Just by swabbing the doorknobs and light switches, you can tell which family lives in which house. When a family moves, the microbial community in their new house becomes rapidly colonized toward that of their old home. Experimental evidence suggests that individuals raised in a household of thin people may be protected against obesity—no fecal transplant necessary.[2211,2212] (Instead, people may be sharing gut bacteria from kitchen stools!)

A famous study published in *The New England Journal of Medicine* found that a person's chances of becoming obese increased by more than 50 percent if they had a friend who became obese, suggesting one's social network can also have a big effect.[2213] This was chalked up to peers affecting each other's norms and behaviors, such as when a group of friends go out to eat the same fattening food together. Given the evidence implicating the role of gut bacteria in obesity, however, this "raises up the possibility that cravings and associated obesity might not just be *socially* contagious," a group of scientists speculated, "but rather truly infectious, like a cold."[2214] A more positive spin was captured by a pair of Harvard obesity researchers in their editorial in a journal called *Cell Host & Microbe* they entitled "Eat Well, or Get Roommates Who Do."[2215]

FOOD FOR THOUGHT

What we eat can change the composition of our gut flora—for good or for ill—within twenty-four hours. The most important thing we can do to foster the growth of good gut bacteria is keep them well fed with their favorite foods—the fiber and resistant starch concentrated in whole grains and legumes. On page 556, I talk about my daily morning BROL bowl, a prebiotic blend you can add to soup, eat as a sweet or savory porridge, or use in all manner of culinary creations. The road to health is paved with good intestines!

RICH IN FRUITS AND VEGETABLES

Do the Studies Bear Fruit?

There is convincing evidence that increasing consumption of fruits and vegetables reduces the risk of three of our leading causes of death—heart disease, stroke, and high blood pressure—and probable evidence it helps protect us from cancer, our other top killer.[2216] What about obesity? Wouldn't it be a refreshing change from all the restrictive "eat less" messaging to hear a positive "eat more" message? Sometimes proscriptions can backfire and make people want what's been labeled taboo even more[2217]—just ask Eve. Can we flip this "forbidden fruit" effect on its head and start encouraging more fruit?

Studies that followed a combined total of a half million people and their diets over the years have found that those who tend to eat the most fruits or vegetables seem to have 17 percent lower odds of weight gain or abdominal obesity.[2218] Another study found that over a ten-year period, those who ate more than about three servings of vegetables a day lost as much weight as those who walked four or more hours a week.[2219] However, people who consume more fruits and vegetables also tend to be more educated and practice other healthy lifestyle behaviors.[2220] The ten-year study did adjust for education, smoking habit, and a few dietary factors, such as meat intake, though.[2221] Three Harvard cohort studies went even further. Following more than one hundred thousand men and women for up to twenty-four years, researchers adjusted for a dozen other dietary aspects and took into account lifestyle factors from sleep habits to hours spent watching television. They, too, found consumption of both fruits and vegetables was associated with weight loss over time.[2222]

Although randomized controlled trials are necessary to prove cause and effect, observational studies like these offer the ability to examine dietary influences over the longer term—years or even decades. There have also been some exciting short-term interventional studies, like the study I mentioned earlier in which people lost weight after adding three apples or pears to their daily diets.[2223] Certain other fruits were not as successful, though. Adding three grapefruit halves, around three kiwifruits, or half a mango a day didn't result in significant weight loss (although it didn't result in weight gain either). Other benefits were noted—for example, grapefruits lowered blood pressure,[2224] kiwifruits improved DNA repair,[2225] and daily mango consumption improved blood sugars[2226]—but rather than being studies demonstrating "eat more, weigh less," they ended up being "eat more, weigh the same."

Though a compilation of interventional fruit-and-veggie studies found that most did result in weight loss, they often included other dietary changes, such as swapping out desserts for added fruits.[2227] More recent systematic reviews of the evidence have been more muted in their enthusiasm, finding the overall average of weight reduction to be small[2228] or concluding that simply telling people to eat more fruits and vegetables is in fact fruitless without also having them cut down on things like junk.[2229]

On the Juice

Issues have been raised about both the quality and quantity of vegetables prescribed and/or provided in studies. On average, the difference between the "high" and low fruit-and-vegetable groups in studies ended up only being about one and a half servings a day.[2230] Beyond the problem of inadequate "dosing," sometimes the interventions involved processed fruit and vegetable products containing added fat and sugar.[2231] For example, one study in which the added-fruit-and-veggie group actually gained weight counted french fries and fruit juice toward their daily intake goals.[2232] Even nonfried potatoes, like mashed, and other starchy vegetables may not have the same weight-reducing potential as nonstarchy veggies,[2233] and fruit juice can carry the same sugar load as soda[2234] and the same amount of fiber: zero. Even "high pulp," "extra pulp," and "most pulp" orange juices are not significant sources of fiber. It's all pulp fiction.

Just as population studies have found that greater whole fruit consumption is associated with lower risk of type 2 diabetes yet more fruit *juice* consumption is linked to higher risk,[2235] consuming whole fruits can facilitate weight loss, while drinking fruit juice may promote weight gain.[2236] Even children given 100 percent fruit juice as toddlers tend to be at higher risk of becoming overweight.[2237] This could be in part because juice may be a "gateway drink" to soda consumption.[2238] Either way, the American Academy of Pediatrics, the American Heart Association, and the Institute of Medicine have all recommended that fruit juice be restricted, encouraging whole fruit consumption instead.[2239]

How can 100 percent fruit juice be fattening but, at the same time, whole fruit slimming? It's apparently not just the fiber. Liquid calories in general may be less satiating. If you feed people four hundred calories of fruit juice, they go on to eat 75 percent more of a test meal of mac 'n cheese than if you had instead fed them four hundred calories of whole fruit, even if the equivalent amount of fiber had been stirred into the juice.[2240]

Could it be because you can down juice in no time, but it takes a while to actually chew through the fruit? That extra time might give your appetite control mechanisms more of a chance to kick in. Researchers put that exact question to the test by measuring satiety after subjects slowly sipped a pound of apple juice in the same time it would take to eat a pound of apples (which is 17.2 minutes, it turns out). Even with the rate of consumption equalized, the apples, not just their juice, were more satiating.[2241]

Some fruit juices, however, don't seem to cause the same weight gain. Why? To understand that, you need to understand why the body handles the sugar in fruit differently from that of corn syrup and table sugar.

Breaking Down the Walls

How can adding fruits and vegetables to our diets result in weight loss? The obvious answer is that they would displace other foods. Since produce tends to furnish so few calories, swapping in fruits and vegetables for the same weight or volume of most anything else would lower caloric intake. However, some studies have shown weight loss with more fruits and veggies *even with no change in overall calories*.[2242] How do we explain that?

In foods, there are intracellular calories and extracellular calories—in other words, calories that are confined inside cells and calories that are free to be absorbed directly. Processed plant foods like fruit juice, refined grains, and sugar are letting it all hang out, and their calories are free for the taking. In contrast, all the calories in *whole* plant foods are not only trapped inside cells—they're also trapped inside cell walls. Animal cells are encased only in easily digestible membranes, which allow the enzymes in our gut to effortlessly liberate the calories within a steak, for example. Plant cells, on the other hand, have walls that are made out of indigestible fiber.

Our bodies do their best to chew through those walls—literally—to get to all the goodness inside, but in the end, it's not about what we eat but what we absorb. The way you measure how many calories a food has is to burn it and see how much energy it releases. When it comes to whole plant foods, the combustible calories significantly exceed the metabolizable calories—that is, the calories that actually make it into your bloodstream.[2243] So, by eating extra fruits and vegetables, on paper, it looks like you're taking in more calories, but when researchers have actually put it to the test and taken careful measurements, they've found that you can actually end up with fewer calories in your system.[2244]

Vegetables may offer the additional advantage of changing the expression of the genes that control our metabolisms. Greens can affect your genes. If you take biopsies of fat from people before and after a few weeks of feeding them extra vegetables, the expression of hundreds of genes is ramped up or down. By correlating those changes to the same ones you get losing weight through caloric restriction, you can uncover the weight-loss pathways and processes that appear affected by the bump in veggie intake.[2245] Give people on a weight-loss diet one to two cups of vegetable juice (low-sodium V8), for example, and they lose more weight than those given none.[2246] Vegetables tend to contain less sugar than fruit, though.

What About All the Sugar in Fruit?

Fruit's influence on obesity has been called a "paradoxical effect" thanks to its sugar content.[2247] Fruit contains sugars such as fructose, which is also found in table sugar and corn syrup. If sugar is bad for us, how is fruit so good for us?

If you directly compare the effects of a diet restricting fructose from both added sugars and fruit to one that only restricts fructose from added sugars, the diet that kept the fruit did *better.*[2248] People lost more weight with the extra fruit present in the diet than when all fructose was restricted across the board.

Is it just the dose? To get the average intake of added sugars in the American diet[2249] in fruit form, you'd have to eat about six and a half cups of apple slices a day[2250] or nearly eight cups of watermelon.[2251] Even if you did, though, it wouldn't have the same effect as getting that same amount of sugar from processed sources. As the *Harvard Health Letter* put it, the problems associated with fructose and sugar in general "come when they are *added* to foods." Fruit, on the other hand, is not just harmless but described as "beneficial in almost any amount."[2252] *Almost* any amount? Can we eat ten servings of fruit a day? How about twenty? That's actually been put to the test.

Seventeen people were made to eat twenty servings of fruit a day for up to six months. Despite their extraordinarily high fructose intakes—presumably the equivalent of drinking about eight cans of soda a day—the investigators found the subjects actually lost weight and their blood pressures improved,[2253] insulin levels dropped, and cholesterol and triglycerides got better.[2254] This is the opposite of what one might expect eating the same amount of fructose in added sugars. Why do our bodies handle the sugars in fruit differently from the sugars added to foods and beverages?

If you drink a glass of water with three tablespoons of table sugar mixed in, which is like a can of soda, you get a big spike in blood sugar within the first hour. Your body freaks out and releases so much insulin you actually overshoot the mark such that, by the second hour, you end up relatively hypoglycemic, dropping your blood sugar below where it was even before you had consumed anything. In response, your body dumps fat into your bloodstream, which can have a variety of adverse effects, such as increasing insulin resistance.[2255] That's one of the reasons we shouldn't be drinking soda, aka liquid candy. But what if you added nature's candy—berries?

What if you eat blended berries in *addition* to the sugar? What would happen if you were to repeat the same experiment but add nearly an *additional* tablespoon of sugar—this time in fruit form, the way nature intended, rather than table sugar? Still, downing four tablespoons of sugar instead of three should cause an even bigger blood sugar spike, right? Not only did that not happen, there was no hypoglycemic dip afterward. Blood sugar simply went up and down without that overshoot and without the surge of fat into the blood.[2256]

Initially, the researchers attributed the difference in response to the thickening effects of the berries, as the soluble fiber in the berries would presumably have a gelling effect. Compared with just guzzling straight sugar water, the berry addition might slow both the rate of stomach emptying and the release of sugars in our intestines. To test to see if it was the fiber, researchers repeated the experiment with berry *juice,* which had nearly all the sugar but none of the fiber. A clear difference was observed early on in the blood sugar response. At the fifteen-minute mark, the blood sugar spike was significantly reduced by the blended berries, but not by the berry juice, although the rest of the beneficial responses were almost the same between the whole fruit and juice, suggesting there's more at play than just the fiber.[2257]

Just Beet It

Fiber content isn't the only difference between table sugar and the source of most table sugar these days, sugar beets.[2258] There are also the thousands of phytonutrients that are stripped away in the sugar-refining process. It turns out some of the polyphenols in fruit can block the transport of sugars through the intestinal lining, slowing absorption.[2259] In fact, adding fruit can actually blunt the insulin spike from high-glycemic foods. For example, white bread creates a big insulin spike an hour after eating it. Eat that same white bread with some berries, though, and even though you just effectively added more sugar, you're able to blunt the spike, because the sugar was in fruit form.[2260] So if you're going to make pancakes or muffins, make them blueberry.

We can finally explain why some juices are better than others. Cloudy apple juice has more polyphenols, which may help explain why whole apples lower cholesterol compared to clear apple juice but not compared to cloudy apple juice.[2261] Have people drink cups of cloudy apple juice every day, and they lose body fat compared to a polyphenol-free control beverage with the same number of calories.[2262] Similar results were found for Concord (purple) grape juice. Have people drink two cups of a grape-flavored drink like Kool-Aid every day for a few months, and they gain a few pounds, but not when the same number of calories were added in the form of grape juice. Sorry, Welch's (the study's funder), but whole grapes would have probably done even better.[2263]

Free the Fruit

In a study entitled "Not Enough Fruit and Vegetables or Too Many Cookies, Candies, Salty Snacks, and Soft Drinks?" public health researchers suggested fruit and vegetable promotion campaigns were distractions from the larger problem of excess junk.[2264] Many urban populations may suffer less from "food deserts," where corner stores lack fresh produce, than from "food swamps."[2265] "It may be politically more expedient to promote an increase in consumption of healthy items rather than a decrease in consumption of unhealthy items," they concluded, "but it may be far less effective."[2266]

To find out which approach worked better, a group of overweight women were randomized to one of two dietary approaches: Avoid high-fat foods or eat more fruits and vegetables. The advice was bolstered with group and individual sessions with a dietitian to try to keep the respective groups on track. Though the group just given the positive messaging to eat more fruits and vegetables lost weight over a period of six months, the restrictive-messaging group lost significantly more.[2267] Win-win, but obviously not either-or.

We don't have to choose between adding fruits and veggies or subtract-ing fattening foods. All the strategies in this book aim to complement each other.

Given the myriad benefits, how can we get more people to eat more fruits and vegetables? Well, we could make them free. Offering free fruits and veggies in a cafeteria setting nearly quintupled the likelihood of people reaching their daily recommended intakes.[2268] Does this translate into weight loss? A study in Norway tested out a free fruit program among schoolchildren. Compared to control schools, a year of free fruit for ten- to twelve-year-olds resulted in a 40 percent lower prevalence of being overweight seven years later.[2269]

Concerns have been raised, however, that by subsidizing healthy food, people might just have more money to spend on junk.[2270] To test this, a small group of low-income, overweight individuals were provided supermarket gift cards worth forty dollars each month. Half were randomized to cards that could buy any food at the grocery store, and the other half to cards good only for fruits and vegetables. After three months, the buy-anything group gained weight, whereas the subsidized-fruit-and-veggie group lost weight, ending up nearly ten pounds lighter than the control group.[2271] Unfortunately, this study appears to be the exception.

A recent study in Toronto found that providing free produce boosted fruit and vegetable intake about 50 percent more than just advising people to eat more of them. Even then, however, the free-fruit-and-veg group only ended up consuming about a total of three servings a day and, not surpris-ingly, lost no more weight after six months than the control group.[2272] The recommended *minimum* number of daily servings of fruits and vegetables a day is seven to thirteen, but most Americans don't even get five.[2273] After the Centers for Disease Control and Prevention realized that even a recommen-dation of five daily servings seemed "unachievable," it changed the National Cancer Institute's "5 A Day Program" to "Fruits & Veggies—More Matters." (It also considered the slogan "Appetite for Life" to emphasize how our food choices are truly life or death, but such messaging was thought perhaps too "rational," needing a "stronger emotional appeal."[2274])

Ideally, on a population scale, fruits and vegetables should be better promoted. The National Fruit & Vegetable Alliance gave failing grades to the federal government for inadequate produce marketing and nutrition education,[2275] and the private sector may be even worse. The U.S. Federal Trade Commission subpoenaed dozens of food, beverage, and restaurant companies to release information about their marketing expenditures that focus on children and adolescents.[2276] The findings? Fruit and vegetable promotion constitutes less than half a penny of each dollar spent.[2277]

Garlic Press

In the Harvard cohorts, the categories of berries and apples/pears appeared to stand out on the fruit side in terms of foods associated with the most weight loss, and cauliflower and tofu/soy did so on the vegetable side.[2278] As I've noted, apples and pears were put to the test in a randomized controlled trial and shown to produce weight loss even compared to same-calorie controls.[2279] Have there been any similar such studies on other fruits and vegetables?

Garlic can reduce the body fat of rats[2280] and mice[2281] even at the same caloric intakes (so it wasn't because they didn't like the taste), but rodent studies found the same for tomatoes,[2282] and that didn't seem to necessarily translate to people.[2283] There was a study in which a few cloves of crushed raw garlic a day appeared to have a waist-slimming effect, but without a control group, you don't know if the subjects may have just lost the weight because they were under observation.[2284] Garlic is so potent, though. What if you stuffed it into a pill and designed not just a randomized controlled study but one that's double-blind with a placebo by giving people coated tablets containing garlic powder versus sugar pills?

One such study tried giving people with metabolic syndrome placebo or actual garlic tablets adding up to a half teaspoon of garlic powder a day. And it worked, resulting in a drop in both weight and waistlines within six weeks.[2285] A half teaspoon of garlic powder costs less than four cents. What about trying garlic supplements, like the fancy aged garlic extract ones you may have seen advertised. No weight-loss benefits were found.[2286,2287]

How about just a quarter teaspoon of garlic powder a day? About one hundred overweight men and women were randomized to two 400 mg garlic powder tablets a day or placebo, and those unknowingly taking the two cents' worth of daily garlic powder lost nearly six pounds of straight body fat over the next fifteen weeks.[2288] The only caveat (besides possible decreased kissability) is that garlic can have blood-thinning effects, so it should be stopped a week before elective surgery.[2289] It may also overly detoxify and interfere with the efficacy of an HIV drug known as *saquinavir* (sold as Invirase or Fortovase).[2290]

FOOD FOR THOUGHT

Does it matter when you eat your fruits and vegetables? In my Negative Calorie Preloading section that's coming up in part IV, I explore the benefits of making them the first choice for your first course. There's even a public health campaign in Japan called "Eat Vegetables First at Meals."[2291] Just changing the order of foods you eat can have meaningful metabolic impact. Compared to the exact same meal eaten in a different order, eating vegetables first can decrease blood sugar and insulin excursions in diabetics[2292] and prediabetics,[2293] resulting in significantly better blood sugar control over the long term.[2294] However, this may be due in part to the fact that those randomized to receive advice to eat vegetables first ended up eating more vegetables overall.[2295] This may also help explain why children who eat vegetables first during a meal may have less than 50 percent of the odds of being overweight compared to those who ate meat/fish first.[2296] So the best time to eat them may in fact be anytime you can.

Just as keeping candy out of plain view can help keep junk out of sight, out of stomach,[2297] increasing the visibility and accessibility of healthy snacks may help. Those randomized to keep a bowl of fruit on the kitchen counter instead of inside the fridge ended up closer to meeting their daily needs.[2298] What about vegetables? Serving greater quantities of veggies was found to significantly increase vegetable intake by preschool children,[2299] as well as adults.[2300] One of the "Top Ten Tips for Weight Loss" used in the studies I discuss on page 430 is "Do not heap food on your plate (except vegetables)."[2301]

For the most delicious produce, explore local farmers' markets, community-supported agriculture, and pick-your-own orchards, or garden yourself. Fruits and vegetables today are bred to survive long-distance shipping, not necessarily to taste their best.[2302] Even heritage breeds can lose flavor after traveling eight thousand miles from New Zealand. Did you know the "fresh" apple you buy at the grocery store may be ten months old?[2303] It's wonderful that we can get produce year-round, thanks to new storage technologies, but if you've never eaten an apple picked straight off a tree, you are missing out.

My favorite fruit in the whole world can't even be sold commercially because it's too fragile. Have you ever had a pawpaw, North America's largest native fruit? Think luscious tropical banana-mango custard. For a few weeks in September across the Midwest and mid-Atlantic, you can forage for them in the wild or find them at farmers' markets (unless I get there first). See you at the next pawpaw festival!

RICH IN LEGUMES

The Hispanic Paradox

According to a national dietary survey, those who eat beans tend to be healthier and have less obesity risk, lower body weight, and smaller waist sizes.[2304] This finding has been used to explain what's known as the *Hispanic paradox*: Despite higher poverty rates and disparities in health care and education,[2305] Hispanic Americans tend to live longer than everyone else.[2306] Hispanics have a 24 percent lower risk of premature death, thanks to lower risks of nine of the fifteen leading causes of death, including notably less cancer and heart disease.[2307]

What's powerful enough to overcome lower socioeconomic status, education level, health literacy, insurance coverage, and disproportionate employment in high-risk occupations?[2308]

Public health researchers suggest it may be "time to spill the beans"[2309]— or, more broadly, the legumes. Legumes, including beans, split peas, chickpeas, and lentils, can be considered "potent tools in the prevention and treatment of chronic disease."[2310]

Just because people who eat beans tend to be slimmer and healthier[2311] doesn't necessarily mean legumes deserve the credit. Each bean burrito may mean one less beef burrito. Researchers were able to show a variety of metabolic benefits randomizing people to swap out two servings of meat for legumes three days a week,[2312] but is the benefit from what is being eaten or what is being replaced? In the Harvard studies, the food category most associated with weight loss over time was soy food products, with nearly ten times the weight reduction associated with vegetable consumption.[2313] But how many people are eating bacon double-cheese tofu burgers? Indeed, bean consumption is associated with less saturated fat and cholesterol intake,[2314] so it may just be a marker for a healthier diet in general. Nevertheless, the Harvard studies controlled for a whole array of dietary and lifestyle factors yet still found a significant link between beans and better health.

Dozens of randomized controlled trials have found that soy can lower cholesterol[2315] and blood pressure,[2316] but what about non-soy legumes? Compilations of more than sixty randomized controlled trials have found that other beans also lower cholesterol,[2317] as well as benefit blood sugars and lower insulin levels,[2318] but consumer surveys suggest most Americans are unaware of these benefits.[2319] One could say they don't know beans about beans!

The Lentil Effect

What about interventional studies on beans and weight control? In the famous "satiety index" study that compared the hunger-slaking power of dozens of different foods, both fiber and protein content were associated with appetite-suppressing effects.[2320] This would seem to make legumes ideal candidates,[2321] and indeed, we've known for more than thirty years that meals featuring beans can disproportionally delay the return of hunger.[2322] Does this then translate into reduced caloric intake throughout the day?

What do you think happened when people were given a cup of chickpeas or the same number of calories of white bread and butter? Those who had eaten the chickpeas ate nearly two hundred fewer calories of a meal served a few hours later.[2323] Navy beans may work even better than chickpeas, and lentils best of all.[2324] How do legumes fare compared to something a little more substantial than Wonder Bread, though?

Researchers compared patties made with fava beans and split peas to protein-matched patties made out of meat. The title of the study gives it away: "Meals Based on Vegetable Protein Sources (Beans and Peas) Are More Satiating Than Meals Based on Animal Protein Sources (Veal and Pork)." Even lower-protein patties in which most of the mashed beans and peas were replaced with potato held their own against the meat.[2325] The researchers suggested this may help explain why intake of animal protein has been associated with subsequent weight gain, but consumption of plant protein hasn't.[2326] Beans are free of the baggage inherent to animal protein sources, such as saturated fat and cholesterol, and instead offer a bonus in the form of fiber, which likely explains their satiety benefits.[2327]

It's no wonder legumes are more satiating than white bread. Both fiber and water have no calories, so to get the same number of calories in bean form, you have to feed people more food. You can imagine how eating a cup of chickpeas would be more filling than eating two pieces of white bread, which you could probably squeeze into a little ball in your fist. Only a minority of studies showed bean consumption actually cut down on subsequent caloric intake at later meals, though, but that may be because the researchers simply might not have waited long enough.[2328] The satiating power of legumes is thought to arise from the effects of the slowly digesting resistant starch and fiber lower down in the intestines, which may not be reflected in studies lasting fewer than three hours.

In 1982, an extraordinary discovery was published. It had already been demonstrated that beans cause an "exceptionally" low blood sugar response, half that of other common foods.[2329] What was discovered was that eating legumes could benefit your metabolism hours later[2330] or even the next day. Eat lentils for dinner, and eleven hours later, your body reacts differently to breakfast.[2331] Even when made to drink straight sugar water the next morning, your body is better able to handle it. At the time, the researchers dubbed it the "lentil effect," but subsequent studies found chickpeas appear to work just as well. It has since been christened the "second meal effect."[2332]

How is that even possible? Remember how we feed our gut bacteria and they feed us right back? Good gut flora can take fiber and produce valuable short-chain fatty acids that get absorbed into our bloodstreams and circulate throughout our systems. So if we eat a bean burrito for dinner, by the next morning, our gut bacteria are eating that same burrito, and the by-products they create may affect how our breakfasts are digested and how full we feel.

This second-meal effect can include changes in appetite. Eat half a can of brown beans at dinner, and you feel less hungry after breakfast the next day than had you instead eaten the same number of calories in non-bean form the night before.[2333]

Researchers solved the mystery of the second-meal effect by giving people rectal infusions of the number of short-chain fatty acids our good bacteria might make from a good beany burrito. The stomach responded within minutes.[2334] So I guess if you forgot to eat any kind of beans for dinner and needed to blunt the effect of your breakfast donut, it's *theoretically* not too late, but, in general, I encourage people to take their food by mouth.

Adding Beans vs. Portion Control

Does all this talk of legumes translate into weight loss? Let's feed people some beans and find out. If you feed overweight and obese individuals three-quarters of a cup of canned navy beans a day for a month, they end up dropping about an inch off their waists.[2335] The study had no control group, though, so we don't know if the subjects would have slimmed down without the daily dose of beans.

As we've discussed, designing dietary trials can be challenging when trying to come up with a proper control. If you simply ask people to add chickpeas to their diets and then analyze their subsequent dietary changes, the single biggest change they make is to reduce their consumption of non-chickpea legumes.[2336] If the subjects are just swapping out one bean for another or eating fewer vegetables to compensate, one would not expect the full benefit to materialize. This may help explain why the interventional trials on legumes for weight control have been disappointing overall, showing on average only a small effect in people randomized to add an average of one serving of legumes to their daily diets.[2337]

The better-designed trials yielded better results, though.[2338] For example, in one study, more than one hundred participants were randomized to either increase legume intake by at least one cup per day or to instead add whole-grain foods to their diets, so both groups would be bumping up their fiber intakes with healthy foods. After three months, the whole-grain group lost a little weight, but the legume group lost significantly more, resulting in about an inch off their waists.[2339]

My favorite bean study was published in 2012 out of the University of Toronto. (I assume everyone has a favorite bean study?) The researchers recognized that calorie cutting is the cornerstone of most weight-loss strategies, but the majority of people who lose weight by eating smaller portions gain it back. Starving ourselves almost never works long term. Therefore, the researchers concluded, "it is important to identify foods that can be easily incorporated into the diet and spontaneously lead to the attainment and maintenance of a healthy body weight."[2340] *Spontaneously* is the key word there—in other words, lose weight without really trying. They figured legumes might be a good candidate, so, for the first time ever, beans were pitted head-to-head against caloric restriction.

The legume group was asked to eat about three-quarters of a cup of lentils, chickpeas, split peas, or navy beans a day, and the calorie-restriction group was tasked with cutting five hundred calories out of their daily diets. So, in effect, the bean group was asked to eat more food and the calorie-cutting group was asked to eat less. After two months, both groups slimmed about an inch off their waists.[2341]

Increasing diet quality appeared to work as well as decreasing diet quantity.

Starch Blockers

Eating legumes achieved weight loss even in studies meant to be weight-neutral like cholesterol- or blood sugar–lowering trials.[2342] Part of the reason may be because nearly 20 percent of bean starch slips through our small intestines undigested, so beans can end up contributing fewer calories than are listed on the can's label.[2343] Some of the starch in legumes is tightly packed into double-spiraled crystals, which our digestive enzymes have trouble infiltrating, and there are also compounds in legumes that directly target our starch-munching enzymes.[2344] This is where the concept of starch blocking comes from.

Crude bean extracts, commercialized as "starch blocker" supplements, have a sordid history. By the early 1980s, the American public was swallowing a million starch-blocker tablets a day for weight loss.[2345] Despite a lack of human testing, hundreds of such products had flooded the market.[2346] Finally, data from clinical trials started to trickle in, and the findings were universally negative, with emblematic titles such as "'Starch Blockers' Are Ineffective in Man"[2347] or simply "Starch Blockers Do Not Block Starch Digestion."[2348] And that was the problem. Apparently, the bean compounds were not stable in pill form.[2349] Starch-blocker pills were all yanked from the market in 1982 by the Food and Drug Administration.[2350]

Subsequently, manufacturers were able to create a more active product,[2351] so, at the very least, it could be put to the test. A compilation of studies on the newer generation of starch blockers found they could reduce body fat compared to placebo.[2352] Unsurprisingly, the majority of studies were funded by the manufacturers themselves. Funding bias aside, the bigger concern is the lack of industry regulation that too often calls into question the purity, safety, and label accuracy of dietary supplements.[2353] So while I can't recommend starch blockers in pill form, I can recommend them in food form. The starch-blocking capacity of whole beans survives cooking and may therefore play a role in the prevention and treatment of obesity.[2354]

What About Lectins?

In 2017, a book called *The Plant Paradox* was published, purporting to expose "the hidden dangers in 'healthy' foods that cause disease and weight gain." The so-called dangerous, disease-causing, and weight-gaining foods included beans, whole grains, and tomatoes. What? In a rehashing of the since discredited[2355] "blood type diet" from decades ago, the author accuses lectins of contributing to chronic disease. *The Plant Paradox* was written by an M.D., but if you've seen any of my medical education videos, you'll know that's effectively an *anti*-credential when it comes to writing diet books. Graduating from medical school basically advertises to the world that you've received likely little or no formal training in nutrition. Dr. Atkins was, after all, a cardiologist.

The thesis of the book doesn't even seem to pass the sniff test. If lectins are bad for you, then beans would be the worst. In that case, shouldn't bean counters find legume lovers have shortened lives? The exact opposite seems to be true: Legumes have been found to be perhaps "the most important dietary predictor of survival in older people" around the world.[2356] As Dan Buettner points out in his Blue Zones longevity work, lectin-packed foods like legumes are the "cornerstones" of the diets of all the healthiest, longest-lived populations on the planet.[2357]

When I heard about *The Plant Paradox,* my first thought was, *Let me guess. He sells a line of lectin-blocking supplements.* And what do you know? "SHIELDING YOUR BODY FROM LECTINS" for only $79.95 a month, his website assures. That's like $1,000 a year. But wait. There's more. The dozens of supplements he hawks on his website could add up to nearly $20,000 a year if taken as recommended. He must be making a fortune stoking, then preying on people's fears. Oh, did I not mention his skin care line? He'll generously sell you a jar of his "Firm + Sculpt" cream for the low, low price of only $120—discounted if you subscribe to his "VIP Club."

In the 1800s, a compound was discovered in castor beans, which we would come to know as the first of a class of lectin proteins—natural compounds found throughout the food supply, but concentrated in beans, whole grains, and certain fruits and vegetables.[2358] Every decade or two, it seems, a question is raised as to whether dietary lectins may be causing disease. It's easy to raise hysteria about lectins. After all, that first one, found back in 1889, went by the name *ricin,* which is known to be a "potent homicidal poison" used by the Kremlin to assassinate anti-Communist dissidents— or (*Breaking Bad* spoiler alert!) by rogue chemistry teachers.[2359] Ricin is a lectin. Thankfully, however, many lectins are nontoxic, such as those found in tomatoes and other common foods,[2360] and even the ones that can cause problems, like those found in raw kidney beans, are utterly destroyed by proper cooking.[2361]

What would happen if kidney beans were eaten raw? Because of the lectins, you would be doubled over with nausea, vomiting, and diarrhea within hours.[2362] But how would you even eat raw kidney beans? The only way they're sold uncooked is as dried beans, which are as hard as rocks. In the first outbreak reported in the medical literature, "an impromptu supper was made" with a bag of beans dumped in a skillet and soaked in water overnight, but never cooked.[2363] You can't even just throw them in a slow cooker. Dried kidney beans have to be boiled. According to some researchers, they should be soaked in water for at least five hours and then boiled for at least ten minutes.[2364] I'm no Iron Chef, but ten minutes? Kidney beans wouldn't be done in only ten minutes. Cooking presoaked beans for a couple of minutes can destroy the lectins, but it takes about an hour of boiling before the beans are soft enough to eat, when they're easily flattened with a fork.[2365] So the lectins would be long gone before they're palatable.

(continued)

The same goes for pressure cooking. Without presoaking, it takes forty-five minutes in a pressure cooker to get rid of all the lectins in kidney beans, but an hour to make the beans edible,[2366] so, again, they'd be lectin-free before you ate them. Even twelve hours at 65°C (150°F), which is about the temperature of hot tea, won't do it, though, but you could tell they weren't cooked enough because they'd be firm and rubbery. Folks have, however, tried putting undercooked kidney beans in something like a "raw" vegetable salad, and people have gotten sick. There have been dozens of such incidents reported, but each could have been "easily prevented" had the beans been cooked properly[2367] or if canned beans had been used instead. Canned beans are cooked beans. The canning process is a cooking process. None of the confirmed incidents was ever due to canned beans.

The purported "plant paradox" is that, on the one hand, whole, healthy plant foods are the foundations of a good diet, but on the other hand, we supposedly need to avoid lectin-containing foods since they can supposedly lead to inflammation. But feed people four servings a week of beans, split peas, chickpeas, and lentils, and you can get a whopping 40 percent drop in C-reactive protein,[2368] a leading indicator of systemic inflammation. More beans equals *less* inflammation. Greater consumption of each of the major categories of whole plant foods—fruits, vegetables, whole grains, beans, and nuts—is associated with living significantly longer,[2369] so there's really no paradox after all.

FOOD FOR THOUGHT

On any given day, only about 8 percent of Americans eat beans.[2370] This may be due in part to an unfamiliarity with how to prepare and incorporate them into our diets. Some people seem intimidated by legumes, imagining overnight soakings and long cooking times, but they can be as easy to prep as a few twists of a can opener.[2371] Rather cook them from scratch? Harvard's Institute of Lifestyle Medicine recommends starting with lentils: Combine three cups of water for every one cup of lentils. Bring to a boil and then simmer for twenty minutes until soft. Drain and enjoy. I encourage you to make extra and freeze them in portions.

Split red or orange lentils are even easier. They're ready in five minutes, quicker than boiling pasta.[2372] Once they've softened, rinse them to cool, then mix with herbs and lemon juice for a basic legume salad. Another favorite of mine is to cook lentils a little longer so they thicken into almost a purée before adding spices like curry, turmeric, cumin, and garam masala for a thick, savory, and healthy Indian-inspired sauce.

Once you're ready to branch out, I'd recommend an electric pressure cooker. Add dried beans and water, press one or two buttons, and beans are cooked to perfection without any presoaking necessary. The cooker even shuts itself off automatically. It couldn't be easier or more foolproof. I used to buy canned (BPA-free, of course) beans by the case, so my electric pressure cooker easily paid for itself, given how incredibly inexpensive dried beans are. It's not that I'm unwilling to splurge the few extra cents for canned—I just prefer the texture of home-cooked beans. I now find canned beans can be a little mushy, which is fine for making hummus, bean dips, or some soup I'll end up blending, but if I'm eating the actual beans, I've become spoiled for a slightly firmer bite.

There's a reason legumes have earned the hallowed distinction of being officially recognized in the federal dietary guidelines as belonging to both the vegetable group and the protein group. They're loaded with protein, iron, and zinc, as you might expect from other protein sources like meat, but legumes also offer nutrients concentrated in the vegetable kingdom, such as fiber, folate, and potassium. You therefore get the best of both worlds with beans, all the while enjoying foods that are naturally low in saturated fat and sodium, and completely free of cholesterol.

Fearful of flatulence? Stop by your local library and check out the Clearing the Air About Beans and Gas section in the beans chapter in *How Not to Die*. The bottom line (no pun intended) is that most people either don't experience any gastrointestinal side effects after adding beans to their diets or the symptoms dissipate within the first few weeks.[2373]

SATIATING

Built for Gluttony

The importance of satiety is underscored by a rare genetic condition known as *Prader-Willi syndrome*. Those born with this disease have impaired signaling between their digestive systems and their brains, so they don't know when they're full. With no sensation of satiety, they can accidentally eat so much they fatally rupture their stomachs. Without satiety, food could be a death sentence.[2374]

Protein is often described as the most satiating macronutrient.[2375] People tend to report feeling fuller after eating a protein-rich meal compared to a carbohydrate- or fat-rich one. But does that feeling last? From a weight-loss standpoint, satiety ratings only matter if they end up cutting down on subsequent caloric intake,[2376] and even a review funded in part by the meat, dairy, and egg industries acknowledges this does not seem to be the case for protein.[2377] Hours after consumption, that protein eaten earlier doesn't tend to end up cutting calories.

Fiber, on the other hand, contributes to suppressing hunger up to ten hours after it's eaten[2378] and can reduce subsequent meal intake.[2379] Why? Its site of action is twenty feet down in the lower intestine. Remember the ileal brake from the High in Fiber-Rich Foods section? Secretly infuse nutrients into the end of the small intestine, and people spontaneously eat as many as hundreds of fewer calories at the next meal[2380] because of a signal to our brains that we are full from head to tail.

We were built for gluttony. It's a hedge against times of scarcity. Stumbling across a rare bounty, those who could stuff themselves the most to build up the greatest reserves would be most likely to pass along their genes. You might say it was the survival of the fullest. So we are hardwired to eat not just until our stomachs are full but also until our entire digestive tracts are occupied. Only when our brains sense food all the way at the end of our lower intestines may our appetites dial down fully.

Fiber-depleted foods rapidly get absorbed early on, though, so not much ever makes it down to the lower gut. Given how little fiber the average American eats, it's no wonder we're so hungry and always overeating: Our brains keep waiting for the food that never arrives. Indeed, this is why, even after a stomach-stapling surgery that leaves just a tiny, two tablespoons–sized stomach pouch, people can still eat enough to regain most of the weight they initially lost. Without sufficient fiber transporting nutrients all the way down our digestive tracts, we may never feel fully satiated.[2381]

Two Hundred Pounds Without Hunger

Anyone can lose weight eating less food. Anyone can be starved thin. Starvation diets are rarely sustainable, though, since hunger pangs drive us to eat. We feel unsatisfied on low-calorie diets. Unsatiated. We do have some level of voluntary control, but our deep-seated instinctual drives may win out in the end.

For example, you can consciously hold your breath. Try it right now. How long can you go before your body's self-preservation mechanisms take over and overwhelm your deliberate intent not to breathe? Your body has your best interests at heart and is too smart to allow you to suffocate yourself—or starve yourself, for that matter. But if our bodies were really that smart, how could they let us become obese? Why don't our bodies realize when we're too fat and allow us the leeway to slim down? Could it be that our bodies *are* actually aware—and actively trying to help—but we're somehow undermining those efforts? How could we test this theory to see if that's true?

So many variables go into choosing what and how much we eat. There are psychological, social, cultural, aesthetic, and other factors. To strip away all of that and stick just to the physiological, Columbia University researchers designed a series of famous experiments using a "food dispensing device."[2382] The term *food* is used very loosely here. Their feeding machine was a tube hooked up to a pump that delivered a mouthful of bland liquid formula every time a button was pushed. Research subjects were instructed to eat as much or as little as they wanted at any time. In this way, eating was reduced to just the rudimentary hunger drive. Without the usual trappings of sociability, meal ceremony, and the pleasures of the palate, how much would people be driven to eat?

Put a normal-weight person in this scenario, and something remarkable happens. Day after day, week after week, with nothing more than their hunger to guide them, they ate exactly as much as they needed, perfectly maintaining their weights. They required about three thousand calories a day, and that's just how much they gave themselves. Their bodies just intuitively seemed to know how many times to press that button to get food.[2383]

What happened when obese people were put in a similar scenario? Driven by hunger alone with the enjoyment of eating stripped away, they wildly undershot and gave themselves as little as 145 calories a day. Fewer than 200 total calories for the entire day! The obese subjects could eat as much as they wanted, but they just weren't hungry. It's as if their bodies knew how grossly overweight they were and so dialed down their natural hunger drives to almost nothing. One research subject started out at four hundred pounds and steadily lost weight. After 252 days, even after switching to drinking the "food" out of a cup at home, he lost two hundred pounds.[2384]

Initially, this groundbreaking discovery was interpreted by some to mean that obesity is not caused by some sort of metabolic disturbance that drives people to overeat. Instead, overeating appeared to be a function of the meaning people attached to food beyond its use as fuel, whether as a source of pleasure or perhaps relief from boredom or stress.[2385] Obesity, then, seemed more psychological than physical. However, subsequent experiments with the feeding machine suggest quite the opposite.[2386]

If you take a lean study subject and covertly double the calorie concentration of the formula, they unconsciously cut their consumption in half to continue to perfectly maintain their weights. Their bodies somehow detected the change in calorie load and sent signals to their brains to press the button half as often to compensate. Do the same thing with obese persons, and nothing changes. They continue to undereat just as much as before. Their bodies appeared incapable of detecting or reacting to the change in calorie load, suggesting a physiological inability to regulate intake.[2387]

Could the brains of obese people somehow be insensitive to internal satiety signals? We don't know if it's cause or effect—that is, maybe that's why they're obese in the first place, or maybe the body knows how obese it is and is shutting down the hunger drive regardless of the calorie concentration. Indeed, the obese subjects continued to steadily lose weight eating out of the machine regardless of the calorie concentration. It would be interesting to see if they regained the ability to respond to changing caloric intake once they reached their ideal weights. Either way, what can we take from these studies to facilitate weight loss out in the real world?

Hyperpalatable Hijacking

At first glance, it might seem like a no-brainer that removing the pleasurable aspects of eating would cause people to eat less, but remember, that's not what happened. The lean study subjects continued to eat the same amount, taking in thousands of calories of the bland liquid formula. Only those who were obese dropped from eating thousands of calories a day down to just hundreds, and this happened inadvertently without them even feeling the difference. Only after eating was disconnected from the reward was the body able to start rapidly reining in the weight.

We have two separate appetite control systems: the homeostatic system and the hedonic system. The homeostatic pathway maintains our calorie balance by making us hungry when energy reserves are low and abolishing our appetites when energy reserves are high. In contrast, our hedonic, or reward-based, regulation can overwhelm our homeostatic pathways in the face of highly palatable foods.[2388] This makes total sense from an evolutionary standpoint.[2389] In the rare cases in our ancestral history when we'd stumble across some calorie-dense food, like a cache of unguarded honey, it would make sense for our hedonic drives to take over the driver's seat to speed us toward devouring the scarce commodity. Even if we didn't need the extra calories at the time, our bodies wouldn't want us to pass up the rare opportunity.

Nowadays, such opportunities are not so rare anymore. With sugary, fatty foods everywhere we look, our hedonic drives may end up in perpetual control, overwhelming the intuitive wisdom of our bodies.

The Spice of Life

How did we evolve to solve the daunting task of selecting a diet that supplies all the essential nutrients? Dietary diversity. By eating a variety of foods, we increase our chances of hitting all the bases. If we ate solely for pleasure, we might just stick with our favorite foods to the exclusion of all others. Thankfully, we have an innate tendency to switch things up.

For example, we end up eating more calories when provided with three different yogurt flavors than just one, even if that one and only one is our chosen favorite.[2390] So variation can trump sensation. This appears to be something we're born with. Studies on newly weaned infants dating back nearly a century show that babies naturally choose a variety of foods even over their one preferred food.[2391] This tendency seems to be driven by a phenomenon called *sensory-specific satiety.*[2392]

Within minutes, the pleasantness of the taste, smell, texture, and appearance of an eaten food drops off compared to the uneaten foods.[2393] It's like how the first bite of chocolate tastes better than the tenth bite. Our bodies tire of the same sensations and seek out novelty by rekindling our appetites every time we're presented with new foods. This helps explain the "dessert effect," where we can be stuffed to the gills but get a second wind when dessert arrives.[2394]

What was adaptive for our ancient ancestors to maintain nutritional adequacy, however, may be maladaptive in the age of overabundance and obesity.

Feed people a four-course meal, and they eat 60 percent more calories than when presented with the same dish served at each of the four courses.[2395] It's not just due to boredom. Our bodies have different physiological reactions. Give people a squirt of lemon juice, and their salivary glands respond with a squirt of saliva. But give someone a squirt of lemon juice ten times in a row, and they salivate less and less each time. What happens if you switch to lime juice? Their salivation jumps right back up.[2396] We're hardwired to respond differently to new foods.

On the same plate,[2397] at the same meal,[2398] or even on subsequent days,[2399] the greater the variety, the more we tend to eat. Give overweight kids the same mac 'n cheese dinner five days in a row, and they end up eating hundreds of fewer calories by the fifth day compared to kids who got a variety of different meals each day.[2400] Even just switching the *shape* of food can lead to overeating. Give kids the same mac 'n cheese but change the elbow macaroni to spiral noodles, and they end up eating significantly more of the new pasta shape.[2401] Even *perceived* variety may get people to eat more. Give people a bowl filled with ten different colors of M&M's, and even though all the colors taste the same, people reportedly eat 43 percent more than if there were only seven colors of the candies offered.[2402] The greater the difference, the greater the effect. Alternating between sweet and savory foods can have a particularly appetite-stimulating effect. In this way, adding a diet soda to a fast-food meal can lead to overconsumption.

The staggering array of modern food choices may be one of the factors conspiring to undermine our appetite control.[2403] There are now tens of thousands of different foods being sold.[2404] In fact, the wide variety available at our groceries is one of the most successful ways to make rats fat. When researchers first tried to make rats fat in a lab, it didn't work. The richer the rat chow, the less the rats ate to maintain their weights. Attempt after attempt failed. "We therefore used a more extreme diet," the researchers recalled. "We fed rats an assortment of palatable foods purchased at a nearby supermarket (e.g., cookies, cheese, marshmallows, chocolate.)" And what do you know? On what became known as the *supermarket diet* (and later the *cafeteria diet*), the animals rapidly gained weight.[2405]

It's kind of like the opposite of the original food-dispensing device. Instead of the all-you-can-eat bland liquid, researchers offered free all-you-can-eat access to elaborate vending machines stocked with forty trays with a dizzying array of beverages and foods like pastries and french fries. Participants seemed to find it impossible to maintain energy balance, consuming an average of 127 percent of their calorie requirements.[2406]

Our understanding of sensory-specific satiety can be used to get people to gain weight, but how can we use it to our advantage? For example, would limiting the variety of unhealthy snacks help people lose weight? Two randomized controlled trials attempted, yet failed, to show significantly more weight loss in the reduced variety groups, but they also failed to get people to make much of a dent in their diets at all. Just cutting down on a few snack types seems insufficient to make much of a difference.[2407,2408] A more drastic change may be needed.

Meatball Monotony and Veggie Variety

Sensory-specific satiety may be one of the reasons meal replacements and fad "mono diets" like the cabbage soup diet and the oatmeal diet can result in better adherence and lower ratings of hunger compared to less restrictive diets.[2409]

An all-potato diet would probably take the (Yukon) gold for blandest and most monotonous and satiating. In fact, in "A Satiety Index of Common Foods," the landmark study I mentioned in the Rich in Legumes section in which dozens of foods were put to the test, the most satiating food researchers found was the boiled potato.[2410] Two hundred and forty calories of boiled potatoes were found to be more satisfying in terms of quelling hunger than the same number of calories of any other food they tested. No other food even came close.

No doubt the low calorie density played a role. To feed people 240 calories of potatoes, they had to feed them nearly a pound of spuds, compared to just a few cookies, but that's kind of the point. They did have to feed people even more apples, grapes, and oranges, though, yet each of those fruits was still about 40 percent less satiating than the potatoes.[2411]

The mono diet is the poster child for unsustainability—and thank heavens for that. Over time, eating just one thing day after day can lead to serious nutrient deficiencies—like blindness from vitamin A deficiency in the case of white potatoes.[2412] The satiating power of potatoes can still be brought to bear, though. Boiled potatoes beat out pasta and rice in terms of a satiating side dish, cutting as much as about two hundred calories of intake off a meal.[2413] Fried potatoes or even baked fries, however, do not appear to have the same satiating effect.[2414]

To exploit sensory-specific satiety for weight loss while maintaining nutrient abundance, you could limit the variety of unhealthy foods you eat, while expanding the variety of healthy foods.[2415] In that way, you can simultaneously take advantage of the appetite-suppressing effects of monotony, while diversifying your fruit-and-vegetable portfolio. Studies have shown that a greater variety of calorie-dense foods like sweets and snacks is associated with excess body fat, but a greater variety of vegetables appears protective.[2416] When presented with more diverse options of fruits,[2417] vegetables,[2418] and vegetable seasonings,[2419] people may consume a larger quantity, crowding out less healthy options.

For the first twenty years of the *Dietary Guidelines for Americans,* it recommended generally eating "a variety of foods." In the new millennium, the guidelines have gotten more precise, specifying a diversity of healthier foods only. As dietitians at Harvard and NYU concluded in a paper on dietary variety as an overlooked weight-loss strategy, "Choose and prepare a greater variety of plant-based foods," recognizing that a greater variety of less healthy options could be counterproductive.[2420]

FOOD FOR THOUGHT

How can we respond to industry attempts to lure us into temptation by turning our natural biological drives against us? Should we never eat really delicious food? No, but it may help to recognize the effects hyperpalatable foods can have on hijacking our appetites and undermining our bodies' better judgment. We can also use some of those same primitive impulses to our advantage by monotonizing our choices of the bad and diversifying our choices of the good. Try picking out a new fruit or vegetable every time you shop.

In my own family's home, we always have a wide array of healthy snacks on hand to entice the finickiest of tastes. The contrasting collage of colors and shapes in fruit baskets and vegetable platters beats out boring bowls of a single fruit because they make you want to mix it up and try a little of each. And with different dipping sauces, the possibilities are endless!

RECIPE FOR SUCCESS

Below are the seventeen ingredients for an optimum weight-loss diet laid out in worksheet form.

In that first blank column, you can place a dietary pattern, a meal, or even an individual food. Try penciling in some of the new diets you've heard about. How do they rate? How many boxes can you tick off? A paleo diet, for example, might nail the fruit-and-vegetables box but fail the legumes one.

	anti-inflammatory	clean	↑fiber	↑water	↓glycemic	↓fat	↓sugar	↓addictive	↓calorie density	↓meat	↓refined grains	↓salt	↓insulin	↑microbiome	↑fruits & vegetables	↑legumes	↑satiating

The next time you sit down for supper, look at your meal and see how many checkmarks it earns. You can imagine how a typical fast-food meal might get a big goose egg—zero out of seventeen—whereas a healthy Mediterranean meal might hit eleven or more due to its vegetable-centric nature. A traditional Mediterranean bean-and-vegetable stew would be anti-inflammatory, low on the food chain, and high in fiber, trapped water, and veggies, have a low glycemic load and insulin index, be free of habit-forming ultraprocessed foods, and could be low in added fat, sugar, meat, salt, and refined grains. The beans check off legumes and microbiome-building, and soups are particularly satiating and low in calorie density. So that one stew could potentially knock off all seventeen optimal weight-loss ingredients. If you had it with bread dipped in oil, though, the meal as a whole might fail to meet the glycemic and insulin response criteria, as well as the added fat, refined grains, and sodium conditions, but it would still be better than most meals people eat.

Every meal is a new opportunity to tick as many boxes as you can. Imagine looking over a Chinese takeout menu. Some items, like General Tso's Chicken—deep-fried meat served in a sugary sauce atop white rice—may not include any of the optimum weight-loss ingredients, whereas a dish from the vegetable section—like broccoli with garlic sauce—might incorporate at least half of them. At a quick-service Mexican joint, a bean burrito bowl salad could let you tick off most of them, especially if you hold the white rice, but nothing beats the control you have at home to prepare a healthy dish without added salt, sugar, and fat.

To reverse engineer the optimal weight-loss diet, we can figure out what constitutes the ideal meal by ranking individual foods—and the more boxes they check, the better. Most fruits and vegetables would top the list at sixteen out of seventeen. By my count, legumes, whole grains, and nuts and seeds together would hit fifteen, fourteen, and thirteen, respectively, but refined grains and animal products would slip down into single digits. Ultraprocessed fatty and sugary snacks might only score one or two, and a product that's both, like Slim Jim's maple-flavored bacon jerky, might completely flop.

Note that some of these criteria are much more important than others. For example, while the value of eating anti-inflammatory foods remains theoretical, there are multiple randomized controlled trials validating the benefits of reducing calorie density. Read through the sections and decide which are most convincing to you and may be easiest to fit into your daily routine.

To varying degrees, any one of these criteria alone may facilitate weight loss. Even just cutting out added sugars without making any other changes at all, for example, could cause you to lose weight.

Now imagine if you tried putting them all together.

III. The Optimal Weight-Loss Diet

INTRODUCTION

Beyond the Seventeen Ingredients

Diets don't work almost by definition. Going on a diet implies that, at some point, you will go off the diet. Short-term fixes are no match for long-term problems.[2421] Lifelong weight control requires lifelong lifestyle changes. That's why there are four other factors that need to be considered alongside my seventeen efficacy criteria, bringing us to twenty-one total ingredients for an optimal weight-loss diet. See the chart on the next page.

First, a diet has to be sustainable. Consider water-only fasting, for example. No diet works better. It's 100 percent effective, but also 100 percent fatal if you manage to stick with it. This is why an optimal weight-loss diet needs additional building blocks to ensure long-term viability.

As well as being efficacious and sustainable, it needs to be safe. Books touting liquid protein diets in the 1970s sold millions of copies, but the diets started killing people.[2422] Safety is about losing weight without losing your health.

Any long-term eating pattern must also be nutritionally complete, containing all essential vitamins and minerals. A vegan diet, for example, can fail at this criterion, as it lacks vitamin B12, which is not made by plants but by microbes that blanket the earth. In today's sanitized modern world, we now chlorinate

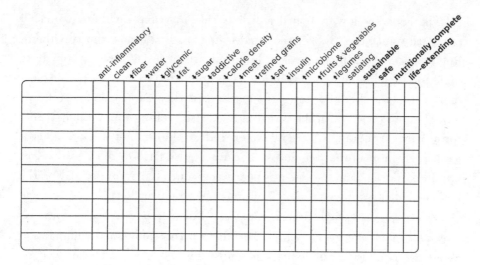

the water supply to kill off any bacteria, so we don't get a lot of B12 in our water anymore—but we don't get a lot of cholera either, which is a good thing! Without that vitamin, though, vegans eventually risk blindness,[2423] psychosis,[2424] paralysis,[2425] and death,[2426] which is why B12 supplements or B12-fortified foods are critically important for anyone adopting a plant-based diet.[2427]

And finally, our chosen diets should be life-extending. At the very least, what we eat shouldn't cut our lives short and ideally should be healthy enough to improve our life spans. There's no point in losing weight if it causes you to lose it all.

Low-Carb Diets Don't Hold Water

So what diet contains the most of the twenty-one ingredients for weight loss? Let's start with the classic dichotomy: low-carb versus low-fat. A meta-analysis of forty-eight randomized trials of various branded diets found that those advised to eat low-carb diets and those told to eat low-fat diets lost nearly identical amounts of weight after a year (averaging 7.25 kg and 7.27 kg, respectively, about 16 pounds).[2428] High attrition rates and poor dietary adherence complicate comparisons of efficacy,[2429] but you can see how both approaches tick off important checkboxes. The four largest calorie contributors in the American diet are (1) refined grains, (2) added fats, (3) meat, and (4) added sugars.[2430] Low-carb diets cut down on #1 and #4, and low-fat diets tend to cut down on #2 and #3.

The hook for low-carbohydrate diets that may explain their recurring popularity since the 1860s is the rapid water loss that can accompany them. Put people on a ketogenic, eight-hundred-calorie-a-day, low-carbohydrate diet, and they lose ten pounds in ten days, compared to only six pounds lost on the same number of calories of a higher-carb diet. Same calories, yet four more pounds gone. What the bathroom scale isn't telling you, though, is that those four extra pounds were all water. Indeed, in the first week of a ketogenic diet, most of the weight lost is in water, not fat. On those same eight hundred calories a day, *fat* loss was nearly the same (163.4 grams a day on the ketogenic diet compared to 166.7 grams on the regular diet).[2431]

When you eat carbohydrates, your body bulks up your muscles with glycogen for quick energy. Eat a high-carb diet for three days, and you may add about two pounds of muscle mass on your arms and legs.[2432] Those glycogen stores drain away on a low-carb diet and pull water out with them. The ketones also need to be flushed out of the kidneys on a ketogenic diet, accounting for the diuretic effect.[2433]

The thrill of seeing the pounds drop so quickly on the scale, though, keeps many keto crazy. When the diet fails, the dieters often blame themselves, but the intoxication of the initial rapid weight loss may tempt them back. It's like getting drunk again after forgetting how terrible the last hangover felt. This has been dubbed the *false hope syndrome*. The diet business thrives off two things—preposterous promises and repeat customers—and one leads naturally to the other.[2434]

Heartbreakers

The authors of the meta-analysis that found the same weight loss for both low-carb and low-fat diets concluded, "This supports the practice of recommending any diet that a patient will adhere to in order to lose weight."[2435] That seems like terrible advice. Would they recommend the Last Chance Diet, which evidently consisted of a "liquid formula made from leftover byproducts from a slaughterhouse,"[2436] that was linked to at least sixty deaths?[2437] An ensuing failed lawsuit, *Smith v. Linn,* from one widower set the precedent for First Amendment protection for deadly diet books.[2438]

The health impacts of a typical low-carb ketogenic diet like Atkins are vastly different from a low-fat, plant-based diet like Dean Ornish's. Not only would they have diametrically opposed effects on cardiovascular risk factors in theory (based on fiber, saturated fat, and cholesterol contents),[2439] but when low-carb diets were actually put to the test, they were indeed found to impair artery function.[2440] Over time, blood flow to the heart muscle itself has been shown to improve on an Ornish-style diet while it diminished on a low-carb diet.[2441]

It is possible to construct a healthy low-carb diet[2442] or an unhealthy low-fat diet (a diet of cotton candy would be *zero* fat), but heart disease tends to progress on typical weight-loss diets[2443] and actively worsen on low-carb diets,[2444] but may be reversed by a healthy plant-based diet.[2445] Given that heart disease is the number one killer of men and women, "recommending any diet that a patient will adhere to in order to lose weight" seems irresponsible.

Making Daily Allowances

When people diet, they often increase their risk of not meeting all their essential nutrient requirements. Ketogenic diets tend to be so nutritionally vacuous that one assessment estimated that in order to get a sufficient daily intake of all essential vitamins and minerals, you'd have to eat 37,500 calories a day.[2446] Choosing a healthier diet may be easier than adding about fifty sticks of butter to your morning coffee.

A comparison of dietary quality of popular weight-loss plans scored Ornish's low-fat, plant-based diet the highest and Atkins's low-carb, more ketogenic diet the lowest.[2447] In general, using a variety of nutritional quality indexes, researchers found that the more plant-based people eat, the healthier their diet scores.[2448] Ironically, even though plant-based eaters are restricting entire categories of foods, they end up getting more nutrition. A paper entitled "A Vegetarian Dietary Pattern as a Nutrient-Dense Approach to Weight Management" found that those eating more plant-based were getting higher intakes of nearly every nutrient: more fiber, more vitamin A, more vitamin C, more vitamin E, more of the B vitamins thiamine, riboflavin, and folate, and more of the minerals calcium, magnesium, and iron.[2449] This came as no surprise. The *Journal of the American Dietetic Association* editor in chief responded, "What could be more nutrient dense than a vegetarian diet?"[2450]

These days, it seems that most published cases of classic nutrient-deficiency syndromes showing up in U.S. emergency rooms are people eating crazy diets. An American servicemember hospitalized for a muscle tear due to scurvy reported eating only two things: chicken without the skin and candy bars.[2451] Ironically, one of the healthiest eating patterns, an exclusively plant-based diet, is perhaps the most life-threateningly incomplete, lacking B12, a vitamin made by bacteria, as I mentioned earlier. In our modern sanitary world, vitamin B12 is found reliably only in animal products, supplements, and B12-fortified foods. Vegetarians and vegans are recommended to take supplements containing at least 50 mcg of cyanocobalamin (the most stable form[2452]) a day or at least 2,000 mcg once a week[2453] (or brush twice daily with a B12-fortified toothpaste[2454]).

We're getting closer to the optimal weight-loss diet, but we aren't quite there—yet.

Having It Both Ways

Just because a weight-loss technique is effective doesn't mean it's healthy. Smoking is the classic example. I will not be including a chapter on choosing the best cigarettes, nor will I explore how best to infect yourself with tuberculosis or develop an addiction to methamphetamine. The goal of weight loss is not to lighten the load for your pallbearers.

Thankfully, you don't need to mortgage your long-term health for short-term weight loss. We can have the best of both worlds. Think about the foods that ranked highest in the ideal weight-loss criteria—whole plant foods such as fruits and vegetables. As I explored in *How Not to Die,* these are the very same foods that in some cases may help prevent each of our top fifteen killers: (1) heart disease, (2) lung diseases, (3) iatrogenic ("death by doctor") causes, (4) brain diseases, (5) digestive cancers, (6) infections, (7) diabetes, (8) high blood pressure, (9) liver diseases, (10) blood cancers, (11) kidney disease, (12) breast cancer, (13) suicidal depression, (14) prostate cancer, and (15) Parkinson's disease.

The best-of-both-worlds eating pattern may therefore be a whole food, plant-based diet.

PLANT YOURSELF

A plant-based diet is defined as an eating pattern that minimizes the intake of meat, eggs, dairy, and processed junk and maximizes consumption of whole plant foods, such as fruits, vegetables, legumes (beans, split peas, chickpeas, and lentils), whole grains, nuts and seeds, mushrooms, and herbs and spices.[2455] Plant-based is often confused with vegetarian or vegan, but it can have very different health implications. Vegetarian (meat-free but may include eggs and dairy) and vegan (free of any animal-derived ingredients) diets may exclude animal products for religious or ideological reasons without necessarily focusing on healthy choices.

An exhaustive collation of pooled meta-analyses and systematic reviews on the chronic health effects of different food groups has been published, and 96 percent of the reviews on whole plant foods associated them with effects that were protective or neutral. At the same time, 77 percent of the reviews on animal-based foods and 90 percent of those on refined grain and sugary drinks linked them to having deleterious or neutral effects. So, when it comes to diet-related diseases, such as cancer, diabetes, or heart, bone, or liver conditions, nine out of ten study compilations show that whole plant foods are, in the very least, not bad, whereas eight or nine out of ten of the reviews on animal products or processed foods show them to be not good.[2456]

Easy as Pie

Just because a diet is healthy and effective doesn't mean it's sustainable. Obviously, diets can only work if people can stick with them. When Dean Ornish, the first to prove heart disease could be reversed with a plant-based lifestyle program, criticized the authors of a famous Mediterranean diet study for exaggerating the benefits—noting there was no reduction in heart attack rates or overall mortality[2457]—the authors replied, acknowledging Ornish-type diets might be superior but the "major problems . . . are its poor palatability and the marginal long-term compliance."[2458] Excuse me? In reality, Ornish and others got extraordinary adherence with healthy plant-based diets, with no differences noted in any measured acceptability scores. For example, study participants reported the same level of enjoyment compared to their regular diets.[2459] They even got success in barbecue country, rural North Carolina.[2460] Stricter diets may meet greater acceptance because they may work better. Ornish and colleagues showed that greater adherence meant greater disease reversal.[2461]

Even those who are young and healthy with no health issues appear to have little problem sticking to a plant-based diet. There was a crossover study in which women were instructed to eat plant-based foods for a few months to see how it would affect their menstrual cycles. But then they were to switch back to their baseline diets to note the contrast, a so-called A-B-A study design where you reverse the experimental variable. The problem is that some participants felt so good eating healthfully—they were losing weight without any calorie counting or portion control, they had more energy, their periods got better, and they experienced better digestion and better sleep—that some refused to go back to their regular diets, which kind of messes up the study.[2462] Because they didn't comply with the protocol and go back to their baseline diets, their data had to be thrown out. So, ironically, the plant-based diet worked a little too well.

Leaner and Greener

With enough portion control, anyone can lose weight. Lock someone in a room, and you can force them to lose as much body fat as you want. Chaining someone to a treadmill could have a similar effect. But what is the most effective weight-loss regimen that doesn't involve caloric restriction or exercise (or a felony)? If you look throughout the published, peer-reviewed medical literature at all the randomized controlled trials, what is the single most successful strategy? If you've been paying close attention, you should be able to hazard a guess.

Let's run through the ingredients for an optimal weight-loss diet. Which eating pattern contains the most anti-inflammatory foods? Which is cleanest, the lowest in potentially obesogenic pollutants? Which diet is highest in fiber- and water-rich foods, yet lowest in addictive and processed foods, glycemic and insulin loads, calorie density, fat, meat, refined grains, salt, and sugar? Which is friendliest to our microbiomes, satiating, and rich in fruits, vegetables, and legumes, while, at the same time, is safe, sustainable, nutritious, and healthy?

It should come as no surprise that the most successful intervention to date is a whole food, plant-based diet.[2463] And as we'll see, unlike entirely too many weight-loss methods where you're forced to essentially mortgage your health to achieve short-term gains, plant-based diets offer the best of both worlds: effectiveness and healthfulness.

Any diet that results in reduced caloric intake can cause weight loss. Dropping pounds isn't so much the issue; the problem is keeping them off. A key difference between plant-based nutrition and more traditional approaches to weight loss is that people are encouraged to eat ad libitum, which is, as I've noted, Latin for *at one's pleasure*. In other words, people on a healthy enough plant-based diet can eat as much as they want. No calorie counting, no portion control—just eating. The strategy is improving the quality of the food rather than restricting the quantity of the food.

We've known for more than thirty years that those eating predominantly plant-based diets weigh, on average, about twenty to thirty pounds less than the general population.[2464,2465] The largest such study, which involved more than ninety thousand people, found that the more plants people ate, the lower their weights seemed to drop.[2466]

To review again, a body mass index of 30 or higher is considered obese, 25–29 is overweight, and under 25 is "normal." Well, not so normal anymore. Given that the average American today is overweight, a BMI under 25 is more of an *ideal* weight. In the ninety-thousand-person study, the average BMI of nonvegetarians was 28.8, bordering on obesity.[2467] Semi-vegetarians or flexitarians, those who ate meat a few times a month but not every week, were at a BMI of 27.3. Those who ate no meat except fish came in at 26.3, and vegetarians were at 25.7. *Vegetarian diet* may seem a contradiction in terms, since how many vegetarians are on diets? But in the United States, even the average vegetarian is overweight. Only those eating purely plant-based diets were, on average, at an ideal weight with an average BMI of 23.6.[2468] However, as I've said again and again, it's certainly not all or nothing.

Those who eat meat regularly may still benefit from eating more plants. One study found that whole plant foods constituted about 10 percent of the diets of obese individuals, 20 percent of the diets of those overweight but not (yet) obese, and closer to 30 percent for ideal-weight individuals.[2469] When whole plant foods made up about 40 percent of the diet, weight gain tended to decline with age rather than creep up.[2470] Although 40 percent might not sound like a lot, because unprocessed plant foods tend to be so low in calorie density, getting 40 percent of your calories from whole plant foods may mean they take up 75 percent of your plate.

Tracking people over time, those who already eat plant-based diets or even just move toward eating more plants tend to gain less weight.[2471] Every additional year of eating purely plant-based is associated with a 7 percent drop in obesity risk among adults.[2472] In school-aged children, meat, eggs, and dairy consumption has been associated with higher odds of obesity, whereas plant-based equivalents like veggie burgers were not, and whole plant foods like grains, beans, and nuts appeared to be protective.[2473]

These kinds of data led the former chair of the nutrition department at Loma Linda University[2474] (as well as Dr. Benjamin Spock,[2475] perhaps the most esteemed pediatrician of all time) to suggest raising our kids plant-based to help combat the childhood obesity epidemic. Getting diabetes as a child can cut nearly twenty years off their life.[2476] What parent wouldn't go to the ends of the earth to add decades to their children's lives? We need to realize that we are making life-and-death decisions at the grocery store when we buy food for our families.

Heftier Diets, Lighter Bodies

Obesity rates among vegans may run as low as 2–3 percent,[2477] which makes it difficult to tease out the health effects of plant-based eating. Are the lower disease rates associated with plant-based eating due directly to the diet itself or indirectly to the ease of weight loss and maintenance? To find control groups of individuals eating typical diets who were as slim as a group of whole-food vegans, studies have had to recruit long-distance endurance athletes running an average of forty-eight miles per week for twenty-one years. Apparently, people who run the equivalent of almost two marathons a week for two decades can be as slim as a vegan no matter what they eat! What's more, the purely plant-based eaters in the studies were sedentary, exercising for less than an hour a week.[2478] So run two thousand miles a year, and your weight may rival that of some vegan couch potatoes? What's their secret?

The simplest explanation is that those eating more plant-based may just be eating fewer calories—as many as 464 fewer calories a day, in fact.[2479] That would certainly do it. That's nearly the 500-a-day caloric restriction recommended in the federal dietary guidelines for weight loss.[2480] But this calorie reduction was achieved without significantly changing the amount of food eaten. Some studies show that those eating purely plant-based diets are actually eating nearly a half pound more food a day compared to nonvegetarians.[2481] That's the beauty of foods with low calorie density: more food, less weight.

Metabolic Boost

Yes, those eating plant-based may be eating fewer calories, but they may also *need* fewer calories. Heavier people have higher calorie requirements because of the energy it takes just to move around all that extra mass, so it could go both ways. Higher caloric intake can lead to obesity, and obesity can also lead to higher caloric intake. But in fact, some studies have found that those eating more plant-based had the same[2482,2483] or even higher caloric intakes,[2484,2485] which makes it even more curious that plant-based eaters are slimmer.

A study in Israel, for example, found that vegetarians weighed about twenty pounds less than nonvegetarians, yet they appeared to be eating about four hundred more calories every day.[2486] As we saw in the High in Fiber-Rich Foods section, it's not what you eat but what you absorb, and the Israeli vegetarians were eating extraordinarily healthy diets, averaging nearly seventy grams of fiber a day. This could help explain why those eating more whole plant foods seem to lose more weight even at the same estimated caloric intake.[2487] Interestingly, a similar paradox arose in rural China at even half the fiber intake.[2488]

Before the Westernization of their diets, the rural Chinese got about 90 percent of their protein from plants. Even the least active "office workers" ate 30 percent more calories than Americans, yet were 25 percent leaner.[2489] Of course, they may have been biking to the office or something, but the calories still didn't seem to add up. It turns out that those eating more plant-based may effectively be burning more calories in their sleep.

In 1994, researchers discovered that those eating more plant-based for at least two years had an 11 percent higher resting metabolic rate.[2490] Their metabolisms just seemed to be revved up naturally, which could help account for the greater weight loss. However, three subsequent studies failed to replicate this finding, but the reported fiber intakes of those studies averaged only eleven grams a day,[2491,2492,2493] which is less than what is consumed on the Standard American Diet. The only way for vegetarians to get that little fiber is to center their diets around highly processed junk. (The rural Chinese, in comparison, were getting thirty-three grams a day.) The latest study, which involved a more respectable fiber intake, found a 22 percent higher resting metabolic rate, which translates into burning off hundreds of extra calories a day without doing a thing. The researchers concluded that this "underlines the need to encourage people to follow a plant-based diet."[2494]

Eat Seven Pounds, Lose Seven Pounds

All the studies that have consistently shown that those who eat more vegetarian meals tend to be slimmer could have been confounded by other diet or lifestyle factors. Even the studies that take such factors as physical activity, smoking, and socioeconomic class into account may not control for other dietary aspects. For example, vegetarians and vegans tend to drink less soda, eat fewer sweets, and use less added fats.[2495] Maybe any eat-less-junk-food diet would have similar benefits. You don't know until you put it to the test.

A meta-analysis of a dozen randomized controlled trials involving more than a thousand research subjects found that those placed in the more plant-based groups lost significantly more weight.[2496] This included studies that compared plant-based nutrition to other diets also emphasizing healthier eating. A larger systematic review of clinical trials lasting at least a month or more found that those who stuck to the more plant-based diets lost about ten pounds, and this was without any instruction for exercise or caloric restriction. Even more remarkably, weight loss wasn't even the specific goal for most of the studies. They were just set up to test the effects of plant-based diets on conditions like arthritis, diabetes, or painful periods, and the weight loss appeared to be just an inadvertent, happy side effect.[2497]

Just like in the observational studies showing the more plant-based people ate, the leaner they appeared to be, the same trend was uncovered when people were randomized to different degrees of plant-based eating.[2498] Those randomized to eat purely plant-based lost more weight than those just avoiding meat, as well as those eating pesco-vegetarian, semi-vegetarian, or full omnivore. By the end of the six-month study, those randomized to eat a completely plant-based diet lost twice as much weight compared to those who ate any fish or other meat, with 7.5 percent of their body weights lost, compared to about 3 percent.[2499] That may only translate into a few pounds of steady weight loss a month, but, again, this was achieved without added exercise, calorie counting, or portion control. Subjects on the plant-based diet were instructed to eat however much they wanted, whenever they wanted. That's the kind of diet one can stick to long term.

Those who follow a whole food, plant-based diet for years can lose dozens of pounds.[2500] In Dr. Dean Ornish's landmark heart disease reversal study, those randomized to the plant-based lifestyle group dropped an average of twenty-four pounds even though most weren't obese or explicitly attempting to lose weight, and they did so while eating as much as they wanted.[2501] They did, however, have the added motivation of a heart disease diagnosis to stick with the program.

Residential plant-based programs, where you may stay in a spa-like setting for a week, can be very successful for the time you're there. For example, participants in Dr. John McDougall's live-in program lose an average of three pounds a week eating unlimited, all-you-can-eat buffets.[2502] One whole-food immersion demonstrated more than seven pounds lost in one week eating nearly seven pounds of food a day.[2503] Live-in programs can be great for optimizing clinical benefits because they can exert greater control over people's diets, but not only are such programs expensive, participants are dumped right back into their toxic food environments at home—the very ones that caused the problems in the first place.

Hans Diehl, the first director of research at the Pritikin Center, recognized the limitations of the live-in approach. Inspired by the amazing results he was seeing (including those of a certain beloved Grandma Greger), he developed a volunteer-run education program that could be offered in the community. He called it *CHIP*, the Coronary Health Improvement Project.

The Weight-Loss Program That Got Better with Time

Residential lifestyle programs can cost thousands of dollars in addition to missed work time, whereas CHIP was designed to be cheap. And what good is it to spoon-feed people an ideal diet only to unleash them back home to their cupboards of cookies? CHIP offers evening classes to teach people how to eat and stay healthy within their home environments. The focus of the program is what CHIP calls the Optimal Diet, one centered around whole plant foods. The program isn't dogmatic. Instead, it simply encourages people to move along the spectrum toward incorporating more "foods as grown" into their diets.[2504]

CHIP doesn't provide meals—just advice and encouragement, empowering people with knowledge.[2505] Within a month on the program, blood sugars, cholesterol, and blood pressures dropped enough for many participants to drop their antidiabetic, cholesterol-lowering, and blood pressure—lowering medications. Better numbers on fewer drugs, along with an average six-pound weight loss.[2506] But what about long term? The only true test of any lifestyle intervention is whether or not it actually changes your lifestyle. So researchers followed up with CHIP participants after eighteen months to see if any of the healthy habits stuck.

By the end of the four-week educational program, people were averaging about three hundred fewer calories per day, even though they were explicitly told to eat as much as they wanted.[2507] There was no calorie or carb counting and no portion control. Instead of eating less food, they just ate healthier food. Great news, but that three hundred fewer daily calories was the case immediately after four weeks of classes. Where were the participants eighteen months later?

Those familiar with weight-loss studies know how this works. You can excite anyone in the short term to lose weight using nearly any kind of diet, but what happens six months later or a year later? Most tend to gain it all back, or even more. CHIP participants, who had been eating about three hundred fewer calories a day during the program, were eating *four hundred* fewer calories eighteen months later.[2508] Hold on. What kind of diet can work even *better* the longer you're on it? The participants were eating even fewer calories more than a year *after* finishing the educational program. That's one of the strengths of a diet centered around whole plant foods. Many weight-loss programs restrict caloric intake by limiting portion sizes or using meal replacements, which can result in hunger and dissatisfaction, thereby contributing to poor compliance and weight regain.[2509] The satiety-promoting, all-you-care-to-eat, plant-based, whole-food dietary approach may therefore be a potent tool for sustainable weight loss.

The CHIP program has since become perhaps the most well-published community-based lifestyle intervention in the medical literature,[2510] with studies involving more than five thousand participants.[2511] People didn't just lose weight and improve their physical health; they achieved significant improvements in feelings of stress and sleeping disorders. After four weeks on the program, there was a greater than 50 percent drop in reported insomnia, restless sleeping, easy emotional upset, and feelings of fearfulness or depression.[2512] With randomized controlled trials showing both physical[2513] and mental health[2514] benefits, CHIP's name was changed from the Coronary Health Improvement Project to the Complete Health Improvement Program.

Dr. Diehl put it best when he said:

> As a society, I think we are largely at the mercy of powerful and manipulative marketing forces that basically tell us . . . what to eat. . . . Everywhere we look, we're being seduced to the "good life" as marketers define it, but . . . this so-called "good life" has produced in this country an avalanche of morbidity and mortality [disease and death]. . . . What I would like to see in America is not this "good life" but the "best life." The best life is a simpler lifestyle—one characterized by eating more whole foods, foods-as-grown.[2515]

All in It to Win It

Dieting comes with an expiration date—the time at which we go off the diet (and all too often back to the habits that got us into trouble in the first place). Permanent weight loss requires permanent dietary changes. Healthier habits just need to become a way of life. That means the new eating pattern has to be one you can stick with and also, ideally, be health-promoting overall. If it's going to be lifelong, you want it to lead to a long life. Is it too much to ask for one diet to be effective, sustainable, and life-extending?

Might there be an inherent conflict between efficacy and sustainability? Wouldn't smaller changes be easier to maintain? Even in the barbecue capital of Memphis, Tennessee, researchers got about an 80 percent six-month compliance rate with a purely plant-based diet, with no adherence benefit found for adding a small daily portion of meat and dairy.[2516] As we've discussed, completely avoiding some problem foods may paradoxically sometimes be even easier than attempting to moderate their intakes.[2517] This is readily apparent in the substance-use literature, where entirely avoiding alcohol is more effective and, ironically, easier for a problem drinker than just cutting down.[2518]

Studies recommending greater dietary changes can produce greater changes in behavior.[2519] For example, in that study randomizing people to four different degrees of plant-based eating—(1) entirely plants, (2) just meat-free, (3) meat-free except for fish, or (4) flexitarian with some meat— all four diets ended up with similar acceptability and adherence, even among those who were initially unhappy with their assignments.[2520] In fact, even among those who ended up being noncompliant, those assigned to the completely meat-free groups ended up making more changes (and losing significantly more weight) than the omnivore controls.[2521] So rather than "All things in moderation," a better aphorism may be "Big changes beget big results."[2522] That old adage "Shoot for the moon—if you fail, you will land among the stars" was obviously written by someone without even the vaguest understanding of astronomy, but the reverse does make decent dietary sense. So *shoot for the stars!*

Success breeds success. After a few weeks of eating more healthfully, you may *feel* so much healthier that your resolve is reinforced. When surveyed, those who choose to eat plant-based for health reasons say it's mostly for general wellness or disease prevention, or to improve their energy levels or immune function. They report it gave them a sense of control over their health, helped them feel better emotionally, and improved their overall health. Most who made the transition for a specific health problem (most commonly for high cholesterol, weight loss, high blood pressure, or diabetes) say it helped them a great deal.[2523] But let's not just take their word for it. Let's put it to the test.

The Best Diet for Weight Loss

In 2017, a group of researchers in New Zealand published the BROAD study, a twelve-week randomized controlled trial bringing a whole food, plant-based diet to the poorest region of the country with the highest obesity rates. Overweight individuals were randomized to receive either standard medical care or semiweekly classes offering advice and encouragement to eat a low-fat diet centered around fruits, vegetables, whole grains, and legumes. The researchers had the subjects focus solely on diet rather than increasing exercise in order to isolate out the effects of striving to eat more healthfully. No meals were provided, and the intervention group was merely informed about the benefits of plant-based eating and encouraged to incorporate it into their own lives, families, homes, and community.[2524]

Even without any restrictions on portions and being able to freely eat all the healthy foods they wanted, the plant-based intervention group lost an average of nineteen pounds by the end of the three-month study. (The weight of the control group didn't change significantly either way.) Nineteen pounds is a respectable weight loss, but what happened next? At the end of the twelve weeks, class was dismissed and no more instruction was given.

The researchers were curious to find out how much weight the subjects had gained back after being released from the study, so everyone was invited to return at the six-month mark to get reweighed. The plant-based intervention group had left the three-month study nineteen pounds lighter. Six months later, though, they were only down about . . . twenty-seven pounds! The plant-based group had been feeling so good both physically and mentally, and had been able to come off so many of their medications, that they were sticking with the diet on their own and the weight had continued to come off.[2525]

What about a year later? Even in studies that last a whole year, where participants are coached to stay on a particular diet the entire time, by the end of the year, any initial weight lost in the first few months tends to creep back. The BROAD study's intervention had only lasted three months, yet after it was over, the participants who had been randomized to the plant-based group not only lost dozens of pounds, they kept them off.[2526]

They achieved greater weight loss at six and twelve months out than any other comparable trial in which caloric intake wasn't limited or regular exercise mandated—and that was months after the study had already ended. A whole food, plant-based diet achieved the greatest weight loss ever recorded at six and twelve months compared to any other such intervention published in the medical literature.[2527] The record-breaking study can be read in full for free at www.nature.com/articles/nutd20173.

The Best of Both Worlds

Obviously, with very-low-calorie starvation diets, you can drop people down to any weight, but quick fixes tend to quickly unravel,[2528] whereas the whole point of whole food, plant-based nutrition is to maximize long-term health and longevity. I mean, even if, for example, low-carb, ketogenic diets were found to be as effective (and they don't appear to be),[2529] the point of weight loss is not to fit into a skinnier casket.

Beyond just the increased rates of constipation, headache, bad breath, muscle cramps, general weakness, and rash reported on low-carbohydrate diets,[2530] people whose diets simply tend to sway that way appear to live significantly shorter lives.[2531] On the other hand, eating plant-based[2532] or even just trending in the direction of eating more healthy plant foods is associated with increased likelihood of living longer.[2533] Those who start out more plant-based but then add meat to their diets at least once a week not only appear to double or triple their odds of diabetes, stroke, heart diseases, and weight gain but suffer an associated 3.6-year drop in life expectancy.[2534]

Thank goodness it's hard to stick to something like a ketogenic diet, since the long-term, adverse health effects could be devastating. Whereas low-carb diets have been shown to impair artery function[2535] and worsen heart disease,[2536] whole food, plant-based diets have been shown to actually *reverse* heart disease.[2537]

So what appears to be the most effective weight-loss diet just so happens to be the only diet ever proven to reverse heart disease in the majority of patients. If that's all a plant-based diet could do—reverse the number one killer of men and women—shouldn't that be the default diet until proven otherwise? And the fact that it can also be effective in treating, arresting, and even reversing other leading killers like high blood pressure and type 2 diabetes would seem to make the case for plant-based eating simply overwhelming. Only one diet has ever been shown to do all that: a diet centered around whole plant foods.

We don't have to forsake our health to lose weight. The single healthiest diet may also be the most effective diet for weight loss.

Health by Design

Isn't it all a bit too convenient? The same foods that check off the most ideal weight-loss ingredients are the same foods that rack up the most points on health and longevity? And whole plant foods aren't just heart-healthy, but brain-, kidney-, and liver-healthy too. What are the odds?

This becomes clearer when we think about some of the underlying physiology. Yes, whole food, plant-based nutrition is the only diet proven to reverse heart disease in the majority of patients, opening up arteries without drugs or surgery. However, the heart muscle isn't the only organ that requires blood flow to bring in oxygen and nutrients and to clear out waste products. Perhaps it's no coincidence then that the diet found best to improve blood flow can support the health of all our organ systems. There are other causal factors such as inflammation that could explain why such an anti-inflammatory diet could affect multiple disease conditions at once, including obesity.

It may also be instructive to take an even further step back and look at our ancestral history. Millions of years before we learned how to sharpen spears, mill grains, or boil sugarcane, our entire physiology is presumed to have evolved in the context of eating what the rest of our great ape cousins eat—leaves, stems, and shoots (in other words, vegetables), fruits, seeds, and nuts.[2538] The Paleolithic period, when we started using tools, only goes back about two million years. We and other great apes have been evolving since the Miocene era, more like *twenty* million years ago.[2539] So for the first 90 percent of our hominoid existence, our bodies evolved on mostly plants.[2540]

We've known for more than a century that you can clog the arteries of herbivores like rabbits by feeding them meat, eggs, and dairy,[2541] but it's virtually impossible to induce atherosclerosis in a carnivore with cholesterol because that's part of their natural diets.[2542] Similarly, rats eating rat food don't get fat, but give them Oreos and it's a different story. Perhaps it's no wonder that our bodies may thrive best on the diet we were designed to eat. So maybe we should go back to our roots. (Pun intended!)

IV. Weight-Loss Boosters

INTRODUCTION

Offering maximum nutrition with minimum calories, a diet centered around whole, healthy plant foods is the best form of girth control. Whole food, plant-based nutrition best checks off the criteria for the optimal slimming diet. It's the tried-and-true recipe with the most ideal weight-loss diet ingredients—so why isn't this the end of the book?

Just eating healthfully enough should do it. Obese individuals randomized to eat plant-based at home lose nearly a cubic inch of deep visceral belly fat a week.[2543] Start packing your diet with real food that grows out of the ground, and the pounds should come off naturally, taking you down toward your ideal weight. The average person eating completely plant-based has a BMI down around the perfect range,[2544] but there is a bell curve. Even if the average is on target, some people naturally fall to either side, so I wanted to offer an array of tools that can drive or boost further weight loss for any stubborn pounds that remain.

That was the reason all the chapters in *How Not to Die* on the leading killer diseases were longer than just the three words: *Eat more plants.* Yes, those who go all in end up with perfect blood pressures and perfect cholesterol levels *on average,* for example, but if you're doing everything right and your numbers are still off, I wanted to go through all the dietary tweaks you could use to optimize your condition. That way, you could create a portfolio of specific foods to help with each specific condition. I want to do the same thing with this book.

My hope with part IV is to give you an arsenal of weapons in your fight against fat.

The average, purely plant-based person has an ideal BMI, which greatly incentivizes sticking with that way of eating, but if that's not where you end up or if you just want to get there quicker, are there specific plants that have an edge? And not some tabloid-y, fat-busting "breakthrough" extrapolated from test-tube data or mouse models but from actual randomized, controlled clinical trials showing objective outcomes?

Yes, there are specific foods shown in interventional studies to cause you to burn more fat, suppress your appetite, rev up your metabolism, block the absorption of calories, and effectively take away even more calories than they provide. What's more, the *context* in which we eat matters too. The same number of calories eaten at a different time of the day, in a different meal distribution, or after different amounts of sleep can translate into different amounts of body fat. Distinct forms of the exact same foods can be distinctly fattening. Combining certain foods together can have a different effect from eating them apart.

What we eat matters most, but how we eat and when can also make a difference.

In part II, we learned that a calorie is not necessarily a calorie. One hundred calories of chickpeas has a different impact than one hundred calories of chicken or Chiclets, based on their different effects on factors like absorption, appetite, or our microbiomes. Here in part IV, we go a step further and see that even the exact same foods eaten differently can have different effects.

Importantly, these tricks and tweaks serve to supplement a healthy, lifelong eating pattern, not replace it. Eliminating obesity requires treating the cause, the underlying diet, but this section is for those who want all the extra help they can get.

ACCOUNTABILITY

Scared Skinny

What is the most effective obesity treatment ever published in the medical literature that doesn't involve surgical fixes like jaw-wiring? The Trevose Behavior Modification Program.[2545] Named after a town in Pennsylvania, the program has been running all-volunteer, self-help support groups since 1970, offering lifetime treatment at no cost. The most demonstrably successful weight-loss program in history is free? Why haven't more people heard about it? Probably because it *is* free and doesn't have a massive promotional budget like billion-dollar corporation Weight Watchers, which spends hundreds of millions on advertising every year.[2546]

After two years on Weight Watchers, the average weight loss is about six pounds.[2547] After two years in the Trevose program, the average weight loss is thirty-nine pounds.[2548] No Weight Watchers trial has ever lasted longer than two years,[2549] but after five years in the Trevose program, participants were still down thirty-five pounds.[2550] Although that was only applicable to the 22 percent of patients who stayed in the program for five years,[2551] as many as 70 percent drop out of commercial weight-loss programs like Weight Watchers within just *three months*.[2552] What appears to be the secret to the Trevose Behavior Modification Program's success? Extreme accountability.

The Trevose program has been likened to "weight-loss boot camp,"[2553] but its rigor is in the rules, not the methods. The program utilizes the standard array of traditional techniques—calorie cutting, exercise, weekly weigh-ins, and group support—but what sets it apart is the strictness of its enforcement. If members fail to attend meetings or meet their weight-loss goals, they are kicked out immediately and can never return. The program accepts almost anyone with one critical exception: No past participants are allowed. There are no second chances, no bargaining, no do-overs, no excuses. When people sign up, they understand it is for a once-in-a-lifetime opportunity.[2554]

Weighing In

Trevose's tough-love approach may not be for everyone, but some of its key principles such as social support may be universal. A randomized trial found that group therapy tends to produce greater results than going it alone, even among those who initially expressed a preference for individual treatment.[2555] Similarly, health coaches can also help people stay engaged and accountable.[2556] Self-monitoring, another important takeaway, is considered the cornerstone of behavioral change for weight loss.[2557] Without awareness of your progress, how can you ever reach your goals?

There are now high-tech wearable activity trackers to monitor our exercise to facilitate weight loss,[2558] but the best device for monitoring caloric intake remains the humble bathroom scale. Until recently, though, frequent self-weighing for weight control was actively discouraged. Clinicians were afraid dieters might be discouraged by the slow rate of weight loss[2559] or, even worse, suffer negative psychological effects.[2560] However, evidence has since accumulated that suggests frequent weighing is a safe and effective tool for weight control.[2561]

Self-weighing was identified as a core weight-control strategy, along with exercise and a low-calorie, lower-fat diet, in the National Weight Control Registry, the largest study of individuals successful at long-term maintenance of weight loss.[2562] Of the thousands of registrants who, on average, lost about seventy pounds and kept it off for years, 79 percent weighed themselves on at least a weekly basis.[2563] Over time, a decrease in self-weighing frequency was associated with greater weight gain, but which came first? Did the lack of monitoring allow the weight to creep up, or did the creeping weight produce an ignorance-is-bliss, head-in-the-sand ostrich effect preventing you from weighing yourself?

Findings from more than a dozen such prospective studies have consistently shown regular self-weighing to be associated with successful weight loss and maintenance,[2564] but they are all stricken with the same nagging question. Does self-weighing lead to more weight loss, or might weight loss lead to more victory-lap weighing? Could there be a third factor related to both? Those with the self-discipline to weigh themselves every day may also have the self-discipline to stick more closely to a diet.[2565] What's the only way to prove cause and effect? That's right: Put it to the test.

Randomized controlled trials have shown that those assigned to daily weighing, accompanied by weekly email messaging tailored to their progress, lost more weight,[2566] were better able to resist weight gain,[2567] and maintained more weight loss.[2568] The control groups, however, received no continued monitoring, so it's hard to separate the effect of the weighing from the effect of the regular email contact. Just providing obese individuals with a scale and telling them to weigh themselves every day without giving them any useful instruction or feedback doesn't appear to help significantly.[2569]

Self-monitoring has been shown to be an effective behavioral technique for helping people eat more healthfully, exercise more,[2570] and drink less alcohol,[2571] but unlike in those cases, self-weighing is monitoring an *outcome* rather than specific behaviors.[2572] If people don't know what to do about the fact that they're gaining weight, getting on a scale may not help at all. Self-weighing is merely a feedback tool to allow for personal accountability and to offer reinforcement, both positive and negative, for whatever strategies are being employed.[2573]

The evidence supporting frequent self-weighing as a part of weight-management interventions is now considered so strong[2574] that it's been incorporated into the official weight-management guidelines put out by the Obesity Society, as well as the American Heart Association and the American College of Cardiology.[2575] The National Institutes of Health calls regular self-weighing "crucial" for long-term weight control.[2576]

So how often should we weigh ourselves? There is insufficient evidence to support a specific frequency of weighing, whether weekly or daily.[2577] One study found that twice daily—upon waking and again right before bed—appeared superior to once a day (about six pounds versus two pounds of weight loss over twelve weeks).[2578]

Early on, concerns were raised that self-weighing might be a double-edged sword, potentially putting one at risk for depression about body image issues.[2579] Thankfully, there does not appear to be an association between self-weighing and mood, self-image, or disordered eating.[2580] Although there may be a negative impact for normal-weight adolescents,[2581] self-weighing among overweight and obese adults appears to actually improve psychological health and well-being.[2582] Among those adults needing to lose weight, self-weighing seems to be associated with less depression, less disordered eating, and less body dissatisfaction, but this may be confounded by the fact that regular self-weighing improves weight loss.[2583]

FOOD FOR THOUGHT

Weigh yourself regularly to monitor your progress. If you are able to splurge, consider treating yourself on your weight-loss and mainte-nance journey with a Wi-Fi and/or Bluetooth-enabled wireless scale that can automatically transmit your data and graph your trajectory. You can even have the information sent to a friend or support group for added accountability.

AMPING AMPK

The Fat Controller

The universal energy currency in all of biology is a molecule called *adenosine triphosphate,* commonly known as *ATP.* The *tri* in triphosphate means *three,* as in tricycle or, in this case, ATP's three phosphates, where energy is stored. Plants make ATP with energy from the sun, and animals make it by burning fat, carbohydrates, and protein. The energy is spent by releasing the phosphates, which transforms ATP to AMP—adenosine *mono*phosphate, with *mono* meaning *one*—which then can be juiced up with two more phosphates back to ATP, and the cycle continues. In this way, every cell in our bodies and in every living thing is like a little rechargeable battery; AMP molecules are charged up with phosphates to ATP using sunlight or food and then drained back down to AMP to do the cell's work. This brings us to AMPK, or *AMP-activated protein kinase.*

A kinase is a type of enzyme. What might be the function of an enzyme activated by AMP? A buildup of AMP means the rechargeable battery is running low. It's akin to the fuel gauge in your car reading empty. As the needle creeps toward the *E,* what do you do? Add more fuel. But instead of having an extra gas can in your trunk, you may have junk in the trunk—fat stores on your body. So that's what AMPK does: It flips the switch in your body from storing fat to burning fat. That's why AMPK is not only known as the *master energy sensor*[2584] in our bodies but also the *fat controller.*[2585]

The discovery of AMPK is considered one of the most important biomedical breakthroughs in the last few decades.[2586] But can it be used to lose weight? If we could find a way to boost its activity, our bodies would burn more fat. The two obvious ways to deplete our energy stores to activate AMPK are exercise and fasting. Put people on a bike and start taking muscle biopsies while they cycle, and you can detect a near tripling of AMPK activity within twenty minutes.[2587] That makes sense. The muscles use up the ATP to contract, so AMP builds up and AMPK is activated. That's one of the ways exercise leads to weight loss.

AMPK activation also leads to mitochondrial biogenesis, meaning the formation of extra mitochondria, the power plants within our cells where fat is burned and ATP is created.[2588] So AMPK doesn't just cause more fat to be shoveled into the furnace—it also causes more furnaces to be built. In this way, AMPK helps explain why endurance training eventually enables us to run faster and farther. So might an AMPK activator be like the fabled exercise in a pill? Indeed, an AMPK-activator drug given to sedentary mice for a month boosted their running endurance by 44 percent.[2589] After one such drug was discovered at the famed Tour de France,[2590] AMPK activators were banned by the World Anti-Doping Agency.[2591]

Even more so than performance boosters, Big Pharma has interest in the obesity market. Obese individuals are often "unwilling to perform even a minimum of physical activity," wrote a group of pharmacologists, "thus, indicating that drugs mimicking endurance exercise are highly desirable."[2592] The thought is that AMPK activation could mimic caloric restriction, effectively fasting in a pill.[2593] When we stop eating, our energy gets depleted, so AMPK is activated and switches us over to start burning through our own fat stores. Might AMPK activation thereby allow us to reap the fat-burning benefits of exercise and fasting without the sweat and hunger?

Losing weight through AMPK activation is not that simple, since in our brains it revs up our appetites, which makes sense. Our fat stores can't last forever, so, in addition to tapping into our tummy fat, AMPK drives us to eat more to make up for the energy deficit. AMPK is one of the reasons we get hungry after a workout (or when we starve ourselves). That's the way the antipsychotic drug Zyprexa makes people gain weight—by boosting AMPK activity in the brain.[2594] So, for weight control, we'd ideally suppress the activity of AMPK in the brain but ramp it up throughout the rest of our bodies,[2595] which is exactly how nicotine appears to work.

Pepper Uppers

Smoking cigarettes may be one of the worst things you can do your body, but it's also one of the most reliable ways to lose weight.[2596] This is thought to be due to the contrasting effects nicotine has on AMPK activation in the brain and body.[2597] Randomized, double-blind, placebo-controlled studies show that nicotine reduces appetite[2598] and caloric intake.[2599] At the same time, fat biopsies taken from smokers show more than five times the AMPK activation compared to fat taken from nonsmokers.[2600] No wonder people tend to gain weight when they quit smoking,[2601] a phenomenon that can be blunted with nicotine gum.[2602]

Is there any way to get the weight-loss benefits of smoking without having to worry about the whole dying-a-horrific-death-from-lung-cancer thing? If you may remember from my Parkinson's disease chapter in *How Not to Die,* tobacco isn't the only plant with nicotine. Tobacco is a member of the nightshade family, along with tomatoes, potatoes, eggplants, and bell peppers, and they all contain nicotine as well.[2603] This is why smokers can't be identified just by looking for the presence of nicotine in their toenail clippings. Because nicotine is in the food supply, nonsmokers grow out some nicotine into their nails too.[2604]

The total amount of nicotine we eat in our daily diets is hundreds of times less than we would get from a single cigarette, though. So while we've known for at least twenty years that there's nicotine in ketchup, it's been dismissed as insignificant.[2605] We then learned that just one or two puffs of a cigarette could saturate half of our brains' primary nicotine receptors.[2606] Even the minuscule nicotine exposure from secondhand smoke may protect against Parkinson's,[2607] and we can get about the same nicotine exposure eating some vegetables in a nonsmoking restaurant that we'd get working in a smoky one.[2608]

Researchers have found that consumption of nightshade vegetables, particularly peppers and maybe tomatoes and potatoes[2609] as well, is associated with a significantly lower risk of Parkinson's disease among nonsmokers.[2610] If there is enough nicotine in these vegetables to affect Parkinson's risk, might there be enough to tweak AMPK activation? In other words, might a peck of peppers make Peter Piper less peckish?

Green pepper juice does have anti-obesity effects on mice,[2611] and a sweet pepper extract was shown to have an appetite-suppressing[2612] and abdominal fat–reducing effect on human subjects.[2613] Though there has yet to be an interventional study with actual foods to see if nightshade vegetables have a particular benefit, why not give them a try? Nonsmokers using nicotine gum can risk long-term addiction,[2614] but I've never heard of anyone becoming a stuffed pepper addict.

Raising the Barberries

More than one hundred plant products have been found to activate AMPK. Nicotine is one, and berberine, which can be found in barberries, is another.[2615] In *How Not to Die,* barberries held the distinction of making it onto two of my favorites lists, as one of my top picks for berries and also for herbs and spices.

Barberries first came across my radar as the single most antioxidant-packed dried fruit I could find. There are some exotic fruits that beat them (with Dr. Seussian names like *whortleberries*), but in terms of what I could find in stores, barberries trumped dried pomegranate seeds and goji berries, two other top contenders.[2616] Barberries are readily and inexpensively found at Middle Eastern groceries, as they're used to make a signature Persian rice dish.

Their taste is described in the medical literature as "pleasantly acidulous,"[2617] which is doctor-speak for *sour*. I had just been sprinkling them on my oatmeal because they're so tasty, but evidently they've played a prominent role in traditional systems of healing around the world for thousands of years. In fact, one pharmacology journal flamboyantly described barberries as an "herbal remedy that has no match in serving [the] human race."[2618] And I thought they were just kind of tangy.

A common problem with the herbal medicine literature is that there is often a long, impressive list of traditional uses but little or no science to back up the claims.[2619] The science that does exist is often either petri dish or lab animal data with questionable clinical applicability. Who cares if barberries have a "menstruation induction effect in guinea pig"[2620] (except maybe the guinea pig)? You end up with scientists injecting herbs into the penises of rabbits in hopes of coming up with the next Viagra,[2621] but few human studies.

That changed recently. I produced a video for NutritionFacts.org that discussed a clinical trial of barberries for acne. Teenagers randomized to take about a teaspoon of dried barberries, roughly eight cents' worth, three times a day for a month experienced a dramatic 45 percent drop in inflamed pimples compared to the placebo control group.[2622] That's great news for zits, but what about barberries for weight loss?

Purified berberine, the purported active ingredient in barberries, has been shown successfully to induce weight loss in randomized controlled studies,[2623,2624,2625] earning it a patent as a "weight-loss agent."[2626] But because the supplement industry is so poorly regulated, you never know what's in the bottle. An analysis of fifteen berberine supplements on the market found that 60 percent failed to match what was claimed on their labels.[2627]

The closest we have to a whole-food barberry intervention for weight loss is a trial from 2018. Diabetics randomized to drink about a cup of barberry juice each day for two months lost about six pounds more than those in the control group (and also had better blood sugars and pressures). Unfortunately, the researchers didn't use a placebo, like barberry-flavored Kool-Aid. The control group didn't get any intervention at all, which is problematic because we know that anytime doing *something* is compared to doing *nothing,* the placebo effect can come into play. At the same time, the barberry group received an extra ninety calories every day through the juice, yet still ended up losing more weight than the no-juice group.[2628]

A note of caution: Barberries are classified as unsafe to eat during pregnancy and are not recommended for consumption while breastfeeding.[2629] The reason so many different plants produce compounds that end up activating AMPK may be because they are trying to fend off nibbling herbivores by producing compounds that impair animal metabolism. Cyanide, for example, is an AMPK activator too. Cyanide can kill by completely blocking energy production, whereas compounds like berberine are thought to just impair our mitochondrial function, making energy production less efficient.[2630] It's this inefficiency that may be what's driving the weight loss.

Is there any way to activate AMPK without mucking with our mitochondria? Alcohol is another plant product that shouldn't be used during pregnancy and activates AMPK, but by a totally different mechanism. Alcohol is detoxified in the body into acetic acid, which our bodies have to use ATP to metabolize.[2631] AMPK is therefore activated naturally in response to the energy expenditure.[2632] The problem is that before alcohol gets fully converted into acetic acid, there's a toxic intermediate called *acetaldehyde,* which is a known carcinogen. That may be why alcohol consumption is understood to increase the risk of at least a half dozen different cancers,[2633] including breast cancer, even among light drinkers.[2634]

If only there were a way to skip the toxic step and take in acetic acid directly.

Take an Acid Trip

In a review on the role of AMPK in burning off excess body fat, an investigator concluded that "it is crucial that oral compounds with high bioavailability are developed to safely induce chronic AMPK activation . . . [for] long-term weight loss and maintenance."[2635] There is no need to develop such a compound, though, since you can already buy it any grocery store in the form of vinegar.

Acetic is derived from the Latin word *acetum,* meaning *vinegar.* By definition, vinegar is just a dilute solution of acetic acid in water.[2636] The acetic acid is absorbed and metabolized with ATP, and we get a natural AMPK boost. Enough of a boost to lose weight at the typical dose you might get dressing a salad? Evidently, vinegar has been used to treat obesity for centuries,[2637] but only recently has it been put to the test.

Researchers in Japan performed a randomized, double-blind, placebo-controlled trial on the effects of vinegar intake on the reduction of body fat in 155 overweight men and women. The subjects were randomly split into one of three groups: a high-dose vinegar group drinking a beverage containing two tablespoons of apple cider vinegar a day, a low-dose group drinking a beverage with one tablespoon of apple cider vinegar a day, or a placebo control group drinking an acidic beverage developed to taste the same as the vinegar drink but prepared with a different kind of acid so it didn't have any *acetic* acid. The researchers monitored the subjects' diets and gave each of them a pedometer to make sure the only significant difference among the three groups was the amount and type of vinegar they were getting every day.[2638]

By the end of the first month, there was already a significant drop in weight in both the high-dose and low-dose vinegar groups compared to placebo, with the high-dose group doing better than the low-dose one, and both vinegar groups continued to lose weight each month. In contrast, by month three, the do-nothing placebo group had gained weight (as overweight people tend to do), whereas the vinegar groups had dropped weight significantly. Like any weight-loss strategy, it only works if you do it. A month after the vinegar was stopped, the weight crept right back, but that's just additional evidence that the vinegar was working.[2639]

Was the weight loss simply statistically significant or actually significant? That's for you to decide. During the three-month trial, compared to the placebo group, the group taking one daily tablespoon of vinegar steadily lost about a pound a month and the group taking two daily tablespoons were down a total of about five pounds. Five pounds may not sound like a lot, but that weight loss was achieved for just pennies a day without removing anything from their diets.[2640]

The vinegar groups also got slimmer, losing about an inch off their waistlines compared to placebo, suggesting they were burning abdominal fat. The researchers went the extra mile by putting the subjects through a CT scanner. That way, they could directly measure the amount of fat before and after the trial, both the superficial fat under the skin that makes for flabby arms and contributes to cellulite, and the visceral fat, which is the fat that builds up around our internal organs and bulges out our bellies. Visceral fat is the killer fat, which is what the placebo group was putting on. Both vinegar groups, however, experienced a *drop* in visceral fat, removing about a square inch off the CT scan slice.[2641]

Perhaps, a competing research group suggested,[2642] the vinegar drinks were just so unappealing they were ruining the subjects' appetites, while somehow the placebo drink wasn't (despite being developed to taste similarly). The diets of all three groups were analyzed, and there were no significant changes in the caloric intakes of any of the groups. So same diets, yet more weight loss in the vinegar groups. That sounds like AMPK activation ignited the fat stores, but you don't know until you put it to the test.

Experiments in a petri dish on human cells (from umbilical cords, a convenient source of human tissue) show that acetic acid can amp up AMPK,[2643] but there's only one way to find out if that's what is happening in our bodies. Another randomized, double-blind, placebo-controlled trial of vinegar was performed by a research group in Korea (this time using pomegranate vinegar). The researchers found the same visceral fat loss on CT scan but took the further step of taking abdominal fat biopsies from study subjects. The fat in those on the vinegar drink was found to have nearly three times the AMPK activation compared to fat taken from those on the placebo drinks, confirming the suspected mechanism.[2644]

The CT scan and biopsies make for very expensive studies, so I was not surprised to learn that they were funded by companies that sell vinegars. On the one hand, that's good, since, otherwise, studies like this might not be performed, but on the other hand, financial conflicts of interest always raise the concern as to whether the funding source somehow manipulated the results. The nice thing about companies funding studies about *healthy* foods, though, is that there's less of a downside. I mean, what's the worst that can happen? Even if we discover one day there was vinegar company meddling and all the findings extolling the virtues of vinegar turn out to be bogus, worse comes to worst, you just would have been eating tastier salads.

Optimal Vinegar Dosing

Treating obesity wasn't the only old-fashioned medicinal use for vinegar. Before the advent of blood sugar–lowering medications, vinegar was used as a folk remedy for diabetes.[2645] Nobody bothered to formally test this, though, until 1988.[2646] After all, how much money can be made from vinegar? Apparently, millions of dollars, according to the Vinegar Institute,[2647] but a single diabetes drug can pull in billions, like Rezulin did before it was pulled from the market for killing too many people, that is (by causing liver failure).[2648] The pharmaceutical company Pfizer still made out like a bandit, though, having to pay out less than a billion dollars to the grieving families for covering up the hazards of its drug.[2649]

In a study refreshingly *not* funded by a vinegar company, two daily tablespoons of apple cider vinegar mixed into a drink reduced fasting blood sugars in prediabetics an average of sixteen points within one week, which is better than what you'd tend to see with antidiabetic drugs like Glucophage or Avandia.[2650] The vinegar was found to be safer, cheaper, and more effective. No wonder vinegar has been used medicinally since antiquity.

Adding just two teaspoons of vinegar to a high-glycemic meal (a bagel and juice) reduces the blood sugar spike by 23 percent.[2651] A meta-analysis of eleven such studies found that vinegar taken with a meal significantly improves both blood sugar and insulin responses, and it didn't seem to matter what kind of vinegar was used.[2652] Originally, we thought this was because vinegar may be delaying the stomach-emptying rate,[2653] but subsequent evidence revealed that taking vinegar at bedtime results in lower blood sugars the next morning,[2654] so it can't just be some stomach-slowing effect. The mystery was solved when a research team in Greece demonstrated that vinegar consumption improves the uptake of blood sugar by our muscles,[2655] an AMPK effect also seen with exercise.[2656]

Adding vinegar to white bread doesn't only lower blood sugar and insulin spikes—it also increases satiety, the feeling of being full after a meal.[2657] When study subjects ate about four slices of white bread, they rated their satiety a three on a scale of one to ten, so they were just a little full. Two hours later, however, they ended up hungrier than even before they had eaten the four slices. When they ate that same amount of bread with some vinegar, though, they felt twice as full, with a satiety rating of around six out of ten, and, even two hours later, still felt nearly as full as they had when they had just eaten the four pieces of bread plain.[2658]

Many cultures have taken advantage of this synergy. Vinegar is mixed with high-glycemic foods like white rice in Japan, for example, to make sushi. Sourdough breads may lower blood sugar and insulin spikes[2659] by the same mechanism.[2660] You do the same thing when you add vinegar to white potatoes to make potato salad.[2661] So if you are going to eat a high-glycemic food like white bread, dip that baguette in some balsamic.

There are some important caveats when it comes to vinegar, though. First, never drink it straight. It can cause intractable hiccups[2662] and burn your esophagus,[2663] as can apple cider vinegar tablets if they get lodged in your throat.[2664] There's another reason not to take apple cider vinegar tablets: They may not actually contain any apple cider vinegar, as was the case when eight different brands were tested.[2665] Vinegar should also never be left on skin, soaked on a bandage, for example, as it can result in third-degree burns.[2666]

How much vinegar should we take? Though as many as a total of six tablespoons a day were not associated with any short-term side effects, until we know more, I'd recommend sticking with more common culinary-type doses, like two tablespoons a day, which is considered safe.[2667] Acetic acid is metabolized quickly in the body,[2668] so I'd recommend splitting up the daily dose to activate AMPK throughout the day, rather than taking it all at once. Given the additional mealtime benefits on blood sugars, insulin, and satiety, I'd recommend taking it with food. In the clinical trials, the belly fat–burning dose was two tablespoons a day. Splitting that over three meals would be two teaspoons a meal.

Syrupy Sweet

Acetic acid is a type of short-chain fatty acid. Where have we heard that term before? You read about it in the High in Fiber-Rich Foods section earlier in the book. That's what our good bacteria make with the fiber and resistant starch we eat. When we eat whole plant foods, our gut flora can make acetic acid from scratch in our colons by fermenting the fiber. The acetic acid can then get absorbed back into our bloodstreams, so we can use the top-down approach to activate AMPK by consuming vinegar, or the bottoms-up approach by eating fiber.[2669]

Most studies on isolated prebiotic supplements and extracts for weight loss have been disappointing, with one "extreme"[2670] exception, a study on yacon syrup. Fiber and resistant starch aren't the only prebiotics. Our good bacteria also eat fructans, and a syrup made from roots of the yacon plant is a concentrated source. Yacon syrup has a caramel taste and is about half as sweet as honey[2671] but with only one-third the calories[2672] since most of the sugars are strung in the form of fructans, which we can't digest, but our friendly flora can.[2673]

A randomized, double-blind, placebo-controlled trial was performed to see if treating our flora to this bounty would help with weight loss, and the results seem too good to be true. Obese individuals randomized to just about four teaspoons of yacon syrup a day for 120 days lost nearly four inches off their waists and more than thirty pounds, whereas those on the placebo syrup gained weight.[2674]

With such extraordinary results, you'd think half the foods at the grocery store would be boasting "Now Made with Yacon!" on their labels by now. Presumably, the reason that isn't the case is that it doesn't take much to go overboard. The original study had a third part to it: People were randomized into the placebo syrup group, the four or so teaspoons of yacon syrup group, or a third group getting closer to nine daily teaspoons of yacon syrup. That larger dose group never made it into the study. That much yacon syrup may have excited their gut bacteria a little too much, resulting in such severe bloating, diarrhea, flatulence, and nausea that the entire group was excluded.[2675]

Fructans are one of the FODMAPs, which are fermentable sugars like lactose that can cause problems for some people. Those with irritable bowel syndrome, for example, who are placed on low-FODMAP diets tend to feel better. Much of this improvement may just be the placebo effect,[2676] which can run as high as 91 percent in irritable bowel syndrome (meaning just giving IBS sufferers a sugar pill can sometimes make up to nine out of ten patients feel better).[2677] The downside of giving it a try for IBS is that restricting healthy, high-FODMAP foods like apples and onions can deplete our microbiomes. FODMAP restriction has been found to result in a large reduction in beneficial *Bifidobacteria* within a matter of weeks.[2678] That's why even the research group who had come up with the FODMAP-restriction diet only recommends doing it for four weeks before starting to reincorporate the restricted foods back into the diet.[2679]

If a spoonful or two of yacon syrup doesn't cause gastrointestinal upset for you, though, then, from a weight-loss standpoint, it could be a good replacement for something like honey, which, metabolically, was found to have the same effects as table sugar and high-fructose corn syrup.[2680]

FOOD FOR THOUGHT

To amp AMPK, I recommend trying two teaspoons of vinegar with each meal. You might be thinking, *Wait—vinegar for breakfast?* Those aghast at the thought of drizzling vinegar on their oatmeal may have never heard of chocolate vinegar, strawberry vinegar, or any of the dozens of other exotic flavors out there.

See if there's a vinegar store near you where you can sample some of the more interesting varieties. That's one of the fun things I do when I'm on the road. If I'm ever in your city, stake out the vinegar store closest to my hotel and odds are we'll end up going tasting together. Unfortunately, TSA won't let me take them back on the plane in my carry-on, but most stores have an online presence and offer mail order. There are savory varieties like hickory smoke, garlic, and herb vinegars for main dishes and sweet selections like apricot and blackberry ginger—and those are just the ones I happen to have in my kitchen right now!

You can also incorporate vinegar into your meals by always having a side salad or even adding it to tea with some lemon juice. For a bonus, you can slice some bell peppers and sprinkle some barberries on your salad, and, if you sweeten your tea with honey or sugar, try yacon syrup instead.

APPETITE SUPPRESSION

Ch-Ch-Ch-Chia

Not only the name of novelty terra-cotta planter pets that sprout "hair," chia is also the edible seed of a flowering plant in the mint family. It's been eaten for thousands of years,[2681] which suggests it's at least safe to consume,[2682] but does it have any special benefits? It's certainly nutritious, providing a good source of fiber, plant protein, niacin, minerals, and antioxidants—black chia seeds perhaps more so than white[2683]—but that could describe a whole host of whole plant foods. Do chia seeds have any unique properties? Though chia seed hawkers make all sorts of claims, a recent review concluded we need to stick to the science rather than rely on cultural traditions, personal belief, or "inaccurate advertising"[2684] (as redundant a term as the cynic in me has ever heard).

There are, for example, more than fifty thousand videos on YouTube on chia seeds and belly fat, but what does the science say? Eating chia seeds does reduce belly fat—in rats[2685] and perhaps chickens.[2686] Evidently, people don't like smelling or tasting fishy chicken, so by feeding chickens chia seeds instead of fishmeal, you can boost omega-3 levels without it turning into funky chicken, but what happens if you cut out the middlehen and eat chia yourself?

In 2017, a research team in Turkey published a study investigating what happens if two or three teaspoons of chia seeds are added to a yogurt snack.[2687] After eating yogurt with chia, participants reported significantly less hunger compared to those who had had plain yogurt, which then translated into eating fewer calories a couple of hours later at lunch. When I first heard about this study, my initial thought was a bit dismissive: *Give people more food by adding chia to whatever they were eating and they're less hungry? Obviously.* But no. The researchers made sure that each snack had the same number of calories by giving people *less* yogurt to compensate for the added chia seeds. Given that, we can at least say that chia seeds are more satiating than plain yogurt. But hours later at lunch, the yogurt-and-chia group didn't just eat a little less food—they ate about 25 percent fewer calories than the group with chia-free yogurt.

Two teaspoons of chia seeds, which have around thirty-five calories, seemed to work as well as three teaspoons. The yogurt-and-chia subjects, however, ended up eating nearly three hundred fewer calories at lunch, so in effect, the chia could be thought as having "negative" calories. We don't know if the subjects somehow compensated later on by eating more at dinner, but if adding chia to your diet means eating hundreds fewer calories day after day due to their satiating effects, you'd expect to lose weight over time. You don't know, though, until you put it to the test.

Researchers at Appalachian State University's Department of Health, Leisure, and Exercise Science (who knew you could major in leisure science?) randomized overweight individuals to two tablespoons of whole chia seeds before the first and last meals of the day for twelve weeks and found no weight-loss benefit at all over placebo.[2688] What happened? We know from the flaxseed literature that people eating muffins made with whole flaxseeds don't seem to absorb all the benefit compared to when they eat muffins made with ground flaxseeds.[2689] Why? The seed's hard natural hull that enables flaxseeds to last for nearly a year at room temperature in an airtight container may work a little too well to protect the seed inside. If a whole flaxseed misses your teeth, it'll pass right through you.[2690] That's why I recommend grinding them up (or buying them preground).

Chia seeds, in comparison, seem so delicate that I was surprised to learn that, ideally, we should also grind them up to get the most out of them. For example, eating whole chia seeds doesn't appear to bump up our omega-3 levels, but eating ground chia does.[2691] Might that explain why the Appalachian study failed to find an effect? A group of Canadian researchers decided to put ground chia to the test for weight loss in a randomized, double-blind, placebo-controlled trial of about two tablespoons a day versus a fiber-matched control made mostly of oat bran. (This study design helps let us know it wasn't funded by a chia seed company, because the researchers put it head-to-head against an active control, not just a sugar pill placebo.) In this way, they could tell if there was some distinct benefit to chia beyond its fiber content.

All study subjects in both groups were put on a relatively low-calorie diet, so even the control group lost weight, but the chia group lost significantly more. The effect was slight, though: only about three pounds better than placebo after six months and only about an extra inch off the waist.[2692] What's more, the effects in most shorter duration studies didn't even reach statistical significance.[2693]

Fortunately, the flaxseed evidence for weight loss is stronger.[2694]

Just the Flax, Ma'am

Like chia seeds, flaxseeds have been shown to cause appetite suppression,[2695] perhaps in part due to their large soluble fiber content, but does this translate into weight loss? One of the most extraordinary studies on flax was published in 2016. Overweight individuals were randomly assigned to receive either daily ground flaxseeds and lifestyle advice for weight loss, or just lifestyle advice alone. Since simply being enrolled in a study and knowing you'll be weighed repeatedly can get people to lose weight,[2696] it wasn't a surprise that body weight, waist circumference, and body mass index decreased significantly in both groups. There was, however, a significantly greater reduction in the flaxseed group, and not just by a little.[2697]

Over the twelve-week study, the control group who had only gotten lifestyle advice lost nearly seven pounds and about an inch off their waists, while the group who had gotten the same advice along with spoonfuls of flaxseeds a day lost more than twenty pounds on average[2698] and nearly four inches off their waists despite being given, in effect, more food to eat. Those are astonishing numbers for an intervention that added, rather than actively removed, calories from the diet. Was this study just some crazy flax fluke?

Another study pitted flaxseeds against nonalcoholic fatty liver disease. Thanks to the obesity epidemic, that's now the most common liver disease, recognized as a major public health problem around the world. A high-fat diet may be the "most common cause,"[2699] but the fat in flaxseeds (flaxseed oil), compared to lard, was found to be better for the liver—in rats.[2700] That's not particularly helpful. What about using whole flaxseeds in people?

Fatty liver patients were randomized using the same setup: lifestyle modification advice with or without flaxseeds. The flaxseed group was instructed to mix their daily ounce or so of ground flaxseeds with water or juice and to drink it after breakfast. Body weight dropped in both groups, along with liver fat, inflammation, and scarring, but significantly more so in the flaxseed group. Again, approximately twenty pounds were lost in three months after telling people to add something to their diets.[2701] Perhaps that first study wasn't just a fluke—or maybe they both were.

There have been more than a dozen randomized controlled trials of flaxseeds and weight loss, and when stacked up next to one another, the two twenty-pound weight-loss studies do appear to be the outliers.[2702] Still, when all the studies are combined together in a meta-analysis, there was a significant reduction in body weight, BMI, and waist circumference following flaxseed supplementation. No benefit was found for flaxseed oil or flaxseed extract supplements, but randomized controlled trials of the *whole food* do show significant weight loss, though you should expect to drop closer to four pounds over a few months rather than twenty.

What About the Cyanide?

How Not to Die has been translated into thirty-four languages so far. Most of the time, all I have to do is just sit back and admire the creative new cover art, but some countries make publication contingent on a set of demands. The Japanese publisher, for example, wouldn't release the book until I added an extra chapter on how not to die from stomach cancer, a leading killer in Japan. Understandable. The proviso from the Swedish publisher surprised me, though. Given my Daily Dozen recommendation to eat at least a tablespoon of ground flaxseed a day, I was asked to add a section on flaxseed safety.

The Swedish National Food Agency's official website features a page warning people to stay away from ground flaxseed for fear of cyanide toxicity,[2703] which helps explain why that was the subject of the first question I was asked when I gave a lecture in Stockholm. Was the Swedish government on to something? Had I been duped by Big Flax–funded researchers who claimed you could literally eat *pounds* of ground flaxseeds a day—more than 150 tablespoons daily—without worrying?[2704]

First, some background. As many as one in five of the plants we eat produces cyanide. In fact, if you look at the major food crops in the world, more than half are cyanogenic, meaning *cyanide-producing*.[2705] Unlike toxins such as lead, mercury, and arsenic, which are chemical elements that can't be broken down, cyanide is an organic molecule made up of one carbon atom attached to one nitrogen atom. In that configuration, the molecule is indeed potently poisonous, but it can instantly lose its toxicity when it's broken down or complexed into something else. That's the reason we have a cyanide-detoxifying enzyme in our bodies that does just that.[2706] Cyanide

(continued)

is a common defense used by plants to fend off herbivores, so our bodies evolved not one—but five—different ways to get rid of it.[2707]

There is a rare genetic condition, though, called *Leber's disease,* where you're born without the ability to detoxify cyanide and can go blind drinking something like apple cider, for example. Other than that, our bodies evolved to be cyanide-detoxifying machines,[2708] but there's obviously a limit. There have been cases, for instance, of cyanide poisoning after bitter almond ingestion.[2709] Regular almonds, the kind you buy at the store, produce about forty times less cyanide than bitter almonds,[2710] which are used in flavor manufacturing. If you did manage to get your hands on some, though, eating fifty bitter almonds could kill you. So, doing the math, presumably eating two thousand regular almonds at one sitting would also not be a good idea.

You may not be able to readily buy bitter almonds, but you can easily get apricots, and the apricot kernels—the seeds inside the stone—have cyanide levels high enough to present a threat. So when it comes to the Swedish authorities, I am completely sympathetic to regulators wanting to take a precautionary approach, but are flaxseeds like bitter almonds, where just a few ounces could kill you, or are they more like regular almonds where typical dietary intake wouldn't even come close to being harmful?

The claim from flax industry–funded scientists that we can eat literally pounds of ground flaxseeds a day without running into trouble is a back-of-the-envelope type of calculation based on the fact we can detoxify "up to 100 mg of cyanide/day."[2711] I'm not interested in how much we can detoxify "up to," though. From a safety standpoint, you want to know about the worst-case scenario, not the best-case scenario. Can't someone please just give people different doses of flaxseeds and simply measure how much cyanide ends up in their blood? Surprisingly, that wasn't done until 2016.

Researchers finally put flaxseeds to the test under conditions expected to maximize cyanide exposure. They examined more than a dozen different sources of flaxseed and used the one with the single highest levels of cyanide they could find.[2712] Making sure to use raw flaxseeds, since cooking often wipes out all the cyanide,[2713] the researchers also used a 20,000 rpm laboratory grinder to ensure maximal mechanical breakdown to maximize absorption. They then gave the subjects a higher-than-typical dose, four and a half tablespoons, and had them eat it all at once on an empty stomach.[2714] So what did they find?

The range of cyanide blood levels one could estimate to possibly be associated with clinical symptoms of intoxication might be around 20–40 micromoles.[2715] Four and a half tablespoons of the highest cyanide-containing ultraground raw flaxseeds eaten on an empty stomach only raised average cyanide blood levels to 6 micromoles before rapidly coming back down, with the highest individual reading coming in at under 14.

There has to be some amount of flax that takes you over the limit, though, so the researchers tested nine tablespoons and then fifteen tablespoons. Nine tablespoons skirted blood levels right up to 20 micromoles, and fifteen tablespoons, practically a whole cup, put the study subject into the potential toxicity zone for more than three hours.[2716] (So much for the industry's claim that eight cups at a time are safe![2717]) Yet even in that worse-case scenario of one cup of ultraground raw flaxseeds at the highest available cyanide concentration on an empty stomach, there still were no actual symptoms of toxicity.[2718] This is consistent with the fact that there's not a single published report of cyanide toxicity after consumption of flaxseeds anywhere in the medical literature, even in Swedish health spas, where individuals are given up to twelve tablespoons as a "fibre shock."[2719]

Cumin

Used in cuisines around the world from Tex-Mex to South Asian, cumin is the second most popular spice on Earth after black pepper.[2720] It is one of the oldest cultivated plants and has a range of purported medicinal uses, including appetite suppression,[2721] but it wasn't put to the test for weight loss until 2015. A randomized, double-blind, placebo-controlled trial pitted cumin versus placebo versus the "fecal spotting" obesity drug orlistat. The cumin appeared to work as well as the drug, and they both beat out placebo, but only by a few pounds over the eight-week trial.[2722] I'd take cumin over anal leakage any day, but rather than the whole spice, the researchers used two drops of cumin essential oil hidden in capsules three times a day, which is the equivalent of about two daily teaspoons of cumin.[2723] A follow-up study sought to see how low in dosage they could go.

The next year, the same research team tried going down to as low as half a drop of cumin essential oil twice a day and still found a similar weight-loss benefit over placebo. However, the interpretation was complicated by the fact that they also added half a drop of lime essential oil.[2724] A drop or two of cumin oil a day may also improve blood sugar control in diabetics,[2725] but it's so hard to trust the accuracy, safety, and purity of extracts and supplements.[2726] What about just giving the whole spice—powdered cumin—readily available at any grocery store?

Overweight women were randomized to eat calorie-restricted weight-loss diets with or without a teaspoon of added cumin a day (half a teaspoon at both lunch and dinner). Over the three-month study, those in the cumin group lost about four more pounds and nearly an extra inch off their waists, in addition to significantly dropping their triglycerides and cholesterol.[2727] Since cumin can be purchased in bulk for less than a dollar an ounce, a teaspoon would cost less than ten cents a day.

Black Cumin

Black cumin is not actually related to cumin; it's a member of the buttercup rather than carrot family. Also known as *Nigella sativa* or simply "black seed," it's a common spice whose peppery flavor is popular in Indian and Middle Eastern cuisines, but it's also been prized for purported medicinal benefits. Described as a "miracle herb,"[2728] with mentions going back to the Old Testament (Isaiah 28:25, 27), black cumin was found cached in King Tut's tomb, and the Prophet Muhammad evidently is quoted as saying it could "heal every disease except death."[2729] Only in the last fifty years or so has it been put to the test, though, culminating in more than a thousand papers published in the medical literature.

Typical doses used in studies are just one or two grams a day, which is only about a quarter teaspoon.[2730] This enables researchers to perform randomized, double-blind, placebo-controlled trials by stuffing the whole-food spice into capsules rather than using just a component or extract.

Systematic reviews and meta-analyses of randomized controlled trials have found that daily black cumin consumption significantly improves cholesterol, triglycerides,[2731] blood pressure,[2732] and blood sugar control.[2733] Some of the results are quite extraordinary. For example, one study found that menopausal women randomized to a gram a day (less than a quarter teaspoon) of black cumin powder reduced their bad LDL cholesterol by 27 percent within two months.[2734] That's the kind of result you'd expect taking a statin drug, but it was achieved with just a sprinkle of a spice. Black cumin may also help with menopausal symptoms themselves.[2735]

Now, taking black cumin didn't *cure* anything—a month after stopping the spice, cholesterol levels crept back up[2736]—but it does appear to be a cheap, safe, effective, and tasty (if you like spice) treatment for some of our deadliest risk factors. And the side effects? Loss of appetite and weight loss.[2737] Bingo!

A recent systematic review and meta-analysis of randomized, controlled weight-loss trials found that about a quarter teaspoon of black cumin powder every day appears to reduce body mass index within a span of a couple of months.[2738] If it's truly so beneficial to so many facets of health, why don't we hear more about it? Why wasn't I taught about it in medical school? Maybe because there's little profit motive. Black cumin is just a spice. The daily dose used in most of these studies would cost about three cents.

Saffron

Saffron is another spice found to be effective for treating a major cause of suffering—depression in this case—with a side effect of diminished appetite.[2739] When put to the test in a randomized, double-blind, placebo-controlled trial, saffron was found to lead to significant weight loss: five pounds more than placebo and nearly an inch off the waist in eight weeks.[2740] The dose of saffron used in the study was the equivalent of drinking a cup of tea made from a large pinch of saffron threads.[2741]

Suspecting the "active ingredient" might be crocin, the pigment in saffron that accounts for its crimson color, researchers also tried giving people just the purified pigment. That also led to weight loss, beating the placebo by two pounds and half an inch off the waist, but it didn't do as well as the full saffron extract. The mechanism appeared to be appetite suppression, as the pigment group ended up averaging about 85 fewer calories a day, while the saffron group consumed 170 fewer daily calories on average.[2742]

A similar study looked specifically at snacking frequency. The researchers thought perhaps the mood-boosting effects of saffron might cut down on stress-related eating. Eight weeks of a saffron extract did cut snack intake in half compared to placebo and was accompanied by a slight but statistically significant weight loss (about two pounds).[2743] The researchers used about half the saffron dose as the other study.[2744]

Even weight loss of just a few pounds is pretty remarkable given the tiny doses utilized, about 100 mg, which is equivalent to around an eighth of a teaspoon of the spice. The problem is that saffron is the most expensive spice in the world. It's composed of delicate threads poking out of the saffron crocus. Each flower produces only a few threads, such that you need fifty thousand flowers—enough flowers to fill a football field—to make a single pound of spice, so that pinch of saffron could cost up to a dollar a day.

FOOD FOR THOUGHT

In my Daily Dozen checklist of recommendations introduced in *How Not to Die* for fitting some of the healthiest of healthy foods into your daily routine, I already push flaxseeds and spices in general (though I focus on turmeric). For those interested in maximizing weight loss, try expanding your repertoire. Add cumin to hummus and baked beans. Why not enjoy a saffron-infused paella sprinkled with black cumin seeds? An easy way I include black cumin in my family's daily diet is by simply mixing it in with the black peppercorns in the pepper grinder. If you aren't familiar with my chia-based chocolate sauce strawberry dip recipe in *How Not to Die,* don't miss out. It's definitely a tastier alternative than nibbling on your chia pet.

CHRONOBIOLOGY

Is Breakfast Really the Most Important Meal of the Day?

Chronobiology is the study of how our bodies' natural cycles—mental, physical, and emotional—are affected by the rhythms of the sun, moon, and seasons. What does this have to do with losing weight? Consider the question of breakfast. It is widely touted as not only the most important meal of the day in general but specifically in relation to weight loss.[2745] This is not just a pop-culture prescription from checkout aisle magazines but an idea put forward by such prestigious institutions as Johns Hopkins[2746] and NYU.[2747] "Want to trim your waist?" read a headline from the American Dietetic Association. "Try eating breakfast!"[2748] referring to breakfast as perhaps the "best kept waist-trimming secret."[2749] But is it true? The Duke University School of Medicine's health newsletter claimed: "It's always been billed as the most important meal of the day—until now."[2750]

While it is widely presumed that eating breakfast protects against obesity, the belief is held up as a poster child of biased distortion of the scientific record.[2751] No one can argue there isn't an association between body weight and breakfast. Studies have shown that obesity and skipping breakfast tend to go together beyond a shadow of a doubt, in fact, gratuitously so. A meta-analysis found that by 2011, the combined P value had reached 10^{-42}.[2752] In science, *P value* refers to the chance of getting a result that extreme, if in fact there really was no such effect. In other words, the probability that the association found between obesity and breakfast-skipping was just a fluke is lower than the chances of winning the lottery not once but five times—and then getting struck and killed by lightning.[2753] The question is whether the relationship between skipping breakfast and obesity is cause and effect.

To illustrate the difference between correlation and causation, let me share an example of the manipulation of science by the candy industry. The National Confectioners Association has the gall to warn parents that *restricting* candy may make their children fat.[2754] Candy hawkers justify this outlandish claim with a study (that they funded themselves, of course) that showed that candy-consuming children and adolescents were significantly less likely to be overweight and obese.[2755] The industry-funded researchers went on to imply this exonerates candy, but what's more likely? Cutting down on candy led to obesity, or obesity led to cutting down on candy? In other words, the lower candy consumption may reflect the *consequences* of obesity, not the *cause* of obesity, as parents of obese children may try to restrict treats.

Similarly, the finding that those who skip breakfast tend to be heavier can be equally interpreted as saying those who are heavier tend to skip breakfast. Doesn't it seem more likely that overweight individuals might be skipping breakfast in an effort to eat less, rather than eating fewer meals somehow leads to weight gain? On the other hand, maybe skipping breakfast somehow slows your metabolism or causes you to overeat so much later in the day that you end up gaining weight. You can't know for certain which direction the causality goes until you put it to the test.

Sometimes randomized controlled trials are impossible.[2756] To test whether parachutes save lives, you can't exactly boot half the people off a plane without them. However, you could easily randomize people to eat breakfast or skip it to see what happens. It turns out eating breakfast doesn't seem to affect our metabolic rates,[2757] nor does it sufficiently suppress our appetites. Most studies have found that eating breakfast leads to the same, or even greater, caloric intake over the day.[2758] Even when people ate more at lunch after skipping breakfast, they didn't tend to eat an entire breakfast's worth of calories more, so they ended up eating fewer calories overall.[2759] For example, people fed about a 500-calorie breakfast may eat about 150 fewer calories at lunch, compared with those randomized to skip breakfast, but they would still end up with that surplus of around 350 calories over the breakfast skippers.[2760] Does eating breakfast then translate into weight gain over time?

Researchers at Brigham Young University randomized forty-nine women who habitually skipped breakfast to either start eating breakfast or continue skipping it. If breakfast somehow magically leads to weight loss, then the group who renewed breakfast eating should benefit. But, no. Compared to those who continued to skip breakfast, adding the extra meal led to hundreds more daily calories consumed and about a third of a pound of weight gain a week.[2761]

Breakfast of Champions?

Of course, breakfast composition matters. Though a bagel,[2762] cereal,[2763] or eggs[2764] may not sufficiently affect lunch intake, oatmeal might. Researchers at Columbia University randomized individuals into one of three breakfast conditions: oatmeal made from quick oats, the same number of calories of Frosted Flakes, or just plain water. They then measured how many calories people took in at lunch three hours later. Not only did those who ate the oatmeal feel significantly fuller and less hungry, some then went on to consume significantly less at lunch. Overweight participants who had eaten oatmeal for breakfast consumed less than half as many calories at lunch, about four hundred fewer calories, which is more than the oatmeal itself had contained.[2765] So in effect, the oatmeal provided "negative" calories. In contrast, the Frosted Flakes was so *unsatiating* that the cereal group ate as much at lunch as the breakfast-skipping, water-only group.[2766] It's as if the cereal group hadn't eaten breakfast at all!

Sadly, only about 6 percent of Americans are eating oatmeal on any given day.[2767] Not only is oatmeal healthier, it's cheaper too. Some high-end breakfast cereals price out closer to steaks than flakes at eight dollars a pound, whereas that same pound of rolled oats from your market's bulk section may be less than a dollar (and would make ten servings).

A nutritional downside of skipping the morning meal is that breakfast may be the only time Americans consume any whole grains,[2768] which are associated with a lower risk of dying prematurely from cancer, heart disease, and all causes put together.[2769] A Harvard study following hundreds of thousands of individuals for more than a decade found that those consuming breakfast cereals tend to live longer, presumably because of their higher fiber intake (and perhaps fewer bacon-and-egg breakfasts),[2770] though this benefit may be limited to whole-grain cereals.[2771]

And we know that children's cereals are the worst. Breakfast cereals marketed to American kids have been found to contain 85 percent more sugar, 65 percent less fiber, and 60 percent more sodium than those marketed to adults.[2772] Sugary cereals are the number one food advertised to kids,[2773] with the average American child exposed to as many as 750 ads for cereal on TV every year.[2774]

Nutrients are added to breakfast cereals as a marketing gimmick in an attempt to create an aura of healthfulness.[2775] Plastering nutrient claims on the box can create a "nutritional façade," acting to distract attention away from unsavory qualities such as excess sugar content.[2776] If those same nutrients were added to soda, would we feed our kids Coke for breakfast? We might as well spray cotton candy with vitamins too. As one medical journal editorial read, "Adding vitamins and minerals to sugary cereals . . . is worse than useless. The subtle message . . . is that it is safe to eat more."[2777] It's been estimated that a child eating one serving per day of the average children's cereal would consume more than ten pounds of sugar in a year, nearly a thousand spoonfuls of sugar, just from breakfast cereal alone.[2778]

General Mills argues it's those spoonfuls of sugar that can help the

(continued)

medicine go down,[2779] explaining that "if sugar is removed from bran cereal, it would have the consistency of sawdust."[2780] If sugar weren't added, General Mills said its cereals could become "unpalatable."[2781] If you have to add sugar to a product to make it edible, maybe that should tell you something. A characteristic of so-called ultraprocessed foods is this necessity to pack them full of salt, sugar, flavorings, and the like since they have their natural intrinsic flavors processed out and you have to mask any unpleasant tastes introduced during manufacturing.[2782]

The president of the Cereal Institute has argued that without sugary cereals, kids might not eat breakfast at all,[2783] similar to dairy industry arguments that removing chocolate milk from school cafeterias would risk kids skipping lunch.[2784] He also stressed we must consider the alternatives.[2785] As Kellogg's director of nutrition once put it: "I would suggest that Fruit [sic] Loops as a snack are much better than potato chips or a sweet roll."[2786] You know there's a problem when the only way to make your product look good is to compare it to Pringles and Cinnabon.

To Skip or Not to Skip

Where did this idea of breakfast as "the most important meal of the day" come from? Edward Bernays, the so-called father of public relations infamous for his "Torches of Freedom" campaign to get women to start smoking back in the 1920s, was paid by a pork company to design and popularize the emblematic bacon-and-eggs breakfast.[2787] The role of PR specialists, he wrote in his book *Propaganda,* is the "conscious and intelligent manipulation of the organized habits and opinions of the masses."[2788]

Breakfast is big business. Powerful commercial interests such as the breakfast cereal lobby are blamed for perpetuating myths about the importance of that morning meal.[2789] In an editorial about the breakfast controversy published in *The American Journal of Clinical Nutrition,* nutrition scientists are urged to speak truth to power and challenge conventional wisdom when necessary "even when it looks like we are taking away motherhood and apple pie." (The editorial went on to conclude, "Actually, reducing the portion size of apple pie might not be a bad idea, either."[2790])

To lose weight, should we therefore *not* break the fast and instead skip breakfast? Though advice to eliminate breakfast "will surely pit . . . nutritional scientists . . . against the very strong and powerful food industry," skipping breakfast has been described as a "straightforward and feasible strategy" to reduce daily calorie consumption.[2791]

Unfortunately, skipping breakfast doesn't seem to work.

Most randomized controlled studies of skipping breakfast found no weight-loss benefit.[2792] How is that possible if skipping breakfast means skipping calories? The Bath Breakfast Project, a famous series of experiments run not out of a tub but at the University of Bath, discovered a key to the mystery. Men and women were randomized either to fast until noon every day or to eat breakfast, which was defined as taking in at least seven hundred calories before 11:00 a.m. As in other similar trials, the group eating breakfast ate a little less throughout the rest of the day but still ended up with hundreds of excess daily calories over those who had skipped breakfast. Yet after six weeks, both groups ended up with the exact same change in body fat.[2793] How could hundreds of calories a day just effectively disappear?

If more calories were going in with no change in weight, then there must have been more calories going out. Indeed, the breakfast group was found to be engaging spontaneously in more light-intensity physical activity in the mornings than the breakfast-skipping group.[2794] Light-intensity activities include things like casual walking or light housecleaning, not structured exercise per se, but apparently enough extra activity to use up the bulk of those excess breakfast calories. There's a popular misconception that our bodies go into energy conservation mode when we skip breakfast by slowing our metabolic rates. That doesn't appear to be true, but maybe our bodies do intuitively slow us down in other ways.[2795]

The extra activity didn't completely make up for the added breakfast calories, though, suggesting there may be another factor to account for the mystery of the missing morning calories.[2796,2797] Recent breakthroughs in the field of chronobiology—the study of our bodies' natural rhythms—have upended another key piece of nutrition dogma: the concept that a calorie is a calorie. As it turns out, it's not just what we eat but *when* we eat. Because of our circadian rhythms—*circadian* coming from the Latin words for *about* and *day*—morning calories don't appear to count as much as evening calories.[2798]

Slave to the Rhythm

The 2017 Nobel Prize in Medicine was awarded for elucidating the molecular mechanisms of our internal circadian clocks.[2799] For billions of years, life on Earth evolved to the twenty-four-hour cycle of light and dark, so it's no surprise our bodies are finely tuned to that pattern. When people are in total darkness without any external time cues, our bodies still continue to cycle in about a twenty-four-hour circadian rhythm.[2800] In fact, you can even take tissue biopsies from people and show the cells continue to cycle outside the body in a petri dish.[2801] Nearly every tissue and organ in our bodies has its own internal clock.[2802]

An intricate system of intrinsic clocks drives not only some of our behavioral patterns, such as eating, fasting, sleeping, and wakefulness,[2803] but also our internal physiology, including our digestion, body temperature, blood pressure, hormone production, and immune activity.[2804] Most of our genes exhibit daily fluctuations in expression, making the circadian rhythm the largest known regulatory system in our bodies.[2805] This cycling is thought to allow for a level of predictability and functional division of labor so each of our body processes can run at the best time.[2806] At night while we're sleeping, a whole array of internal housekeeping activities can be switched on, such as clearing accumulated waste products from the brain, for example, and as dawn approaches, our bodies can shift back into activity mode.

Anyone who's ever had jet lag knows what throwing off our cycles by even a few hours can do, but now we know our circadian rhythms can literally be the difference between life and death. A study of more than fourteen thousand suicide attempts using poison (such as drinking pesticides) found that those who tried killing themselves in the late morning were more than twice as likely to die than those who ingested a similar dose in the evening.[2807] In the same vein, properly timed chemotherapy can not only end up being five times less toxic but twice as effective against cancer.[2808] The same drugs, at the same doses, but with different effects depending on the time they're given. Our bodies absorb, distribute, metabolize, and detoxify what we ingest differently depending on when the processes are occurring during the twenty-four-hour cycle.

We're just beginning to figure out the optimal timing for different medications. Randomize people suffering from hypertension into taking their blood pressure pills at bedtime instead of the morning, and not only does the bedtime group achieve better blood pressure control and suffer fewer heart attacks and strokes, but they also cut their risk of death in half.[2809] (Sadly, most physicians and pharmacists still tell patients to take their blood pressure meds in the morning.[2810])

If chronotherapy—the optimal timing of drugs—can have such an impact, it may come as no surprise that chronoprevention—the scheduling of lifestyle interventions like mealtimes—can also make a difference.[2811]

No Time to Lose

In the official Academy of Nutrition and Dietetics position paper on effective treatments for obesity, importance is placed on both the quantity and the timing of caloric intake. "Potentially consuming more energy earlier in the day, rather than later in the day," the paper concluded, "can assist with weight management."[2812] Some have gone further and even characterized obesity as a "chronobiological disease."[2813] What evidence do we have to back up these types of claims?

The timing of caloric intake may have shifted slightly over recent decades toward a greater proportion of food later in the day,[2814] which raised the question about a possible role in the rise in obesity. Middle-aged men and women who eat a greater share of daily calories in the morning do seem to gain less weight over time.[2815] A study entitled "Timing of Food Intake Predicts Weight Loss Effectiveness" found that dieters eating their main meal earlier in the day seemed to steadily lose more weight than those eating their main meal at a later time. An obvious explanation for this finding would be those who eat later also tend to eat more. But is that really what's going on?

There does seem to be a relationship between when people eat most of their calories and how many calories they end up eating over the entire day, with those eating a greater proportion in the morning eating less overall.[2816] Could it be that later eaters are just overeating junk on the couch while watching prime-time TV?[2817] A tendency has been found for night owls to consume more fast food and soda, and fewer fruits and vegetables.[2818] In the field of social psychology, there's a controversial concept called *ego depletion,* where self-control is viewed as a limited resource, like a muscle that can become fatigued from overuse. As the day wears on, the ability to resist unhealthy food choices may decline, leaving one vulnerable to temptation.[2819] So is it just a matter of later eating leading to greater eating?

To the surprise of the investigators in the study that showed earlier eaters steadily lost more weight, the early eaters seemed to be eating as much as the later eaters. Despite that, the early eaters ended up about five pounds lighter than the later eaters by the end of the twenty-week study, even though they were apparently eating the same amount of food.[2820] There didn't seem to be any difference in physical activity between the two groups either. Could it be that the *timing* of caloric intake matters? Scientists decided to put it to the test.

Like Night and Day

Mice are nocturnal creatures. They eat during the night and sleep during the day. If, however, you just feed mice during the day, they gain more weight than if you feed them a similar number of calories at night.[2821] Same food and about the same amount of food, but different weight outcomes, suggesting that eating at the "wrong" time may lead to disproportionate weight gain. In humans, the wrong time would presumably mean eating at night.

Weight management recommendations often include advice to limit nighttime food consumption, but this was largely anecdotal since it wasn't studied experimentally until 2013. Researchers instructed a group of young men not to eat after 7:00 p.m. for two weeks. Compared to a control period where they continued their regular habits, after the night-eating restriction, they ended up about two pounds lighter. This is not surprising, given dietary records showing they inadvertently ate fewer calories during that period.[2822] To see if timing has metabolic effects beyond just foreclosing eating opportunities, you'd have to force people to eat the same amount of the same food, but just at different times of the day. The U.S. Army stepped forward to carry out just such an investigation.

In the first set of experiments, Army researchers had people eat a single meal a day, either within an hour of waking or after twelve hours of waking, so they each had just one meal as either breakfast or dinner. The breakfast-only group lost about two pounds a week compared to the dinner-only group.[2823] As with the night-eating restriction study, this is to be expected, given that people tend to be hungrier in the evening. Think about it. If you went nine hours without eating during the day, you'd be famished, but people go nine hours overnight without a meal all the time yet don't wake up ravenous. There is a natural circadian rhythm to hunger that peaks at about

8:00 p.m. and drops to its lowest level at around 8:00 a.m.[2824] That may be why breakfast is typically the smallest meal of the day.

The circadian rhythms of our appetites aren't just behavioral—they're biological. It's not just that we're hungrier in the evening because we've been running around all day. If you stayed up all night and slept through the day, you'd still be hungriest when you woke up that evening. To untangle the factors, scientists use what's called *forced desynchrony* protocols where they confine people in a room without windows in constant, unchanging, dim light and make them sleep in twenty- or twenty-eight-hour cycles to totally scramble them up.[2825] This goes on for more than a week so the study subjects end up eating and sleeping at different times through all phases of the day. It's then possible to see if the cyclical phenomenon is based on internal clocks or is just a consequence of what you happen to be doing at the time.

There's a daily swing in our blood pressures, hormone production, digestion, immune activity, and almost everything else,[2826] but let's look at body temperature for an example. Our core body temperatures usually bottom out around 4:00 a.m., dropping from 98.6°F down to around 97.6°F.[2827] Is this just because our bodies cool down as we're sleeping? No. It can be shown experimentally that it happens at about the same time no matter what; it's part of our circadian rhythms just like our appetites. It makes sense then that if you are only eating one meal a day and want to lose weight, you'd want to eat in the morning when your "hunger hormones" may be less active.[2828]

Okay, but then it just gets weirder.

The Army scientists repeated the experiment, but this time had the participants eat exactly two thousand calories, either for breakfast or dinner, taking appetite out of the equation. (They were also not allowed to exercise.) Same number of calories, so same change in weight, right? No, the breakfast-only group *still* lost about two pounds a week compared to the dinner-only group.[2829] Two pounds of weight loss eating the same number of calories.

Breakfast Like a King, Lunch Like a Prince, Dine Like a Pauper

What about just shifting our daily distribution of calories to earlier in the day? Israeli researchers randomized overweight and obese women into one of two isocaloric groups, meaning each group was given the same number of total calories. One group was given a seven-hundred-calorie breakfast, a five-hundred-calorie lunch, and a two-hundred-calorie dinner, and the other group was given the opposite—two hundred for breakfast, five hundred for lunch, and seven hundred for dinner. Since they were all eating the same number of calories overall, the king-prince-pauper group should have lost the same amount of weight as the pauper-prince-king group, right? But no; the group who ate the most at breakfast lost more than twice as much weight as the group eating the most at the dinner meal. In addition to slimming nearly an extra two inches off their waistlines, by the end of the twelve-week study, the king-prince-pauper group lost nineteen pounds compared to only eight lost by the pauper-prince-king group despite eating the same number of calories.[2830] Eleven additional pounds lost eating the same number of calories. That's the power of chronobiology.

700/500/200 is 50 percent of calories at breakfast, 36 percent of calories at lunch, and only 14 percent at dinner. What about 20 percent of calories for dinner? How would a calorie percentage spread of 50/30/20 compare to eating 20 percent of calories at breakfast, 30 percent at lunch, and 50 percent at dinner? Again, the bigger-breakfast group experienced "dramatically increased" weight loss, about nine pounds difference in just eight weeks with no significant difference in overall caloric intake or physical activity between the groups.[2831]

Instead of eating more than 80 percent of calories at breakfast and lunch, what about just consuming 70 percent compared to 55 percent? Overweight homemakers were randomized to eat either 70 percent of their calories at breakfast, a morning snack, and lunch, leaving 30 percent for an afternoon snack and dinner, or a more balanced 55 percent up through and including lunch. In both cases, only a minority of calories was eaten for dinner. Would it matter if it were 55 percent of calories eaten up through lunch or 70 percent? Yes, there was significantly more weight loss and slimming in the dietary pattern that was more slanted toward the morning. The researchers concluded that one clear communication physicians could give is: "If you want to lose weight, eat more in the morning than in the evening."[2832]

Simply telling people to eat their main meal at lunch rather than dinner may help. Despite comparable caloric intakes, participants in a weight-loss program randomized to get advice to make their main meal lunch beat out those who were instead told to make dinner their primary meal.[2833] The evidence isn't completely consistent, though. A review of meal pattern studies questioned the role that reducing evening intake would facilitate weight loss, citing a study that showed the evening-weighted group did *better* than the heavy-morning-meal group.[2834] Perhaps that was because the morning meal group was given "chocolate, cookies, cake, ice cream, chocolate mousse or donuts" for breakfast.[2835]

Overall, the *what* is still more important than the *when*. Like each of the other Weight-Loss Boosters in part IV, you can use chronobiology to expedite weight loss, but caloric timing can't substitute for a healthy diet. When he said there was "a time for every purpose under heaven," Ecclesiastes probably wasn't talking about donuts.

Burning the Morning Oil

Why do calories eaten in the morning seem to be less fattening than calories eaten in the evening? One reason is that more calories are burned off in the morning due to diet-induced thermogenesis, the amount of energy the body takes to digest and process a meal, given off in part as waste heat. When people are given the exact same meal in the morning, afternoon, and at night, their body uses up about 25 percent more calories to process the meal in the afternoon than at night and about 50 percent more calories to digest it in the morning.[2836] That leaves fewer net calories in the morning to be stored as fat.

Let's put some actual numbers to this. A group of Italian researchers randomized twenty people to eat the same standardized meal at either 8:00 a.m. or 8:00 p.m. After a week, the subjects returned, this time eating the same meal at the opposite time. So each person had a chance to eat the very same meal for breakfast and for dinner. After each meal, the subjects were placed in a "calorimeter" contraption to precisely measure how many calories they were burning over the next three hours. The researchers calculated that the meal given in the morning took about 300 calories to digest, whereas the exact same meal given at night used only about 200 calories to process. The meal itself was about 1,200 calories, so, when given in the morning, it ended up providing only about 900 calories compared to around 1,000 calories at night.[2837] Same meal, same food, same amount of food, but effectively 100 fewer calories when consumed in the morning. So a calorie is not just a calorie. It depends on when it's eaten.

But why do we burn more calories eating a morning meal? Is it behavioral or biological? If you started working the graveyard shift, sleeping during the day and working all night, which meal would net you fewer calories? Would it be the "breakfast" you had at night before you went to work, or the "dinner" you had in the morning before you went to bed? In other words, is there something about eating before we go to sleep that causes our bodies to hold on to more calories, or is it built into our circadian rhythms such that we store more calories at night regardless of what we're doing? Harvard researchers decided to find out.

People were randomized to eat identical meals at 8:00 a.m. versus at 8:00 p.m. while under simulated night shifts or day shifts. Regardless of activity level or sleeping cycle, the calories burned while processing the morning meals were 50 percent higher than the evening meals.[2838] So the difference is explained by chronobiology; it's just part of our circadian rhythms to burn more meal calories in the morning.

How does it make sense for our bodies to race through calories in the morning when we have the whole day ahead of us? Perhaps our bodies aren't so much *wasting* calories as *investing* them. When we eat in the morning, our bodies bulk up our muscles with glycogen, which is the primary energy reserve we use to fuel our muscles. That takes energy, though. In the evening, our bodies expect to be sleeping for much of the next twelve hours, so rather than storing blood sugar as extra glycogen in our muscles, the body preferentially uses it as an energy source, which may end up meaning we burn less of our body fat.[2839] In the morning, however, our bodies expect to be running around all day, so instead of just burning off breakfast, our bodies continue to dip into our fat stores while we use breakfast calories to stuff our muscles full of the energy reserves we need to move around over the course of the day.

This is where the "inefficiency" may come from.[2840] Why does it cost more calories to process a morning meal? Instead of just burning glucose (blood sugar) directly, our bodies are using up energy to string together glucose molecules into chains of glycogen in our muscles, which are then broken back down into glucose later in the day. That extra assembly/disassembly step takes energy, energy that our bodies take from the meal, leaving us with fewer calories.[2841]

So in the morning, our muscles are especially sensitive to insulin, rapidly pulling blood sugar out of our bloodstreams to build up glycogen reserves. At night, though, our muscles become relatively insulin-resistant and resist the signal to take in extra blood sugar. Does this mean we get higher blood sugar and insulin spikes in the evening compared to when we eat the exact same meal in the morning? Yes! In that hundred-calorie difference study, for example, blood sugars rose about twice as high after the 8:00 p.m. meal compared to the same meal eaten at 8:00 a.m.[2842] So shifting the bulk of our caloric intake toward the morning would appear to have the dual benefit of more weight loss and better blood sugar control.

Time Heals Some Wounds

We've known for more than a half century that our bodies' ability to keep blood sugars under control, known as *glucose tolerance,* declines as the day goes on.[2843] If you hook yourself up to an IV and just steadily drip sugar water into your vein throughout the day, your blood sugars start to go up around 8:00 p.m. even though you haven't eaten anything and the infusion rate didn't change.[2844] The same amount of sugar is going into your system every minute, but your ability to handle it deteriorates in the evening before bouncing right back again in the morning. A meal eaten at 8:00 p.m. can cause twice the blood sugar response as an identical meal eaten at 8:00 a.m.[2845]—as if we had eaten twice as much! Our bodies just aren't expecting us to be eating when it's dark outside. Our species may have only discovered how to make fire about a quarter million years ago.[2846] We just weren't built for twenty-four-hour diners.

One of the tests for diabetes is the glucose tolerance test, which measures how fast your body can clear sugar from the bloodstream. You drink a cup of water mixed with about four and a half tablespoons of regular corn syrup and then have your blood sugar measured two hours later. By that point, your blood sugar should be under 140 mg/dL. Between 140 and 199 is considered prediabetic, and 200 and higher is a sign of full-blown diabetes.[2847] The circadian rhythm of glucose tolerance is so powerful that a person can test normal in the morning but prediabetic later in the day.[2848] Prediabetics who average 163 at 7:00 a.m. test as frank diabetics by 7:00 p.m. at over 200.[2849]

In the Low Glycemic Load section, I talked about the importance of choosing lower-glycemic foods for weight loss. Timing is critical, though. Because of our circadian pattern of glucose tolerance,[2850] eating a low-glycemic food at night can cause a higher blood sugar spike than consuming a high-glycemic food in the morning. We're so metabolically crippled at night that researchers found that eating a bowl of All-Bran at 8:00 p.m. caused as high a blood sugar spike as eating Rice Krispies at 8:00 a.m.[2851] High-glycemic foods at night would seem to represent the worst-case scenario.[2852] So if you can't resist eating refined grains and sugary junk, they might be less detrimental in the morning.[2853]

This drop in glucose tolerance over the day may help explain the weight-loss benefits of frontloading calories toward the beginning of the day beyond just the diet-induced thermogenesis effects.[2854] Simply eating an earlier, rather than later, lunch may make a difference. People randomized to eat a large lunch at 4:30 p.m. suffered a 46 percent greater blood sugar response compared to an identical meal eaten just a few hours earlier at 1:00 p.m.[2855] Breakfast versus lunch also seems to make a difference. A meal eaten at 7:00 a.m. can cause 37 percent lower blood sugars than an identical meal taken at 1:00 p.m.[2856] There doesn't seem to be any difference between a meal at 8:00 p.m. and one at midnight,[2857] but eating *that* late can disrupt our circadian rhythms so much that it can mess up our metabolisms the next morning, resulting in significantly higher blood sugars after breakfast.[2858]

The revelations of chronobiology bring the breakfast debate full circle. Skipping breakfast not only generally fails to cause weight loss, but it worsens overall daily blood sugar control in both diabetic[2859] and nondiabetic individuals.[2860] This may explain why those who skip breakfast appear to be at higher risk of developing type 2 diabetes in the first place.[2861]

Breakfast skippers also tend to have higher rates of heart disease[2862] and atherosclerosis in general.[2863] Is this just because skipping breakfast tends to cluster with other unhealthy choices, such as smoking and sicklier eating habits overall?[2864] The link between skipping breakfast and heart disease—even premature death in general[2865]—seems to survive attempts to control for these confounding factors, but you don't really know until you put it to the test.

Does skipping breakfast lead to higher cholesterol, for example? Yes, within just two weeks, there was a significant rise in bad LDL cholesterol in those randomized to skip breakfast.[2866] The Israeli 700/500/200 study found that the triglycerides of the king-prince-pauper group got significantly better, dropping 60 points, while those of the pauper-prince-king group got significantly worse, rising 26 points.[2867]

So consuming more calories in the morning relative to the evening may actually have the *triple* benefit of more weight loss, better blood sugar control, and lower heart disease risk.

Chronodisruption

One of the most important breakthroughs in recent years has been the discovery of peripheral clocks.[2868] We've known about the central clock, the so-called suprachiasmatic nucleus, for nearly a half century.[2869] It sits in the middle of our brains right above where our optic nerves cross, allowing it to respond to night and day. We now know there are semiautonomous clocks in nearly every organ of our bodies.[2870] Our hearts run on a clock, our lungs run on a clock, our kidneys run on a clock. Up to 80 percent of the genes in our livers are expressed in a circadian rhythm,[2871] and our entire digestive tracts are too.

The rate at which our stomachs empty, the secretion of digestive enzymes, and the expression of transporters in our intestinal linings for absorbing sugar and fat—these all cycle around the clock. So, too, does the ability of our body fat to sop up extra calories.[2872] The way we know these cycles are driven by local clocks rather than being controlled by our brains is that we can take surgical biopsies of fat, put them in a petri dish, and still observe their natural rhythm.[2873]

All this clock talk is not just biological curiosity. Our health may depend on keeping these clocks in sync. Think of it like a child playing on a swing. Imagine you're pushing the child, but become distracted by other goings-on in the playground. You stop paying attention to your timing, so you push too early, push too late, or forget to push altogether. What happens? Out of sync, the swinging becomes erratic, slows, or even stops. That is what happens when we travel across multiple time zones or have to work the night shift.[2874]

The pusher in this case is the light cue falling on our eyes. Our circadian rhythms are meant to get a bright light push every morning at dawn, but if the sun rises at a different time or we're exposed to bright light in the middle of the night, this can push our cycles out of sync and leave us feeling out of sorts. That's an example of a mismatch between the external environment and our central clocks. Problems can also arise from a misalignment between the central clock in our brains with all the other organ clocks throughout our bodies. An extreme illustration of this is a remarkable set of experiments suggesting even our poop can get jet lag.

Our microbiomes seem to have their own circadian rhythms. Even though our friendly flora are down where the sun don't shine, there's a daily oscillation in both bacterial abundance and activity in our colons.

Check this out: If you put people on a plane and fly them halfway around the world, then feed their poop to mice, those mice grow fatter than mice fed their preflight feces.[2875] Though it may have just been bad airline food or something, the researchers suggest the fattening flora were a consequence of circadian misalignment.[2876] Indeed, several lines of evidence now implicate chronodisruption—the state in which our central and peripheral clocks diverge out of sync—as playing a role in conditions ranging from premature aging and cancer[2877] to mood disorders and obesity.[2878]

Bright light exposure is the synchronizing swing-pusher for our central clocks. What helps drive our internal organ clocks that aren't exposed to daylight? Food intake.[2879] That's why the timing of our meals may be so important. Removing all external timing cues by locking people away under constant, dim light, researchers showed you could effectively decouple central from peripheral rhythms just by shifting mealtimes. They took blood draws every hour and even took biopsies of the subjects' fat every six hours to demonstrate the resulting metabolic disarray.[2880]

Just as morning light can help sync our central clocks, morning meals can help sync our peripheral clocks. Skipping breakfast disrupts the normal expression and rhythm of the clock genes themselves, which coincide with the adverse metabolic effects.[2881] Thankfully, much of this can be reversed. Take a group of habitual breakfast skippers and have them eat meals at 8:00 a.m., 1:00 p.m., and 6:00 p.m., and their cholesterol and triglycerides improve compared to taking those three meals five hours later, at 1:00 p.m., 6:00 p.m., and 11:00 p.m.[2882] There's a circadian rhythm to cholesterol synthesis in the body as well, which is also strongly influenced by food intake, as evidenced by the fact that cholesterol production drops 95 percent in response to a single day of fasting.[2883]

Working Against the Clock

Night-shift workers have higher rates of obesity, as well as diabetes, cardiovascular disease, and cancer[2884]—graveyard shift indeed!—but is it because they tend to eat out of vending machines or simply because they don't get enough sleep? Highly controlled studies have attempted recently to tease out these factors by putting people on the same diets with the same sleep, but at the wrong time of day.[2885] Redistributing eating to the nighttime not only resulted in elevated blood pressure, inflammation, and cholesterol,[2886,2887,2888] but shifting meals to the evening in a simulated night-shift protocol turned about one-third of the subjects effectively prediabetic in only ten days.[2889] Our bodies just weren't designed to handle food at night.[2890]

Just as avoiding bright light at night can prevent circadian misalignment, so can avoiding eating at night. We may have no control over the lighting at our workplaces, but we can try to minimize overnight food intake, which has been shown to help limit the negative metabolic consequences of shift work.[2891] When we do finally get home in the morning, though, we may disproportionately crave unhealthy foods. In one experiment, 81 percent of participants in a night-shift scenario chose high-fat foods such as croissants off a breakfast buffet, compared to just 43 percent of the same subjects during a control period on a normal schedule.[2892]

Shift work may leave people too fatigued to exercise, but even at the same physical activity levels, chronodisruption can affect energy expenditure. Researchers at the Sleep and Chronobiology Laboratory at the University of Colorado found that we burn 12–16 percent fewer calories while sleeping during the daytime compared to at night.[2893] Just a single improperly timed snack can affect how much fat we burn every day. Study subjects eating a specified snack at 10:00 a.m. burned about six more grams of fat from their bodies than on the days they ate the same snack at 11:00 p.m.[2894] While that's only about a pat and half of butter's worth,[2895] it's astounding that eating an identical snack just given at a different time can make such a difference. What's more, the evening snack group also suffered about a 9 percent bump in their LDL cholesterol within two weeks.

Only a Matter of Time

Social jet lag is the discrepancy in sleep timing between the days we work and the days we're off.[2896] From a circadian rhythm standpoint, when we go to bed late and sleep in on the weekends, it's as if we flew a few time zones west on Friday evening and flew back east on Monday morning.[2897] Travel-induced jet lag goes away in a few days, but what might be the consequences of constantly shifting our schedules every week over our entire working career? To my knowledge, no interventional studies have tested this yet, but population studies suggest those who have at least an hour of social jet lag a week (which may describe more than two-thirds of people[2898]) have twice the odds of being overweight.[2899]

If sleep regularity is important, what about meal regularity? Evidently, the importance of regular meals at roughly the same time every day was emphasized by such luminaries as Hippocrates and Florence Nightingale,[2900] but it wasn't put to the test until the twenty-first century. A few population studies have suggested that those eating meals irregularly were at a metabolic disadvantage, including heavier body weight and wider waistlines,[2901] but the first interventional trials weren't published until 2004. Subjects were randomized to eat their regular diets split up into either six regular eating occasions a day or three to nine daily eating occasions, but in an irregular manner. Researchers found that eating an irregular pattern of meals every day can cause drops in insulin sensitivity[2902] and diet-induced thermogenesis,[2903] as well as cause cholesterol levels to rise.[2904] Obese participants ended up eating more, though, on the irregular meals, so it's difficult to disentangle circadian effects. The fact that overweight individuals may overeat on an irregular pattern may be telling in and of itself, but it would be useful if such a study were repeated using identical diets to see if irregularity on its own has metabolic effects. And, indeed, just such a study was published in 2016.

During two periods, people were randomized to eat identical foods in either a regular or irregular meal pattern. During the irregular period, people had impaired glucose tolerance and lower diet-induced thermogenesis, meaning they had higher blood sugar responses to the same food and burned fewer calories to process each meal. The difference in thermogenesis only came out to be about ten calories per meal, though, and there was no difference in weight changes over the two-week periods.[2905] However, diet-induced thermogenesis can act as a satiety signal.[2906] The extra work put into processing a meal can help with slaking one's appetite, and, indeed, the lower hunger and higher fullness ratings during the regular meal pattern could potentially translate into better weight control if they were maintained over the long term, but this has yet to be tested.[2907]

Keeping Yourself in the Dark

If weakening our circadian rhythms can cause weight gain, might strengthening them facilitate weight loss? Regular morning meals can give our circadian cycles a little daily push,[2908] but the biggest shove comes from our exposure to bright midmorning light (8:00 a.m.–11:00 a.m.). Similarly, exposure to light at night would be analogous to nighttime eating.[2909] Yes, we've had candles to illuminate the darkness for five thousand years, but flames from candles, campfires, and oil lamps are skewed toward the red end of the light spectrum, and the shorter blue wavelengths are the ones that specially set our circadian clocks. Even incandescent electric lighting, which only started a little over a century ago, consisted of mainly low-level yellow wavelengths, but they've been replaced over just the last few decades with fluorescents and LED lights that now contain extra blue wavelengths,[2910] which are more similar to morning sunlight.[2911]

Using wrist meters to measure ambient light exposure, researchers found that increased evening and nighttime light exposure correlated with a subsequent increased risk of developing obesity over time.[2912] This was presumed to be due to circadian misalignment, but is it possible it may instead be a sign they're not sleeping as much, and that's the real reason they grew heavier?

A study of more than one hundred thousand women controlled for this and found that the odds of obesity trended with higher nighttime light exposure independent of sleep duration.[2913] Compared to women who reported their bedrooms at night were either too dark to see their hands in front of their faces or at least too dark to see across the room, those who reported it was light enough to see across their bedrooms were significantly heavier on average.[2914] And it isn't as though they were sleeping with night-lights. Without blackout curtains on the windows, many neighborhoods may be bright enough to cause circadian disruption. Using satellite imagery, scientists have even been able to correlate higher obesity rates with brighter communities.[2915] There's so much light at night these days that, outside of a blackout, the only Milky Way many of our children will likely ever see is inside a candy wrapper.

Begin to See the Light

Insufficient morning light may be the circadian equivalent of skipping breakfast. Indoor lighting is too bright at night, but it may also be too dim to robustly boost our daily rhythm.[2916] Light exposure from getting outdoors in the morning even on an overcast day is correlated to lower body weight compared to typical office lighting,[2917] so some doctors started trying phototherapy to treat obesity. The first case reports began being published back in the 1990s. Three out of four women lost an average of about four pounds over six weeks of morning bright light exposure, but there was no control group to confirm the effect.[2918]

Ten years later, the first randomized controlled trial was published. Overweight individuals were randomized to an exercise intervention with or without an hour a day of bright morning light. Compared to normal indoor lighting, the bright light group lost more body fat,[2919] but it's possible the light just stimulated them to exercise harder. Studies show that bright light exposure even the day prior to exercise may boost performance. In a hand-grip endurance test, exposure to hours of bright light increased the number of contractions until exhaustion from about 770 to 860 the next day.[2920] While light-induced improvements in activity or mood can be helpful in their own right, it would be years more before we finally learned whether the light exposure itself could boost weight loss.

Following unpublished data purporting to show a twelve-and-a-half-pound weight-loss advantage from eight weeks of thirty minutes of daily daylight compared to indoor lighting, researchers in Norway tried three weeks of forty-five minutes of bright morning light compared to a placebo: the same time sitting in front of an ion generator that appeared to turn on but was secretly deactivated. The three weeks of light beat out the placebo, but the average difference in body-fat reduction was only about a pound.[2921] This slight edge didn't seem to correlate with mood changes, but bright light alone can stimulate serotonin production in the human brain[2922] and cause the release of adrenaline-type hormones,[2923] both of which could benefit body fat aside from any circadian effects.[2924] Regardless of the mechanism, bright morning daylight exposure could present a novel weight-loss strategy straight out of the clear blue sky.

Winter Never Comes

SAD doesn't just stand for the *Standard American Diet*. There's a condition known as *seasonal affective disorder* that's characterized by increased appetite and cravings, along with increased sleepiness and lethargy, beginning in autumn when light exposure starts to dwindle. This now appears to simply represent the far end of a normal spectrum of human behavior. We all appear to eat more as the days get shorter. There is a marked seasonal rhythm to caloric intake, with greater meal size, eating rate, hunger, and overall caloric consumption in the fall.[2925]

During the winter, some animals hibernate and, in preparation, double their fat stores with autumn's abundance to deal with the subsequent scarcity of winter.[2926] Genes have been identified in humans that are similar to hibernation genes,[2927] which may help explain why we exhibit some of the same behaviors. The autumnal effect isn't subtle. Researchers have calculated an average difference of 222 calories per day between caloric intake in the fall versus spring, and this isn't just because it's colder, since we eat more in the fall than the winter.[2928] It appears we are just genetically programmed to prep for the deprivation of winter that no longer comes.

It's remarkable in this day and age of modern lighting and heating that our bodies would still pick up on the environmental cues of the changing seasons enough to affect such a major influence on our eating patterns. Unsurprisingly, bright light therapy is used to treat seasonal affective disorder, nearly tripling the likelihood of remission compared to placebo.[2929] Though it's never been tested directly, it can't hurt to take the dog for some extra morning walks each fall to help fend off some of the coming holiday season weight gain.

Resetting the Clock

There are many ways we can preserve, sync, and strengthen our circadian rhythms. We can eat breakfast and get some sun in the morning, and at night, try to avoid eating and exposing ourselves to bright light. But because it is evidently "highly unlikely" that people will change their lifestyles, concludes a review on chronobiology approaches to obesity, "pharmacological modulation of circadian clock function . . . might offer an easier alternative."[2930] One such approach might be melatonin, the so-called darkness hormone.

Melatonin is secreted by a little gland in the center of our heads as soon as it gets dark and shuts off when the sun comes up in the morning. Its rise and fall overnight in the bloodstream helps sync all the circadian clocks throughout the body. Appropriately timed and dosed, melatonin, which is available over the counter, has been found to effectively decrease jet lag symptoms after long flights.[2931] What about taking it before bedtime to reinforce our rhythm for weight loss? It works for rats[2932] and mice,[2933] but what about people?

There are certain antipsychotic drugs notorious for causing weight gain.

Melatonin was put to the test as an adjunct treatment to try to forestall this effect and, in some cases, was able to improve weight outcomes compared to placebo in patients with bipolar disorder[2934] and schizophrenia.[2935] These particular mental illnesses are known to have a chronodisruption component, though, so the melatonin findings can't necessarily be generalized to others.[2936] Combined with Prozac, melatonin was found to have an extraordinary effect on body weight, resulting in about a four-and-a-half-point drop in BMI over twenty-four weeks compared to Prozac plus placebo. At average height, that's a difference of twenty-seven pounds.[2937] Again, though, one can't extrapolate to the general population since Prozac itself appears to interact with melatonin secretion.

There was a study of the effect of melatonin on migraine sufferers, and the melatonin group lost slightly more weight than those who were instead given a placebo or a conventional migraine medication.[2938] However, a trial in which otherwise healthy obese individuals were given 6 mg a day of melatonin or placebo failed to provide evidence of a weight-loss benefit.[2939] Given how poorly regulated the supplement industry is, there are troubling issues with the strength and purity of over-the-counter melatonin, so I recommend that you *not* use melatonin supplements to regulate your sleep schedule.

First of all, the doses found in melatonin supplements are massive. Even just taking a 3 mg dose produces levels in the bloodstream that can be fifty times higher than normal nightly levels,[2940] which raises safety concerns.[2941] After all, melatonin used to be known as an *anti-gonad hormone,* with human-equivalent doses of just a milligram or two reducing the size of sex organs and impairing fertility in laboratory animals.[2942] Obviously, rats aren't people, but considering the pronounced effects of melatonin on reproduction in other mammals, commentators have suggested it might be naïve to assume melatonin wouldn't have some effects on human sexuality. Some have even speculated it may have a role one day as some sort of a contraceptive agent.[2943]

Wouldn't we know about these effects, though? Not necessarily, since there isn't any post-marketing surveillance of dietary supplements for side effects as there is with drugs.[2944] There also isn't the same guarantee of authenticity with dietary supplements. Based on an analysis of thirty-one different brands, the actual melatonin content varied by up to nearly 500 percent compared to what was listed on the bottle.[2945]

Then there are the contaminants.

Two-thirds of melatonin products tested from health food stores were found to contain unidentified impurities.[2946] With no exclusive patent, companies appear unwilling to invest in ensuring purity since the pills are sold so incredibly cheaply.[2947] The concerns raised are not just theoretical. Contaminants present in tryptophan supplements, for example, were thought responsible for a disease outbreak that affected more than a thousand people and resulted in dozens of deaths.[2948] Given the structural similarities between the melatonin impurities and the implicated tryptophan contaminants, melatonin supplements may just be another accident waiting to happen.[2949] Because of all these reasons, melatonin supplements cannot be recommended.[2950]

Dietary Melatonin

It's a shame there's no way we could get the purported benefits of melatonin without the risks—*unless* melatonin were somehow found naturally in certain foods you could eat. And sure enough, melatonin was first discovered in plants in 1995 and has since been found throughout the plant kingdom.[2951] Randomize people to eat more or less vegetables, and you can demonstrate an effect on melatonin levels within the body.[2952]

Eat two bananas or drink the juice of about two pounds of oranges or pineapple, and you can also get a significant bump, and the melatonin levels found in those fruits are pretty modest compared to some other foods.[2953] Cranberries appear to be the most melatonin-rich fruit.[2954] Consume just a single ounce, about a third of a cup, and it's like you took a melatonin supplement with only good side effects.[2955] Unfortunately, Craisins, or dried cranberries, may not have the same affect.

A study of various tart cherry products suggests that the drying process wipes out their melatonin, so there isn't any melatonin in dried cherries and presumably not in dried cranberries either.[2956] The same appears to be the case with juice. The level of melatonin in cherry juice concentrate was also found to be nondetectable, so drinking cranberry juice would presumably also be a wash.

That brings us to pistachios.

Pistachios are not just the most melatonin-rich nut, they are off the charts as the most melatonin-rich food ever recorded.[2957] To get a physiological dose of melatonin, all you have to eat is two. Two cups? Two handfuls? No, just two pistachios. Pistachio nuts were found to contain 0.2 mg of melatonin per gram.[2958] It only takes 0.3 mg of melatonin to cause the normal daily spike our brains give us, so just two nuts would presumably do the trick.[2959] So the best food for jet lag would appear to be appropriately timed pistachios. Sound too good to be true? It may be. A second lab failed to replicate the findings using a different batch of pistachios,[2960] but it can't hurt to give it a try.

FOOD FOR THOUGHT

The proverb "Eat breakfast like a king, lunch like a prince, and dinner like a pauper" evidently has another variant: "Eat breakfast yourself, share lunch with a friend, and give dinner away to your enemy."[2961] I wouldn't go that far, but there does appear to be metabolic benefit to frontloading the bulk of calories earlier in the day. And certainly, if you're going to regularly skip a meal—for example, those practicing intermittent fasting or trying to fit all their food into a certain window through time-restricted feeding—it would probably be safer and more effective to skip dinner rather than breakfast.

Other "recommendations for the prevention of obesity . . . by improving the circadian system,"[2962] based on varying degrees of evidence, include:

- Sleep during the night and be active during the day
- Sleep enough (seven to eight hours a night)
- Early to bed, early to rise
- Avoid bright light exposure at night
- Sleep in total darkness when possible
- Eat dinner at least two and a half hours before going to bed
- Avoid eating at night

I also talked about the potential for shedding light on shedding pounds through bright morning daylight exposure, especially in the fall, and eating regular meals at the same time every day. Any other ways to lose weight like clockwork? You could try eating two pistachios two to three hours before bedtime. Will that help? There's only one way to find out.

EATING RATE

A Solid Grip on Satiety

As I discussed in the Rich in Fruits and Vegetables section, the human body doesn't seem to register calories from liquids as well as it does calories from solid foods for some reason. Take, for example, the famous study of soda versus jelly beans. Researchers had people add twenty-eight extra spoonfuls of sugar to their daily diets in the form of jelly beans or soda and then measured how many calories the study participants ate over the rest of the day to see if their bodies would compensate for all that extra sugar. In the jelly bean group, their bodies registered the extra calories from the handfuls of candy, and the subjects ended up eating less of everything else throughout the day. In the end, they ate pretty much the same number of calories before and after adding the jelly beans to their diets. In the soda group, however, despite all the added calories from the cans of pop they drank every day, they continued to eat about the same amount of the rest of their diets. No wonder they gained weight after a month of drinking soda.[2963] Their bodies didn't seem to fully recognize the extra calories when they were in liquid form and, therefore, didn't compensate by reducing their appetites for the rest of the day. Of course, when it comes to deciding which is a better dietary choice—soda versus jelly beans—the answer is *neither*. When I encourage people to eat beans every day, I'm decidedly not talking about the Jelly Belly variety.

What about solid-versus-liquid *healthy* foods? What if you drink a smoothie for breakfast instead of eating a solid meal? Will your body mistakenly think you effectively skipped breakfast and lead you to eat more later in the day? To answer this, we first have to make sure this solid-versus-liquid-calorie effect is real. Soda and jelly beans don't just differ by physical form; they have different ingredients.

To truly test for a solid-versus-liquid effect, you'd have to use the exact same foods in two different forms. Finally, a study did just that. Researchers looked at what happens if you eat a fruit salad of raw apples, apricots, and bananas and drink three cups of water or, instead, blend the fruit with two cups of water to make a smoothie and drink the third cup of water.[2964] The meals are identical except one is in solid form and the other is in smoothie form. What happened? People felt significantly less full after the smoothie, even though it was the same type and amount of food. In smoothie form, it didn't fill people up as much as eating fruit au naturel.

Originally, we thought it was due to the lack of chewing. The act of chewing itself may send "I've eaten enough" signals that you don't get just by drinking.[2965] In one experiment, people were asked to eat pasta, chewing either ten or thirty-five times per mouthful, until they felt comfortably full.[2966] Those who chewed thirty-five times per bite ended up eating about a third of a cup less pasta than those who had only chewed ten times per bite. So there we have it: not only proof of a solid-versus-liquid effect from the smoothie study but the actual mechanism. As so often happens in science, however, just when you think everything is neatly wrapped up with a bow, a paradox arises.

The Great Soup Paradox

Puréed, blended soup—essentially a warm smoothie of blended vegetables— was sometimes found to be *more* satiating than the same veggies in solid form.[2967] Since the meal in liquid form was more filling than the same meal in solid form, it can't be due to the amount of chewing. How can cold smoothies be less filling than the constituent ingredients eaten in solid form, but warm smoothies are more filling? So filling, in fact, that when people have soup as a first course, they may end up eating so much less of the main course that they eat fewer calories overall, even when the added soup calories are taken into account.[2968] How can we explain this paradox?

Might puréed fruits be less filling than solid fruits, but puréed vegetables more filling than solid vegetables? To test this, Purdue University researchers gave subjects three apples to eat, three cups of apple juice to drink, or a warm, blended apple soup made from a cup of apple juice with two cups of applesauce liquefied in a blender and heated up. Within fifteen minutes of eating the three actual apples, the subjects reported feeling pretty full. Drinking three cups of apple juice, on the other hand, didn't cut hunger much at all. What about the apple soup, which was pretty much just apple juice mixed with applesauce and warmed? The apple soup cut hunger almost as much as the whole apples, even more than an hour later, and in fact beat out whole apples for decreasing overall caloric intake for the day.[2969]

What's so special about soup? What does eating soup have in common with prolonged chewing that differentiates it from drinking a smoothie? Time. It took people about twice as long to eat when they chewed each bite of pasta thirty-five times rather than ten in that previous study.[2970] Now think about how long it takes to eat a bowl of soup compared to drinking a smoothie. Could eating more slowly reduce caloric intake?

Alternatively, maybe we just think of soup as a filling food so the added satiety is more like a placebo effect. Feelings like hunger and fullness are subjective. People tend to report hunger more in accordance with how many calories they think something has rather than the actual caloric content.[2971] Remember that movie *Memento* about a guy who can't form short-term memories? That's actually a real disorder in which people can't remember what had just happened more than a few moments earlier. Tragically, sufferers of anterograde amnesia can overeat to the point of vomiting because they forgot they had just eaten, which shows what poor judges we are of our own hunger.[2972]

The effects of thoughts about foods can extend beyond the subjective. In a famous study entitled "Mind Over Milkshakes," people were offered two different shakes: one described as indulgent, "decadence you deserve," and another labeled as sensible, "guilt-free satisfaction." People had different hormonal responses to the two options even though they were being fooled and given the exact same milkshake.[2973] Just the *thought* of them being different was enough to affect how their bodies responded based on objective blood tests.

Or could it be as simple as soup is most often served hot and warmer foods are more satiating?[2974] How could we figure out if the answer to the soup paradox was time, thought, or temperature? If only that blended fruit salad and water study had a third group in which the smoothie was just eaten cold out of a bowl with a spoon. That would solve the mystery. If it were just preconceived notions about the comforts of soup or its warmth, then fullness ratings would fall down around that of the smoothie. It turns out that the study did include just such a third group, and the participants felt just as full sipping the smoothie with a spoon as they did eating the whole fruit—so the answer is *time*.[2975] The only real reason smoothies aren't as filling is that we gulp them down. If we sip them slowly over time, they can be just as filling as if we had eaten the fruits and veggies whole.

The Twenty-Minute Rule

Schoolchildren have been timed consuming lunch in an average of seven to ten minutes.[2976] Children are often scolded not to wolf down their food, but does it really matter how fast we eat? More than you may realize. People were given soup, but half were given small spoons and told to eat slowly, and the other half were given big spoons and told to eat quickly, and an amazing thing happened: The slow-eating group not only ended up feeling more satiated, but they did so after eating less soup.[2977] They felt fuller eating less food.

Prolonged meal duration can allow more time for our bodies' own "I'm full" satiety signals to develop before too many calories have been consumed.[2978] The slower we eat, the more time our bodies have to catch up. As Harvard's Healthy Weight Checklist puts it: "Slowing down at meals . . . can help avoid overeating by giving the brain time to tell the stomach when it's had enough food."[2979] We evolved for millions of years trying to extract calories from undomesticated fruits and vegetables, which were much tougher and fibrous than produce today. This was long before hot dog–eating contests enabled the human frame to inhale twenty thousand calories in ten minutes.[2980] Our bodies are built to expect us to take our time when eating.

When we eat, anorexigenic hormones such as GLP-1 and PYY, which I discussed in the High in Fiber-Rich Foods section, are released from cells lining our intestines into our bloodstreams. These hormones then have to travel to our brains to flick on the satiety switch to get us to slow down, but this process takes time. Preload studies, where people are fed a first course one, five, fifteen, twenty, thirty, or sixty minutes before the main meal, show that this fullness feedback loop may take about twenty minutes to fully tamp down our appetites.[2981] This, then, explains the soup study results. The fast-soup-eating group was done in fewer than nine minutes, while the slow-soup-eating group stopped after twenty-nine minutes.[2982] Even though the group eating more slowly and with smaller spoons ended up having less soup overall, their brains had time to fully process the meal and were able to give them a stronger sense of satiety.

In smoothie form, you can drink fruits and vegetables at about two cups a minute—ten times faster than it might take to eat fruits and vegetables in solid form.[2983] Liquid calories can be consumed so quickly they can undermine our bodies' ability to regulate food intake at healthy levels. It's not the liquid texture per se but the high rate of consumption at which liquids are normally consumed. Blend all the smoothies you want, but sip them slowly for a half hour or so rather than gulping them down.

Every one of a dozen population studies found that those who eat faster are at higher risk of obesity, approximately doubling their odds.[2984] In a behavioral treatment program for obesity, those who were able to slow their average meal length by just four minutes, from fourteen to eighteen minutes, lost more weight over a seven-month period.[2985] There are lots of ways to extend meal duration, like putting down your utensil between bites, chewing longer, taking smaller bites, or choosing foods that simply take longer to eat.

Merely inserting enforced breaks while eating doesn't appear to work, however. One experiment in which people were interrupted with a buzzer every minute or so and asked to pause eating for up to sixty seconds ended up eating more,[2986] seemingly out of sheer frustration.[2987] Prolonged chewing shows more promise.

Chewing the Fat Away

An obituary from 1919 about health food enthusiast Horace Fletcher proclaimed that he "taught the world to chew."[2988] Also known as the Great Masticator, Fletcher was a health reformer who popularized the idea of chewing each mouthful more than thirty-two times, a chew for every tooth.[2989] That practice wasn't put to the test until nearly a century later in that pasta study when chewing a bite thirty-five times was shown to beat out chewing only ten times and resulted in 12 percent fewer calories eaten at a meal.[2990] A similar study found a similar result, comparing forty versus fifteen chews.[2991] This is not surprising given the twenty-minute rule—the fewer-chews group finished in fifteen minutes, whereas the greater-chews group took nearly a half hour before they felt satisfied, allowing their natural satiety feedback loop time to kick in. The investigators concluded that public health messages to promote "slower eating" are vague, whereas a recommendation to chew food more thoroughly may be more actionable advice.[2992]

Do people who chew less weigh more? One study sent people home with a chew-recording device—a headband with electrodes placed over their jaw muscles—and found that those scoring fewer chews had up to nine times the odds of gaining more than twenty pounds over the subsequent decades.[2993] Of course, the obvious confounding factor to *how* they were eating was *what* they eating. Maybe the high-chew group gained less weight because they were eating lots of fiber-rich foods like vegetables, while the low-chew group was slurping down more calories from Slurpees. Eating an apple may take an average of 186 chews, whereas the same weight in Jell-O may only take 23.[2994]

If you seat people in a room and watch them eat the same food, overweight and obese individuals do seem to chew fewer times per mouthful than those who are normal weight, resulting in a faster eating rate.[2995] If you ask people to double their baseline number of chews per bite, they end up eating about 15 percent less pizza, feeling just as full eating more than one hundred fewer calories.[2996] Even just asking them to chew 50 percent more times than normal may cut their consumption by nearly 10 percent.[2997]

More thorough chewing leads to a slower eating rate, which leads to fewer calories consumed.[2998] In other words, the same fullness with less food. If you have people eat the same amount but chew more, they end up less hungry,[2999] but does that appetite suppression translate into less food eaten hours later? Researchers gave people a fixed amount for lunch and told some to chew as they normally would and the others to chew each bite for thirty seconds. Later that afternoon, the subjects were presented with a snack (essentially Skittles and M&M's) and those who, hours earlier, had chewed each mouthful of lunch for thirty seconds ended up eating only half as much candy.[3000]

But just when we think we have the mechanism figured out, a new enigma arises. The candy study also involved a third group instructed to chew lunch normally but with a ten-second break between each mouthful, which resulted in approximately the same meal duration as the chew-each-bite-for-thirty-seconds group. So the same slowed eating rate would presumably result in the same drop in snack intake hours later, right? No. Only the prolonged-chewing group sufficiently suppressed appetites enough to significantly cut down on snack intake later on, even though both of the slowed eating groups ate lunch over about the same protracted period.[3001] There must be more to the story than just allowing time for our brains to recognize the release in satiety hormones from the digestive tract.

Oral Stimulation

The cephalic phase of digestion starts before food even hits our stomachs. *Cephalic* means *in the head*. There are nerves traveling straight from our brains to our mouths. This is how even the thought of food can get us salivating. And the nerves are a two-way street. Signals coming from our mouths can tip off our brains to what's coming down the pike.[3002]

To test the effect of this mind-to-mouth connection on appetite, you can insert a tube down someone's throat to compare regular eating to slipping the same amount of food directly into their stomachs. Removing the experience of the taste, smell, and texture of the food left people feeling significantly less full even though they ended up with the exact same amount of food in their stomachs.[3003] This wasn't just a psychological effect. Objective measures, such as slowed stomach emptying times, prove that sensations from the mouth translate into physical fullness.[3004]

Another way to study the cephalic phase response is to use sham feeding, known less delicately as the *chew-and-spit technique*. The insulin levels in our blood can be doubled within fifteen minutes just by chewing on some pizza, even though none of it is swallowed.[3005] Based on the signals coming from the mouth, our brains seem to anticipate how much insulin is going to be needed to handle the incoming load and try to get a head start. Incidentally, the mismatch between the sweetness on the tongue and the lack of calories flooding in when drinking diet soda may actually help explain some of the metabolic disruption associated with the consumption of artificial sweeteners.[3006]

In regard to appetite control, the cephalic phase response can be so powerful that fake eating can even trump actual eating. Consider this ingenious study: Subjects were split into two groups—one who chewed and spat out cake for one minute, and another who chewed and spat out cake for eight minutes, the "long oral stimulation" group. Meanwhile, within each group, half had about one hundred calories of "cake-solution" pumped into their stomachs with a tube and the other half had eight hundred calories pumped in. Then, thirty minutes later, everyone was offered a meal to see what effect each manipulation had on appetite. Remarkably, the long-chewing group getting the smaller, hundred-calorie preload ate less than the short-chewing group getting the larger, eight-hundred-calorie preload.[3007] So eight times the oral exposure more mightily tamped down their hunger than getting eight times more actual food in the stomach. Amazing!

You can see how the cephalic phase response would work in concert with the digestive hormone feedback loop. It would take the average person about twenty minutes to eat nine cups of apple slices, whereas drinking the same number of calories of apple juice would take less than two minutes.[3008,3009,3010]

Not only would that twenty minutes allow time for our "stop-eating" hormones to make it up to our brains, but the apples offer eighteen more minutes of oral exposure and ten times the number of oral-stimulation signals racing from the mouth to the brain, letting it know we're chowing down.

Slow Burn

The cephalic phase response also plays a role in diet-induced thermogenesis, the calories your body burns just to process the food you eat. As soon as food hits your mouth, your brain starts priming the pump. You've got to spend money to make money, and it costs the body roughly 10 percent of the calories you eat to get at the other 90 percent. That could add up to hundreds of calories a day, and about half of them are due just to the signals to the brain that arise from contact between food and the inside of your mouth. We know this because if people are tube-fed, diet-induced thermogenesis gets cut by 53 percent[3011,3012] or more.[3013]

Half of just 10 percent of the calories you eat may not sound like a lot, but it could add up to thousands of calories a month.[3014] What are the practical implications of this, though? It's not as if you wake up every morning and have to decide whether or not to tube feed. You can, however, increase oral exposure time by slowing down at mealtime. If you have people eat especially fast (consuming in five minutes what would normally take them fifteen), diet-induced thermogenesis gets cut by nearly a third within fifteen minutes, so you don't get to take full advantage of the effect for weight loss.[3015] In contrast, having people slow down by chewing each bite "until no lumps remain" significantly boosts thermogenesis compared to a rapid-eating group. Using Doppler ultrasound, the researchers were able to correlate these differences to the changes in abdominal blood flow.[3016] As soon as our brains detect food in our mouths, they start rerouting blood to the intestines to deal with the coming influx.

Another study compared chewing thirty times per mouthful versus not chewing at all (effectively drinking the same meal blenderized into a purée). The researchers found the same 50 percent difference in thermogenesis uncovered in the tube-feeding studies. So eating without chewing seemed to register as little as not eating at all. It's almost as if the mouth had been bypassed entirely. The researchers concluded that "thorough mastication [chewing] before swallowing . . . may be useful for preventing obesity."[3017] But was it the act of chewing itself or just the extra time the food was present in the mouth?

Bite-Sized

How could you design an experiment to differentiate among prolonged chewing, oral exposure, and meal duration? A research group in the Netherlands came up with an elegant solution. They had people effectively take either a teaspoon of tomato soup every five seconds or a tablespoonful every fifteen seconds until they were full. Because a tablespoon is three times bigger than a teaspoon, the eating rate was exactly the same at a quarter cup per minute. Note, though, the oral exposure time was completely different. Even though the tablespoon of soup lasted slightly longer in the mouth (three seconds versus two seconds with the teaspoonful), because the tablespoon group was only getting four spoonfuls a minute, the total oral exposure time every minute was only half that of the teaspoon group (twelve seconds versus twenty-four seconds). So it was the same eating rate, but the soup was only in the mouths of the tablespoon group one-fifth of the time and in the mouths of the teaspoon group nearly half the time.[3018] Who ended up eating more soup?

If chewing were the critical factor, then both groups would have presumably eaten the same amount of soup since there was no chewing in either group. (It was creamy tomato.) Similarly, since their stomachs were filling up at the same rate, if it were just the length of the meal, then both groups would get full around the same time. But if the results came down to the amount of time food is physically in our mouths, then the teaspoon group would get fuller faster and end up eating significantly less—and that's exactly what happened. The teaspoon group felt full after about four minutes, but the tablespoon group ate for closer to six minutes and ended up consuming a third more soup.[3019]

The same thing happens when you replicate this experiment with drinks. Researchers had people swallow teaspoon-sized sips of orangeade every other second versus a larger four-teaspoon swallow every eight seconds. Same minute-by-minute drink rate, but twice the oral exposure in the teaspoon-sip group. Again, the smaller-sip group won out, feeling satiated after about one-and-a-half cups compared to the two cups it took when taking larger sips.[3020] Experiments simultaneously varying bite size and oral exposure time with solid food found the same phenomenon: It's better to nibble and savor than chomp and gulp.[3021]

What About Chewing Gum?

If prolonged oral exposure can cause appetite suppression, what about chewing gum as a weight-loss strategy? An article entitled "Benefits of Chewing Gum" suggested as much, but it was written by—no joke— the executive director of the Wrigley Science Institute.[3022] Big Gum likes to point to a letter published in 1999 in *The New England Journal of Medicine,*[3023] where Mayo Clinic researchers claimed chewing gum could burn eleven calories an hour. Critics pointed to the fact that this was based on having people chewing the equivalent of four sticks of gum at a "very rapid cadence"[3024] ("precisely 100 Hz"[3025]) for twelve minutes. That seemed to burn two and two-tenths calories, hence potentially eleven calories an hour.

One might have more confidence in the Mayo scientists' conclusion had they not lacked a fundamental understanding of basic units: 100 hertz would mean one hundred chews per second, which *would* be very rapid indeed![3026] If the eleven calories an hour is true, though, that might mean you could burn more calories actively chewing gum while sitting in a chair than you would *not* chewing gum while upright at a standing desk.[3027] The calorie expenditure isn't only due to our little jaw muscles at work. For some reason, chewing gum revs up our heart rates—as much as an extra twelve beats per minute after chewing two sticks of gum for just five minutes at rest[3028] or three more beats per minute while walking[3029] (proving scientifically that people *can* indeed walk and chew gum at the same time).

Chewing one small piece of gum at your own pace may only burn about three calories an hour,[3030] which would approximate the calorie content of sugar-free gums (typically two to three calories per piece). Chewing off the calories of sugar-sweetened gum, however, which are typically twenty to twenty-five calories each, might take all day.[3031] There's more to the energy balance of gum, though, than just all the chewing.

If the oral exposure of chewing a meal can increase diet-induced thermogenesis, how about effectively extending this period by chewing gum immediately after a meal? Will that trick the body into thinking it's still eating? Chewing a single, three-calorie piece of gum for fifteen minutes after a meal does appear to burn off six to eight calories in extra thermogenesis.[3032] A few calories here and there would be nothing, though, compared to any effect chewing gum might have on portion size if it affected our appetites. So does it?

The results from studies on the effects of chewing gum on hunger are all over the place. Some studies show decreased appetite ratings,[3033,3034] others show no effect,[3035,3036] and one even shows significantly *increased* hunger after chewing gum.[3037] The more important question is whether there are any changes in subsequent caloric intake. Again, the findings are mixed.[3038,3039] One study even found that while chewing gum didn't impact consumption of M&M's, it did appear to decrease the consumption of healthy snacks.[3040] The chewing gum was mint and the healthy snacks included mandarin orange slices, though, so this may have just been an orange-juice-after-tooth-brushing effect.

It can take an hour before the residual taste effect of mint toothpaste dissipates.[3041] This is bad if it cuts our fruit intake, but what about harnessing this power against Pringles? An international group of researchers had people eat Pringles potato chips for twelve minutes, interrupting them every three minutes to swish with a menthol mouthwash. Compared to those in the control group swishing with plain water, the minty mouthwash group cut their consumption of chips by 29 percent. The researchers concluded that "if a consumer finds themselves snacking on too many [potato chip] crisps during a given eating occasion, one potential strategy could be intervening by having a peppermint tea, menthol flavoured chewing gum, or brushing their teeth, to slow down or stop snacking."[3042]

What really matters, though, is weight loss. Even if some little modification like chewing gum can affect the consumption of a single snack, our bodies could just compensate later in the day. The only way to know for certain whether chewing gum can be used as a weight-loss hack is to put it to the test.

(continued)

Researchers at the University of Buffalo randomized study participants to either not chew any gum at all or chew gum before every single eating occasion, which meant they didn't just have to chew gum before each meal but also before each snack or even before each drink if the beverage had calories. This may have been too much for folks, so they actually ended up eating on fewer occasions, switching from eating four times a day on average down to around three. However, they ended up consuming more calories at each of those fewer eating occasions, so they had no overall change in caloric intake and no change in weight.[3043]

University of Alabama researchers tried a different tack, randomizing people to chew gum after and between meals. After two months, compared to those randomized to avoid gum entirely, no improvements were noted in weight, BMI, or waist circumference.[3044] What about those few studies that did show immediate hunger suppression with chewing gum? In one study, for example, people ate sixty-eight fewer calories of pasta at lunch after chewing gum for twenty minutes.[3045] Okay, but other studies showed otherwise.

Different types of gum using different sweeteners could have contributed to the diversity of findings. The study showing chewing gum actually increased appetite, for example, was done with gum sweetened with aspartame. People reported feeling hungrier after chewing the sweetened gum—not only compared to no gum but also compared to chewing the same gum with no added aspartame. True, not a single randomized controlled trial has ever shown a benefit to chewing gum, but they've all used gum containing artificial sweeteners.

Remember that orangeade study demonstrating that sip size matters? The one where subjects taking smaller sips felt satiated drinking less than those taking larger sips of the same beverage? Using an artificially sweetened orange drink instead appeared to blunt the effect.[3046] Since getting repeated pulses of a calorie-free flavor didn't appear to be an appetite suppressant, is it possible a different type of gum, perhaps with a different sweetener, would have a different effect? In that study where people ate fewer calories of pasta at lunch after chewing gum for twenty minutes, the gum used was largely sweetened with sorbitol,[3047] a sweet compound found naturally in foods like prunes.[3048] Like prunes, though, it can have a laxative effect.

Case reports with names like "An Air Stewardess with Puzzling Diarrhoea" unveil what can happen when you eat sixty sticks of sorbitol-sweetened, sugar-free gum a day.[3049] Another was entitled "Severe Weight Loss Caused by Chewing Gum," but not in a good way: A twenty-one-year-old woman ended up malnourished after suffering up to a dozen bouts of diarrhea a day for eight months due to the twenty daily grams of sorbitol she was getting from chewing sugar-free gum.[3050] Most people suffer gas and bloating at ten grams of sorbitol a day, which is about eight sticks of sorbitol-sweetened gum, and at twenty grams, most get cramps and diarrhea.[3051] So be careful how much sorbitol you eat.

The bottom line is that we have no good science showing that chewing gum results in weight loss. Could that be because the studies tended to use gum with artificial sweeteners that may have counteracted any benefits? That's a possibility. The most obvious conclusion from the results to date, however, according even to gum company–funded researchers, "is that chewing gum simply is not an efficacious weight-loss strategy."[3052]

Hard Feelings

We've talked about some of the ways to increase the time food stays in our mouths so we can take better advantage of the cephalic phase response. Whatever you're eating, you can take smaller bites, eat slower, or chew longer. Another strategy is to choose different foods entirely. The *texture* of foods can make a difference. By default, harder foods are consumed in smaller bites, eaten more slowly, and with longer chewing. If you feed people a soft rice salad made with creamy risotto rice and boiled vegetables, they end up eating 17 percent more calories than when given the same salad made with regular rice and raw vegetables. Even just swapping a hard hamburger bun for a soft one can make a difference.[3053] However, this is the opposite of what Big Food tends to dish us. The food industry processes products for maximum consumption rate.[3054] They don't call it *fast food* for nothing.

People overeat more liquid yogurt when presented with a straw versus a spoon because we can gulp faster than we can spoon.[3055] For the same reason, if people are given chocolate milk versus pudding made from nearly identical ingredients but fine-tuned with different thickeners to change the physical state, they will consume more of the liquid than the semisolid food. If the eating speed is standardized, though—for example, if the products are pumped directly into their mouths at the same rate—people can end up feeling just as full either way.[3056] Some studies still suggest a satiety benefit of more solid foods, however, even at the same rate of consumption.[3057] This may be due in part to differences in stomach-emptying rates.

If you put people in an MRI machine to measure how quickly food is draining from their stomachs, you can see that thicker foods tend to drain more slowly. In fact, one hundred calories of a thick milkshake can end up being more satiating than five hundred calories of a thin shake.[3058] Presented with thick or thin porridge, people feel just as satisfied eating about fifty fewer calories of the thick porridge.[3059] So, when making oatmeal, remember that thicker and chewier may be more filling.

Adding dried fruits and nuts can create textural complexity, which has also been found to suppress appetite, based on studies of retro Jell-O salad–like concoctions that mixed in layers of chewy and crunchy bits. The appetite-lowering benefits over more homogenous foodstuffs are thought to be due to enhanced oral-sensory stimulation.[3060]

The Time-Calorie Displacement Program

Whether through increasing viscosity or the number of chews, or decreasing bite size and eating rate, dozens of studies have demonstrated that regardless of how we boost the amount of time food is in our mouths, it can result in lower caloric intake.[3061] Some approaches may be more viable than others. For example, in that study where people had to chew each mouthful for thirty seconds before swallowing, they went on to eat less candy hours later—but they weren't happy about it. The prolonged-chewing group reported enjoying their meal significantly less,[3062] calling long-term amenability into question.[3063] My favorite method for increasing oral exposure time is to choose healthier foods.

As opposed to those made in a factory, foods that *grow* tend to be slow. Thanks in part to the fiber content of whole, healthy plant foods, the default eating rate of more healthful foods just tends to be slower naturally.[3064] Though there are certainly exceptions, like caramel toffee, highly processed foods tend to be consumed quicker. There can be a hundredfold difference in consumption between the fastest and the slowest foods. You could consume an entire two-thousand-daily-calorie-allotment's worth of chocolate milk in four minutes, whereas it would take more than six straight hours to chew through that many raw carrots.[3065,3066,3067]

Even healthy foods can vary drastically. The average eating rate of boiled carrots is ten times that of raw.[3068] This is not to say cooked carrots aren't super healthy, but the longer something takes to eat, the more time those hunger-squashing hormones have to reach your brain and the more direct mouth-brain nerve stimulation there will be to quell your appetite. So, from a weight-loss standpoint, raw carrots clearly beat out boiled.

Directing people toward more slow-food options was formalized into a weight-loss program known as *Time-Calorie Displacement,* also known as *Time-Energy Displacement,* which sounds like a contraption that belongs in a De-Lorean. In the Low in Calorie Density section, I talked about how whole plant foods tend to offer a much greater volume of food for the same number of calories, and more food takes longer to eat, so in effect, healthier foods can often displace less healthy options in both time and space. A greater quantity of food doesn't just physically fill you up more. All that extra eating can allow other satiety mechanisms beyond just stomach-distension time to kick in.

When people were put on a diet packed with fruits, vegetables, whole grains, and beans and allowed to eat all they wanted, they ended up eating 48 percent fewer calories than they might have otherwise.[3069] Part of that was due to the lower calorie density of the plant-heavy diet, but people also spent about 40 percent more time chewing, for seventeen minutes per meal compared to twelve minutes. It's one thing for people to feel just as full on half the calories, but can they be kept satisfied on a thousand-calorie diet if they're eating enough whole plant foods? That's what the Time-Calorie Displacement diet was all about.[3070]

Thousands of people went through the official Time-Calorie Displacement Program[3071] (since renamed the EatRight program).[3072] The weight loss of participants averaged eighteen pounds over six months of active treatment, and body fat was lost while muscle mass was maintained. The critical question, though, is what happened after that? Over an average follow-up of seventeen months post-treatment, 44 percent of patients continued to lose weight, and more than 90 percent stayed under their baseline weights.[3073] In designing the diet, the researchers recognized that nearly any diet can cause weight loss at least short term, but the ends don't always justify the means. Their challenge was to design a "nutritionally sound" diet "conducive to a lifelong pattern of healthful eating."[3074] To that end, the diet encourages people to eat more high-bulk, calorie-dilute foods (vegetables, fruits, whole grains, and beans) and fewer energy-dense foods (meats, cheeses, sugars, and fats).[3075]

In *The Journal of the American College of Nutrition,* a review article was published entitled "Rational Weight Loss Programs: A Clinician's Guide." The Time-Calorie Displacement Program was held up as a prototypical example: safe, effective, health-promoting, and based on sound scientific principles.[3076]

FOOD FOR THOUGHT

A systematic review and meta-analysis of the effects of faster versus slower eating found that no matter how the eating rate was manipulated—whether solid food versus liquid, thick versus thin, spoon versus straw, or just telling people to slow down when they eat—on average, the slower-eating groups had their hunger satiated eating less food.[3077] So choose foods that take longer to eat, and eat them in a way that prolongs the time they stay in your mouth. Think bulkier, harder, chewier foods, such as apples, carrots, or intact grains, eaten in smaller, thoroughly chewed bites. Snack on raw veggies, and fall in love with soup. If possible, extend meal duration so it lasts at least twenty minutes to allow your natural satiety signals to take full effect.

Try eating with chopsticks. Even in experienced hands, they tend to slow eating rate.[3078] If you are going to drink your calories, make your smoothies thicker and sip them leisurely through a skinnier straw (preferably reusable, like the glass straws with silicone tips I love). The notion that eating quickly may lead to weight gain used to be considered an old wives' tale.[3079] As anyone married to one can attest, though, wives—young or old—are most often right in the end.

EXERCISE TWEAKS

The Exercise "Myth"

When trying to lose weight, which is more important: diet or exercise? A national survey found that a "vast majority" of Americans, seven out of ten, believe that food and beverage consumption and physical activity are equally important when it comes to weight loss. About two out of ten favored exercise, and only about one in ten chose diet.[3080] The vast majority of Americans are wrong.

It's easy to understand how people might think diet and exercise play equal roles. After all, our body fat is determined by the balance of calories in and calories out. What people may not understand about this energy-balance equation is that we have much more power over the calories-in side. In fact, on a day-to-day basis, we have full control. We could choose to eat zero calories or ten thousand calories. Most of the calories out, however, tend to be outside our control.

Wild animals typically burn most of their calories on activity,[3081] but thanks in part to our energy-intensive brains, most of our daily calories are used just to keep us alive.[3082] Even if we stayed in bed all day, we'd still burn more than a thousand calories just to fuel our resting metabolic rates—the basics like thinking, breathing, and keeping our hearts pumping. In contrast, even most "active" people exercise less than two hours a week, which may average out to fewer than one hundred calories burned off daily.[3083] That's less than 5 percent of the calories-out side of the equation.[3084] Given that, the two thousand calories we may take in every day can exert twenty times more influence than exercise over our weight destiny.

Though most people believe exercise is a "very effective" way to lose weight,[3085] that has been referred to as a "myth" in the scientific literature.[3086] In fact, it's been labeled as one of the most common misconceptions in the field of obesity,[3087] yet virtually all formal weight-loss guidelines include some sort of exercise recommendation.[3088] What does the science say?

Population studies certainly have found strong correlations between physical inactivity and obesity, but does a sedentary lifestyle lead to obesity, or does obesity lead to a sedentary lifestyle? It probably works a little in both directions.[3089] To prove cause and effect and also to quantify the relationship, you really have to put it to the test.

Can You Outrun a Bad Diet?

Dozens of randomized controlled trials involving thousands of participants have been published on the effects of exercise on weight loss.[3090] How did exercise fare? Surprisingly, physical activity was not found to be an effective strategy.[3091] Think of it this way: A moderately obese person doing moderate-intensity physical activity, like biking or very brisk walking, would burn off approximately 350 calories an hour.[3092] Most drinks, snacks, and other pro-cessed junk are consumed at a rate of about 70 calories a *minute*. Therefore, it only takes five minutes of snacking for someone to wipe out a whole hour of exercise.[3093]

Looking at the studies that tried to use exercise alone to induce weight loss, for example, people only lost about three pounds over an average of about six months.[3094] The experiments ranged from two to twelve months in duration, with people exercising under supervision for fifteen to seventy minutes at a time, two to five days a week, with intensities ranging from light to vigorous. Putting all the studies together, it looks like it took an average of around eight weeks of exercising to get people to lose a single pound. That was exercise alone, though. What about exercise as an adjunct to diet?

When people are randomized into diet-and-exercise interventions ver-sus diet alone, the diet-and-exercise groups do better, but the difference in weight loss only averages about two pounds.[3095] The studies lasted between three and twelve months, and all that extra prescribed exercise seemed to translate into only a few pounds lost. The two-pound difference was *statisti-cally* significant, however, which means we're pretty sure it was a real effect, but losing two pounds over a year's time can hardly be considered *clinically* significant. As a general rule, researchers like to see at least a five- or six-pound drop.[3096]

The longer-term trials performed even worse. In a meta-analysis of eigh-teen randomized controlled studies lasting a minimum of six months, the diet-plus-exercise group failed to beat out the diet-only group at all.[3097] There appeared to be no long-term benefit to encouraging people to add exercise to their weight-loss regimens. What is going on? Maybe exercise is better at just preventing people from regaining weight but not losing it to begin with? The vast majority of randomized controlled trials examining weight-loss maintenance also failed to show an exercise benefit.[3098]

Part of the problem is compliance. It's one thing to tell people (or even ourselves) to adhere to an exercise regimen; it's another thing for them to actually do it. A 2018 review found that, in most cases, the groups of people randomized to work out showed no weight-loss benefit. However, if the people who flouted the instructions are excluded and the analysis is limited just to those who actually put in the time and sweat, a clear advantage to exercising emerges.[3099] Exercise, like diet, only works if you actually do it. Still, though, people tend to experience less weight loss than one would predict based on the number of calories burned.

Exercise can rev up your baseline metabolic rate. For up to forty-eight hours after a single bout of exercise, you can experience an afterburn effect, known technically as *EPOC,* or *excess post-exercise oxygen consumption.* EPOC can bump up our resting metabolic rates as much as 5–10 percent. That may not seem like much, but it can build up. For example, a brisk half-hour walk may only burn 150 calories,[3100] but if it then boosts our metabolic rates by 7.5 percent over the subsequent thirty-six hours, that EPOC effect alone could burn an additional 170 calories or so—more than was burned during the actual walk. So we should be burning *more* calories than expected by exercising, not less. What's going on?

An Hour a Slice

Our gross overestimation of the capacity of exercise to burn off extra calories may be one reason people can rapidly become disillusioned with their new gym membership.[3101] Consider some foods that are CRAP—that is, *calorie-rich and processed,* as I explained on page 18. To walk off the calories found in a single pat of butter, we'd have to add an extra seven hundred yards to our stroll that evening. What about a Snickers bar? We'd need to jog a quarter mile for every single bite. If we eat two chicken legs, we'd better get out on our own two legs and run an extra three miles that day just to outrun the calories—and that's for boiled chicken with the skin removed.

A piece of pizza has about three hundred calories, which converts into an hour of brisk walking per slice. How many kids are jogging two hours a day to burn off their Happy Meals? Who's got time to climb up the Empire State Building's eighty-six flights to burn off a single donut?[3102] That's one reason what we put into our mouths is most important.

Public health researchers have been experimenting with providing this kind of information for public consumption. Labeling fast-food menus with pictograms of exercising stick figures was found to help nudge people toward lower-calorie options. Once they know that supersizing their fries would mean walking about three extra miles that day or that choosing the chicken salad over the garden salad could mean having to run around three miles, people are more likely to make the healthier choice.[3103]

For their calculations, the researchers assumed about 125 calories burned per mile run. We're remarkably efficient animals. It doesn't take much energy for us to move. Take sex, for instance. One of the "Seven Myths About Obesity" identified in *The New England Journal of Medicine* is that a bout of sexual activity burns a few hundred calories.[3104] So you may think, *Hey, I could get a side of fries with that!* But if you hook people up (literally *and* figuratively) and actually measure their oxygen consumption during the act (assuming they don't get too tangled up in all the wires and hoses), having sex only turns out to be the metabolic equivalent of bowling. Given that the average bout of sexual activity may only last about six minutes, a young man might expend approximately twenty-one calories during intercourse. Because of baseline metabolic needs, he would have spent roughly one-third of that just lounging around watching TV, so the incremental benefit is plausibly on the order of fourteen calories.[3105] So maybe he could have *one* fry with that.

Licensed to Eat

Evidently, most overweight individuals choose exercise as their first approach to weight loss.[3106] When unrealistic hopes inevitably clash with reality, the disappointment may lead to abandonment of weight-loss efforts altogether as an exercise in futility. (Pun intended!) Our false expectations may also give us license to overeat. Our pie-in-the-sky notions about the power of exercise may be used to justify an extra slice of pie right here on earth. Some researchers warn that labeling menus with calorie equivalents of exercise could be counterproductive, backfiring if people rationalize their indulgences after a workout.[3107] This concern has actually been put to the test.

Experimental psychologists took a group of men and women, put them on stationary bikes, and had them cycle until they burned either 50 calories or more than 250 calories. Unbeknownst to them, the experimenters effectively manipulated the machines to give false readouts such that, in actuality, both groups burned the same number of calories, about 120; they just thought they had burned more or less than that. The subjects were then offered snacks ten minutes later, ostensibly to measure the "effects of exercise on taste perception and food reward." The real purpose, however, was to covertly measure how much they ate. Those who falsely believed they had burned off more calories on the stationary bike did seem to demonstrate a greater license to eat, ending up eating significantly more calories—mostly in the form of chocolate chip cookies.[3108]

After a workout, people may be tempted to treat themselves for their sweaty sacrifice. To prevent this knee-jerk reaction from undermining our efforts, we should strive to make exercise less of a chore. A paper entitled "Is It Fun or Exercise? The Framing of Physical Activity Biases Subsequent Snacking" described a study in which individuals were randomized to the same amount of physical activity, but with different descriptions. Half were told they were going on a "fun walk," while the other half were told they were going on an "exercise walk." Afterward, researchers covertly measured how much dessert everyone took at a subsequent meal. Those in the movement-as-exercise group reportedly served themselves about 35 percent more chocolate pudding than the movement-as-fun group.[3109]

This is all the more reason to choose activities that are enjoyable, such as walking with friends or while listening to music or a podcast, or watching a video while on the treadmill. Reframing exercise as play rather than work may not only make for a more sustainable regimen, it may make us less likely to consciously or unconsciously feel the need to reward ourselves later at the buffet line.

Even just thinking about exercise may compel people to eat more food. Those randomized to simply read about physical activity went on to give themselves nearly 60 percent more M&M's than those in the control group, adding up to hundreds of extra calories. The researchers concluded that "simply imagining exercising leads participants to serve themselves more food."[3110]

Working Up an Appetite

Expending energy through exercise may not only predispose us *psychologically* to eat more, it also may make us hungrier *physiologically*. As we've discussed, we evolved in the context of scarcity, so our bodies place great value on rapidly replenishing lost fat stores.[3111] This offers another explanation as to why the average weight loss with exercise training is only 30 percent of that pre-dicted.[3112] Calories in versus calories out can be complicated by the fact that changes on one side of the equation can affect the other side too.

Carefully controlled studies show that caloric intake tends to rise over time to match any increase in caloric expenditure, making significant weight loss through exercise alone remarkably difficult.[3113] This doesn't happen over a day or two, though.[3114] After a workout, there may not be an immediate increase in hunger, but averaged over the week[3115] or weeks,[3116] our appetites do tend to increase. This calorie compensation, this attempt to balance it out, isn't perfect, however, so we can end up with a net loss in body fat, par-ticularly at higher exercise levels.[3117]

Here's a concrete example: Overweight men and women were random-ized to an exercise regimen that consistently burned off 1,500 calories a week, which would be about forty-five minutes of brisk walking every day, for instance. After twelve weeks of all that extra exertion, they didn't lose a significant amount of weight. An analysis of the changes that took place in their diets explains why: Yes, they burned 1,500 more calories a week, but they inadvertently started eating about 950 more calories a week. So, at the end of the three months, they were only down about three pounds.[3118]

What would happen if they doubled their workouts? Burning 3,000 calo-ries a week is equivalent to walking briskly about ninety minutes a day, every day, seven days a week. On that kind of regimen, how much more did they end up eating? Their appetites increased, but not enough to keep up with the increased caloric expenditure, so they ended up losing about six pounds over that same period. Though the 1,500 calories-out group had started taking in about 950 more calories, the *3,000* calories-out group had boosted their intakes a similar amount—about 1,000 calories a week above baseline—so they ended up with a much greater calorie deficit. Our bodies try to com-pensate by boosting our appetites, but there is a limit.

The secret to weight loss through exercise may be sheer volume: at least three hundred minutes a week to achieve appreciable fat loss.[3119]

This regulation of our appetites through activity works in both direc-tions. Just as there exists a higher level of exercise where we can start to outpace our appetites and lose weight, there's a lower level of exercise where our bodies lose the ability to sufficiently downgrade our appetites and we gain weight. This "zone of regulation" where our appetites become uncou-pled from our activity levels appears to start at around 7,100 steps a day.[3120]

If you've been a really active person and have to cut back on exercise for whatever reason, you may be surprised that you don't gain much weight, but that's likely because your appetite tends to come down as well. Once you cross that threshold, though, once you dip below logging at least 7,100 steps a day on your pedometer, your appetite doesn't slow much further to match, so the pounds can start to pile on. Your body tries to keep your weight steady by adjusting your appetite, but we just weren't designed to handle such an extremely low level of movement that sadly characterizes about 80 percent of the U.S. population.[3121]

Coming In from the Cold

Swimming and aquatic exercise in general are popular alternatives to land-based activities such as walking or biking.[3122] Buoyancy in water helps take some of the weight-bearing stress off joints, but swimming appears to be less effective for weight loss. Obese women were randomized to an hour a day of walking, cycling, or swimming. Six months later, the walkers lost an average of seventeen pounds, the cyclists lost an average of nineteen pounds, but the swimmers didn't lose an ounce—in fact, they actually gained five pounds. Gauging skin folds to estimate body fat, the measurements slimmed more than 40 percent in the walking and cycling groups, but there was no change at all in the swimming group.[3123] What's going on?

Some exercise boosts appetite more than others. In contrast to walking,[3124] running, or cycling,[3125] swimming can significantly heighten hunger within hours.[3126] This may explain why swimmers tend to have more body fat than runners of equal athletic caliber.[3127] If anything, one might think swimming may lead to even greater weight loss since you lose heat to the water, but swimming didn't seem to work at all.[3128] The cold, it turns out, may be the culprit.

If you exercise in warm water (about 90°F), it doesn't boost your appetite more than exercising on land. After the same workout in cool water (about 70°F), however, people can end up eating more than twice as many snacks an hour later.[3129] Maybe they're just burning off extra calories to stay warm? No, even at the same number of calories expended, people

(continued)

eat hundreds more calories after exercising in colder water. When offered a buffet after burning off about five hundred calories in cool water, people ate nearly nine hundred calories, hundreds more than after exercising in warm water or just resting on dry land.[3130]

Would the same thing happen under different temperatures on land? A team of British researchers sought to find out, randomizing people to walk briskly for forty-five minutes on a treadmill in the cold (at about 46°F) or at closer to room temperature (about 68°F). Participants were then presented with a buffet meal in which their eating was recorded covertly. Caloric intake was significantly greater after exercising in the cold. The researchers concluded that though walking is often prescribed for overweight individuals, "if walking was to take place in a cold environment, such as in winter, then this may stimulate food intake."[3131] In the warmer months, obesity researchers suggest, exercising outdoors may be preferable to an air-conditioned gym.[3132]

All studies to date on the effects of hot and cold environments have found that exercising in cool water or under cool conditions on land leads to an increase in post-workout caloric intake.[3133] What about a quick dip in the pool after you exercise? Australian researchers found that immersion in water—cool or warm—for fifteen minutes after a running session resulted in increased caloric intake. What is it about getting wet that whets our appetites? Maybe they got a chill after getting wet before they could change into dry clothes? This suggests that although a cool shower after a workout may be invigorating, it might be better to stick to a hot one.

Changing the Equation

Throughout millions of years of our prehistory, starvation was a bigger problem than obesity, so our bodies developed a multitude of ways to fight against weight loss. Let's look at the energy-balance equation to see how:

Body Fat = Calories In − Calories Out

In this simplified model of weight basically equaling calories in minus calories out, you can see how the only way our bodies can defend themselves

Calories Out

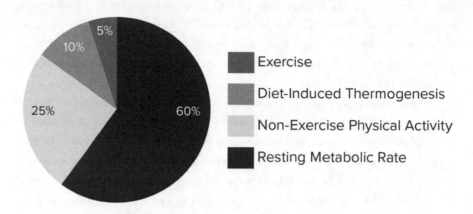

Exercise
Diet-Induced Thermogenesis
Non-Exercise Physical Activity
Resting Metabolic Rate

against weight loss if the calories-out factor goes up (we start exercising, for example) is to simultaneously ratchet up the calories-in factor (that is, boost our appetites).

Let's break down the equation further. *Calories In* means food and beverages; *Calories Out* means metabolism and motion. Motion can be further separated into exercise versus nonexercise physical activity, and most of the calories people expend on movement fall into the nonexercise category. (Leisure-time exercise, such as working out at the gym, typically only accounts for about 5 percent of daily energy expenditure.) Our resting metabolic rates use up at least 60 percent of our daily calories. Remember diet-induced thermogenesis from the Chronobiology section? That takes up about 10 percent of our daily calories. Movement takes up the remaining 30 percent, but if only 5 percent is structured exercise, the other 25 percent is comprised of nonexercise physical activities, such as cleaning the house or caring for children.[3134] The pie chart above illustrates a typical situation.

Our bodies then have a number of options to offset an increase in exercise:

Body Fat = Food + Beverages − Metabolism − Exercise − Other Movement

Since our metabolisms are already remarkably efficient at baseline, there's limited wiggle room to slow them down much further to prevent us from losing weight. What's more, exercise can end up boosting our metabolic rates, both through that EPOC afterburn and by building muscle mass, which takes more energy to maintain.[3135] Even if our bodies can't resist exercise-induced weight loss much by slowing our metabolisms, there's another option besides just boosting our appetites. Can you figure it out by looking at the equation?

An increase in exercise can inadvertently result in a decrease in nonexercise physical activity. When overweight adolescents engaged in an hour of moderate-intensity exercise, they burned off a total of 286 calories. Within that same period, they would have burned off 80 calories just existing. So, at the end of the hour, the exercise group had more than a 200-calorie deficit, and that deficit remained at the end of the day. By the end of the week, though, that calorie-expenditure gap had narrowed to less than 100 calories. The kids had been fitted with high-tech accelerometer devices to measure all their movements over the week. What was happening? The exercise group unintentionally moved less over the few days after the single bout of activity. Simple things like sitting instead of standing or fidgeting less can add up over time and eat away at the gains you make exercising.[3136]

Again, this makes total sense evolutionarily. Our bodies are trying to conserve energy. If you spend one day chasing (or being chased by) a woolly mammoth, your body tries to mellow you out over the next few days to make up for it.[3137] It's like what happens with appetite. You might not feel hungrier the day you exercise, but over the ensuing week, your body tries to fill in the gap.

Let's say that after you wake up tomorrow, you go out and take an hour-long walk in nice weather. (See the Coming In from the Cold box on page 361 to see why this temperature-related caveat is necessary.) Over the rest of the day, you'll likely end up eating and moving just as much as you would have had you slept in instead of gone for a walk. So if you walked off three hundred calories, at the end of the day, you'll be left with a three-hundred-calorie deficit. Your body doesn't like being in the red, though, since millions of years of scarcity-stress has been hardwired into our DNA. As a result, over the next few days, your body starts to chip away at that debt from both directions, nudging you to eat a little more and move a little less such that by the end of the week, all the walked-off calories are back on board. In terms of calorie balance, it's almost as if you hadn't taken that walk at all. This explains why so many exercise interventions fail to result in weight loss over time.[3138]

Over the millennia, those whose bodies failed to defend their fat stores were likely more often felled by famine and long winters. Plopped down into the land of plenty, though, this genetic legacy becomes a handicap. Winners in the ancient fight against famine are today's losers in the battle of the bulge.[3139] But like most handicaps, that just means we may have to work a little harder.

Consider the same scenario as before, but what if you repeat that morning walk every day? Those calorie deficits would start compounding, and your body would be forced to keep up by starting to make withdrawals from your body fat. Perhaps only significant amounts of exercise can cause significant weight loss.[3140] In a review entitled "Why Do Individuals Not Lose More Weight From an Exercise Intervention . . . ," the investigators suggested it was in part "primarily due to low doses of prescribed exercise."[3141]

Is there a magic exercise threshold that allows us to overcome our bodies' attempts to undermine our weight loss?

Nearly everyone seems to agree that the current national[3142] and international[3143] recommendations of 150 minutes a week of moderate-intensity exercise simply aren't enough. That only comes out to be about one hundred calories burned a day, against which our bodies could easily compensate. From an obesity standpoint, this has been considered the "physiological equivalent of bringing a knife to a gunfight."[3144]

At the same time, no one disagrees that there isn't at least some level of exertion that works. Just as extreme inactivity, such as twenty-four-hour bed rest, can reliably increase body fat,[3145] extreme activity like military training[3146] or mountain climbing[3147] can reliably decrease body fat. At about ten times the recommendation—a thousand calories of exercise a day—people lose about a pound a week, down eleven pounds within three months.[3148] The question is, what's the minimum amount of extra physical exertion that we should expect to have a non-negligible effect?

Published recommendations range from the American College of Sports Medicine's 250 minutes a week[3149] up to a USDA-funded paper pushing 250 minutes a day.[3150] I checked with the lead author, and, thankfully, the latter was a typo.[3151] They also had meant to say *weekly*. That fits the Healthy Lifestyle Institute's "200–300 min per week" minimum,[3152] a level that can at least help keep our weight stable, according to the U.S. Department of Health and Human Services Physical Activity Guidelines Advisory Committee.[3153] For significant weight loss, however, the committee recommends closer to a minimum of 450 minutes a week, or more than an hour a day. Note that these times are for moderate-intensity activity, such as walking. For vigorous activity like running or rapid cycling, exercise duration can be cut by more than half.

The National Academy of Medicine, arguably the most prestigious medical authority in the United States, recommends an hour a day for everyone based on the exercise habits of normal-weight individuals.[3154] For those who started out obese but slimmed down and are trying to prevent weight regain, one analysis estimated a threshold of eighty minutes a day was necessary.[3155] This falls into the daily sixty-to-ninety minutes range suggested in one systematic review,[3156] which is what an earlier version of the *Dietary Guidelines for Americans* recommended[3157] before it wimped out.[3158] Such levels of exercise had evidently "not proven manageable."[3159]

Up to 50 percent of Americans self-report that they reach the 150 minutes a week recommendation, but if people are hooked up to accelerometers and their movement is objectively measured, what do you think the real number is? Not the 50 percent self-reported, but less than 5 percent. Indeed, rather than one in two people meeting the 150 minutes a week recommendation, it was only one in twenty.[3160] Some people can pull it off, though. Those in the National Weight Control Registry who successfully lost lots of weight and kept it off for years evidently average about an hour a day, most commonly in the form of walking. About one in six hardly exercised at all, though, showing it is possible to stay slim without the gym.[3161]

The bottom line is that exercise for obesity is neither a "myth"[3162] nor a "magic bullet."[3163] Sufficient, regular exercise can indeed aid in weight loss, just not nearly as much as most people think.[3164] On a population scale, even a 1 percent decrease in body mass index could potentially prevent millions of cases of diabetes and heart disease, and thousands of cases of cancer,[3165] but on an individual level, the weight loss can prove disappointingly small.[3166] We just have so much more control over the calories-in side of the equation than the calories-out. There is, however, a neat trick.

NEAT

Why do some people gain more than others? If you experimentally overfeed a group of people the same amount over the same time period, you might assume there would be *some* variation, but the actual range of variability is truly mind-boggling. In a famous study out of the Mayo Clinic, subjects ate a thousand extra calories every day for eight weeks with no added exercise. In some people, that extra thousand calories translated into only about a spoonful of added daily body fat, whereas others gained more than a third of a cup of body fat every day. By the end of the eight weeks, there was a tenfold variation in fat gain from under a pound in total to more than nine pounds.[3167]

Hold on. Someone ate fifty-six *thousand* extra calories and gained less than a single pound of body fat? There's a law in physics that basically says calories can't just disappear,[3168] so what happened? Let's look at the energy-balance equation again:

Body Fat = Food + Beverages − Metabolism − Exercise − Other Movement

The exercise level for the study subjects was fixed at a steady, low amount, and it turned out their metabolisms didn't change much. So the only way caloric intake could shoot up without depositing as body fat would be if "other movement" shot up as well. And that's what happened. The secret to eating in excess of fifty thousand calories without gaining weight is NEAT: *nonexercise activity thermogenesis.*

NEAT is the heat given off by our regular activities of daily living, such as standing, moving, and fidgeting. On average, fewer than four hundred of those extra thousand calories consumed each day of the study ended up being stored as fat. The bulk was burned off, particularly from a spontaneous increase in movement. One participant inadvertently started moving so much that an extra 692 calories burned off in a day. That's like spending a quarter of your waking hours in motion.[3169]

You'd think overfeeding might lead to the opposite: inactivity. I imagine someone crashed on the couch rubbing their swollen belly. But no—when people are fed a thousand extra calories a day, a strange thing happens. They spontaneously start to move more out of some instinctual drive. This could be in the form of fidgeting or gesticulations, a restlessness leading to frequent standing or pacing,[3170] using up as many as hundreds of extra calories on average over the course of a day.[3171] Basically, NEAT is the sum of calories burned by everything we do that is not sleeping, eating, or sports-like exercise.[3172]

So the primary reason some people gain more weight than others despite eating the same amount of food is that they go weak in the NEAT.[3173] Easy gainers just don't intuitively start moving more to compensate for the extra calories. Indeed, a NEAT deficit has been identified in obesity. Studies show obese individuals tend to remain seated for about two and a half hours longer each day than the average, inactive yet lean, shoestring couch potato.[3174] Normal-weight individuals just tend to get up and move around more.

After fitting "sedentary" people with sensors that tracked their posture and movement, researchers were surprised to find they in fact were walking the equivalent of seven miles a day. That distance was just split up into dozens of stints lasting a few minutes at a time simply ambling around throughout the day.[3175] Remarkably, those small moments of movement can add up to more than two thousand calories a week, which just so happens to be what those overfed study subjects started burning up and about what you'd get from the hour-a-day exercise recommended for weight loss.[3176]

Just by subtly moving around more, your body can drain off as many calories as pounding it out an hour a day at the gym. Remember those extra 692 calories a day burned off by the study subject who had inadvertently started moving more? That's more than you might burn rock climbing for an hour. Given its demonstrated power, if our bodies aren't going to move more unconsciously, then maybe we should make a conscious effort to accrete some NEAT.

Staying One Move Ahead

Since prescriptions for structured exercise have so often failed to result in appreciable weight loss, some obesity researchers have turned to trying to enhance NEAT instead.[3177] After all, remember the pie chart? Nonexercise activity typically burns off at least five times more calories a day than an average exercise program. The reason the Amish have some of the lowest rates of obesity is not a high prevalence of gym memberships. They walk an average of eighteen thousand steps a day just living their lives.[3178]

You don't have to go full horse-and-buggy to enjoy the benefits of nonexercise activity thermogenesis. NEAT means taking the stairs instead of the escalator and parking at the far end of the lot. It means singing, laughing, cleaning, and doing yard work—any activity that creates muscular contractions. Cooking dinner burns five to ten times more calories than sitting in front of the TV.[3179]

Imagine two scenarios of modern life: An office worker drives to work, sits all day at their desk, drives home, and then sits all evening watching television or surfing the internet. If they had gotten home at 5:00 p.m. and went to bed at 11:00 p.m., those six hours of leisure time probably wouldn't expend more than fifty calories, even if they double-thumbed the remote control. What if instead, when our hypothetical office worker got home, they started raking leaves or vacuuming? They would have burned about ten times more calories that same evening[3180] and around twenty times more if they more actively commuted, like biking rather than driving to work.[3181]

Stand to Lose

In *How Not to Die,* I documented the health risks associated with prolonged sitting. The reason nearly all the studies to date on television viewing and mortality have found an association between screen-based entertainment and premature death is thought to be because screen time tends to equal sitting time.[3182] Sitting more than three hours a day may be responsible for more than four hundred thousand deaths every year worldwide.[3183] (Sitting, however, is decidedly *not* the new smoking. Tobacco is responsible for up to more than ten times greater shortening of life expectancy.[3184])

What about standing versus sitting for weight loss? Standing burns three times more calories per minute than sitting.[3185] Even if you're standing still, your postural muscles are tensed and stretched to fight gravity,[3186] so anything you usually do while sitting, try doing while standing, like watching TV or reading the newspaper. A sure sign that I'm speaking at a lifestyle medicine conference versus a more traditional medical event is how many more audience members are standing along the back of the lecture hall.

A standing desk can be as simple as a crate on a table you can use when you pay bills or watch cat videos on your computer. Prolonged standing on a hard floor can be hard on our feet, but using cushioned insoles in our shoes or standing on an "anti-fatigue" mat (or maybe a thick or doubled-over yoga mat) has been shown to help relieve discomfort.[3187] Another potential downside of prolonged standing is increased risk of developing varicose veins,[3188] a cosmetic concern hopefully offset by the decreased risk of obesity[3189] and premature death.[3190]

There are "sit-stand desks" available now that are height-adjustable so you can alternate between sitting and standing. In the short term, they were found to reduce sitting time at work on average by one hundred minutes per workday, but after three months, people appeared to tire of them and only sat about an hour less a day.[3191] Those using sit-stand workstations were also found to compensate a bit at home by sitting down more in their off hours.[3192]

Even without compensation, though, standing for six hours a day rather than sitting may only net about a fifty-calorie deficit daily.[3193] Walking at a treadmill desk, on the other hand, could wipe out more than seven hundred calories a day. Just moving at a snail's pace at about one mile per hour, people burn an extra two calories a minute over sitting.[3194] That means you could erase more than one hundred extra calories an hour while you work or two hundred extra calories at 3 mph.[3195] (My treadmill desk is currently set at 1.8 mph.) If you work 250 days a year and stroll while you work for even just half the workday, you could theoretically burn off thirty pounds of fat a year if your body didn't otherwise compensate for the one hundred thousand annual calorie deficit.[3196] No wonder obesity researchers have called for a "moratorium on the chair."[3197]

Does productivity suffer using a standing or walking desk? With the exception of high-precision mouse tasks, work performance in general appears to be unaffected,[3198] but one study of transcriptionists on treadmill desks found that their speed slowed by 16 percent, though their accuracy was unchanged.[3199]

While I'm a big fan of treadmill desks, I'll admit they can be expensive and noisy. Even if the motor is quiet, the footfalls may be distracting to co-workers. (When I'm on the phone, interviewers sometimes ask me what that "thumping" is.) Stepping devices, also known as *exercise steppers,* are a smaller, cheaper, quieter, and more convenient alternative. They have two pedals you stand on, allowing you to simulate walking up stairs. Steppers appear to burn even more calories in an office setting than walking,[3200] and you can simply slide them under a desk when not in use.

Dynamic Sitting

Sedentary comes from the Latin word meaning *to sit,* but just because you're sitting doesn't mean you're sedentary—just ask any cyclist or rower. The problem is sitting *motionlessly.* That causes blood to pool and stagnate in our legs, which can result in arterial dysfunction. Just like our muscles can atrophy from disuse, it may be *use it or lose it* when it comes to artery function as well. Special cells lining our arteries can detect the tugging, sheer force of the blood flowing past and send signals through the artery wall to maintain proper structure and function.

Significant decrements in artery function can be detected within three hours of sitting,[3201] while three hours of standing, even while motionless, does not produce the same effect. Part of the reason blood flow can be stanched nearly 40 percent by prolonged sitting[3202] is the ninety-degree angle in our knees that kinks our blood vessels.[3203] When that's straightened out by standing, our arteries remain fully functional.

If standing or dynamic workstations are not an option, taking five-minute walking breaks every hour can prevent the stiffening of the arteries that comes with prolonged sitting.[3204] Frequent trips to the watercooler (and then subsequently to the restroom) or taking out the trash during commercial breaks can maintain full artery function.

What are your options if you really can't walk away from your workstation? Exercising your legs for forty-five minutes before sitting down can preserve artery function[3205]—another advantage to an active commute. Researchers concluded that "people should be encouraged to engage in aerobic leg exercise before sitting for extended periods of time and, if this is not possible, sitting should be replaced by standing."[3206]

Just standing intermittently for a few minutes an hour does not appear sufficient to counteract the adverse effects of sitting, and neither does a few minutes of pedaling under your desk with one of those sit-cycle gadgets.[3207] Constant standing works, though, as presumably would constant pedaling, an example of "dynamic sitting." You may have noticed people in an office sitting on large rubber stability balls. That does activate trunk muscles in your core, but it's been found to cause more low-back discomfort and spinal shrinkage,[3208] likely due to the absence of a backrest.

What about a fidget chair that allows for a degree of side-to-side lateral movement of your hips?[3209] Unfortunately, people tend to move so little while seated in them that they only burn about thirteen more calories an hour compared to sitting in a regular chair.[3210] A cheaper way to burn comparable calories while sitting is the use of a fidget bar, a device referred to in the medical literature as an "under-the-table leg-movement apparatus."[3211] It's sort of like a balance beam that hangs under your desk that you can put your feet on to fiddle around, burning up an extra twenty-two calories an hour.[3212] Either fidgety approach could easily add up to burning one hundred calories a day.

(continued)

Does seated fidgeting protect our arteries, though? Researchers had people intermittently fidget just one leg for one minute out of every five, while keeping their other leg still. While artery function in the resting leg dropped, that of the restless leg experienced a pronounced improvement.[3213] This helps explain why frequent fidgeting appears to neutralize the mortality risk of prolonged sitting.[3214] What I liked most about the one-leg fidget study was that the researchers didn't rely on any fancy gizmos. They simply had people tap their heel by bouncing their knee at their own natural cadence, something we can all try to remember to do. Just try not to annoy the person you're sitting beside on the airplane or at the movies.

The Object of the Exercise

Should word get out that exercise is relatively ineffective for weight loss, it could have negative public health implications. The problem with the prevailing bait and switch of "come for the weight loss and stay for the longevity" is that it could end up being counterproductive, which is why some experts suggest we should promote exercise without any mention of weight loss.[3215] The fear is that the relatively unchanging number on the bathroom scale will disillusion people out of exercising altogether, and then they really would miss out on exercise's myriad benefits, which may indeed include living longer. Walking briskly just fifteen minutes a day is associated with a life span gain of about two years, for example, and an hour a day may give us four more years on this earth.[3216]

While the data on exercise for weight loss are relatively weak, the evidence supporting the overall health benefits of physical activity is overwhelming.[3217] For example, forty minutes a day, four days a week, can improve erectile function in men.[3218] Being more fit can mean having more fun, all the while reducing risk of breast cancer,[3219] colon cancer,[3220] diabetes, gallstones, hypertension, heart disease, and stroke.[3221] Exercise can also help minimize the bone loss that can accompany weight loss.[3222]

A single exercise session can improve insulin sensitivity for up to seventeen hours[3223] and may be used to treat prediabetes as effectively as medications.[3224] Exercise *is* medicine. Researchers at Harvard and Stanford found that exercise may work as well as drugs for coronary heart disease patients and even better than some medicines for stroke. They suggested that drug companies should perhaps be required to compare any new chronic disease drugs head-to-head against exercise, as "patients deserve to understand the relative impact that physical activity might have on their condition."[3225]

Visceral Reaction

The number on the scale doesn't tell the full story. When obese diabetics were put through four months of strength training, they didn't achieve any significant weight loss, which is typical. They did, however, lose about eight pounds of body fat! The reason that loss didn't register on the scale is that they *gained* about seven pounds of lean body mass.[3226] They lost fat while gaining muscle, and their blood sugar control improved to reflect that, so it wasn't a wash at all. Far from it. Aerobic exercise can cause a similar fat loss in thirteen weeks, with no significant difference noted between thirty minutes a day and sixty minutes a day,[3227] though those putting in two-hour bouts do separate out from the pack.[3228]

One of the reasons exercise can be such a lifesaver is that, while it may not affect our overall weights, it can help get rid of our most dangerous body fat—that visceral fat slithering around our internal abdominal organs.[3229] A systematic review found that even in the absence of weight loss, exercise may cause a 6 percent drop in visceral fat levels.[3230] Exercise in particular seems to home in and burn off the worst fat first. An average obese person losing about ten pounds through caloric restriction might remove about 13 percent of their visceral fat, but the same amount of weight loss through exercise could wipe out 21 percent.[3231]

What about doing crunches? Thanks to advertising claims from companies trying to sell people various exercise gadgets and workouts targeting the tummy, there's a common perception that we can reduce our waistlines solely by doing abdominal exercises. Seven different abdominal exercises were put to the test, including sit-ups, leg lifts, and abdominal crunches, two sets of ten repetitions each for five days a week. After six weeks, there was no effect on abdominal fat.[3232] All that core conditioning only took about ten minutes a day, so that just doesn't burn enough calories to make a difference. Based on averaging together a dozen or so studies, it may take three months of around three hours of aerobic exercise a week to take an inch off our waists.[3233] One inch may not seem like a lot, but on a CT scan or MRI cross section of our abdomens, that may mean the removal of a respectable five square inches of visceral belly fat.[3234] When it comes to the worst of the worst kind of fat, aerobic exercise appears to beat out resistance exercise.[3235]

HIIT It Off?

What about interval training? High-intensity interval training (HIIT) involves short bursts of vigorous exercise interspersed with periods of low-intensity activity or rest. The idea is that you could burn the same number of calories in a shorter time, thereby improving compliance for those who don't feel they have the time. When it's put to the test in a real-world setting, though, adherence to even just two unsupervised sessions of HIIT a week declines rapidly to less than 20 percent within twelve months. No surprise then that the HIITers experienced no significant weight or body-fat benefit over the standard recommendation of engaging in moderate-intensity activity for thirty minutes a day most days of the week.[3236]

The benefits of HIIT for weight loss appear modest even under more carefully controlled conditions. A meta-analysis of thirty-nine studies found that people only lost about a pound of fat a month,[3237] which is no better than when engaging in continuous, moderate-intensity activity.[3238] The HIIT required about 40 percent less of a time commitment, though, so HIIT participants accomplished in about an hour and a half a week what took the medium-intensity groups closer to two and a half hours—namely, no change in weight, but a loss of a few pounds of body fat over a few months and one inch off the waist.[3239] This suggests that what matters is not the intensity but the total work performed[3240]—but that's not entirely true.

Does walking a mile or running a mile burn more calories? Running burns more than twice as many calories per minute, but you could finish the mile in less than half the time it would take to walk it. So does it all equal out? No, because we were designed to walk at a speed that minimizes the energy cost of transport.[3241] Our bodies try to get from A to B using the fewest calories, and peak efficiency is walking about 3 mph. Walking slower burns fewer calories but takes longer. Walking faster gets you there quicker, but you burn more—and that's what we want. Efficiency is good for conserving energy, but if the aim is to lose weight, you don't want to conserve your fat. You want to get rid of it.

Indeed, have people run a mile at a 6 mph pace in ten minutes versus walk a mile at about a 3 mph pace in twenty minutes, and the runners expend about 110 calories compared to 90 calories spent by the walking group. This is then compounded by the afterburn advantage of higher-intensity activity. During the recovery period, the running group burned about an extra 50 calories compared to more like 20 calories in the walking group. So in total, the runners beat out the walkers by about 50 calories and did so in half the time.[3242]

In a nutshell, continuous high-intensity activity beats out lower intensity, but shorts bursts of high intensity don't appear to beat out continuous, moderate-intensity exercise.

All Walks of Life

Running isn't for everyone, though. Vigorous activity is warned against in certain heart conditions and can be difficult or uncomfortable for the beginner.[3243] Walking, on the other hand, can be easy, safe, and sociable, and may therefore be "ideal as a gentle start-up for the sedentary."[3244] Hippocrates evidently called walking "man's best medicine"[3245] (and it works for women too!).

Pooled together, twenty-two studies of walking for weight loss found that an average of forty-five minutes or so of brisk walking about four times a week for three or four months removes nearly six pounds of body fat and takes about an inch off the waist.[3246] What's the optimum dose? The more the better. The longer you walk and the faster you walk, the more calories you burn—though not as many as might be expected due to compliance and compensation.

When doctors prescribed ninety minutes of walking a day as part of a research protocol, within three weeks, accelerometer data showed people were actually only putting in sixty-five minutes a day, and those prescribed sixty minutes were only walking about forty minutes. Those prescribed thirty minutes, however, were keeping up with their full half hour.[3247] So, though those prescribed more did walk more, asking people to triple their walking time may only end up doubling it.

All the study subjects were told to add the walking on top of their baseline levels of activity, but that only worked to varying degrees. Adding thirty minutes of walking to their routines didn't affect the rest of their daily activity much, but most of the extra steps in the ninety-minute group were effectively

lost since the participants compensated by moving so much less over the remainder of the day. Nearly two-thirds of the added exercise was offset by a
reduction of other daily activities. Still, even with the compensation and compliance, those who set out to do more, did more.[3248] The optimal duration is
as long as possible.

Timing Is Everything . . . Right?

What's the best exercise dose for weight loss? The more the better. What
about the optimal timing? Is it better to exercise in the morning or the evening? Before or after breakfast? A Nobel Prize–winning exercise physiologist
said he always ran a mile every morning before breakfast.[3249] Was that prize-
winning timing?

More than a dozen experiments have been published comparing the
amount of fat burned in a fasted state versus a fed state, and every single one
found more fat was burned on an empty stomach. On average, a single bout
of low- to moderate-intensity activity before a meal burned off three more
grams of fat than the same amount of exercise after a meal.[3250] Same amount
of exercise, but more fat loss just because of timing.

Simply because you burn more fat while exercising doesn't necessarily
mean you end up with less fat at the end of the day. Maybe our bodies offset
the extra fat loss that occurs during exercise with a little extra fat storage
when you finally do eat, balancing out the equation. Researchers in Japan set
out to investigate this possibility by measuring twenty-four-hour fat balance
after one hundred minutes of running either before breakfast or after lunch.
On the exercise-after-lunch day, subjects burned a total of 608 calories of fat
over the course of that day. In contrast, on the exercise-before-breakfast day,
in the same twenty-four-hour period, they burned through nearly 90 percent
more—1,142 calories of straight fat.[3251] So the next day, before-breakfast ex-
ercisers woke up with about a quarter cup less fat after the same amount of
exercise. Remarkable!

Running for one hundred minutes is pretty hard-core no matter whether
you do it before or after breakfast. What about something less intense, like
walking? Study subjects walked for sixty minutes at different times of the
day—before breakfast, after lunch, or after dinner—and also had a control
day when they didn't exercise at all. Over twenty-four hours, they burned
off 432 fat calories after exercising in the evening and 446 fat calories after

walking in the afternoon. On the exercise-free control day, however, they burned through 456 fat calories. It's almost as if the post-lunch and post-dinner walkers hadn't walked at all. What about a pre-breakfast walk? The same amount of exercise before breakfast resulted in 717 calories of fat loss.[3252] Over the course of a day, timing truly does matter.

All such similar studies on both men and women show we burn through more fat on the days we exercise before, rather than after, eating.[3253] After reading the Chronobiology section, though, an alternative explanation may spring to mind. Maybe it's just a morning thing. Is it possible it has nothing to do with meals at all and our circadian rhythms are dictating the difference?[3254] No. Exercising in the morning after breakfast appears no better than exercising in the evening after dinner,[3255,3256] and exercising before breakfast works better than immediately after breakfast, yet both are still in the morning.[3257] It really does seem to be a pre- versus post-meal effect—but why?

Skinny Dip

Carbohydrate is the preferred fuel for our bodies. Whenever you eat sugars or starches, they get broken down and converted into blood sugar. After a meal, blood sugars rise, and our muscles are quick to snatch them up for fuel without having to rely much on our energy stores. If you take a siesta after a meal, your muscles have no immediate need for energy, so the excess blood sugar from that meal can be stored for later use in the muscles in the form of glycogen, which is just a bunch of blood sugar molecules strung together into a mass of branches that can be broken off and used for quick bursts of energy anytime you need them.

If you exercise after a meal, your muscles can siphon off some of the extra blood sugar floating around for energy. When you work out before a meal, though, your muscles have to resort to dipping into your energy stores and end up burning mostly a combination of glycogen and fat.[3258] That explains why you burn more fat during fasted exercise, but what about all the extra fat burned throughout the rest of the day?

Glycogen is more than a store.[3259] It isn't just an energy reserve. Glycogen acts as a sensor capable of activating metabolic pathways. Exercising before breakfast can exhaust as much as 18 percent of your glycogen stores, and that depletion can act as a powerful rallying cry to your fatty tissues to start pulling more of their weight by breaking down more fat. The lower glycogen stores fall, the greater the sustained twenty-four-hour fat loss.[3260]

How long do you have to go without food in order to trigger this effect? Six hours may be sufficient, so before breakfast isn't the only optimal window.[3261] If you timed it right, you could exercise midday before a late lunch or, if you had an early enough lunch, before dinner after you got home from work.

If exercise in a fasted state isn't possible, does it matter what you eat? Insulin release after a meal appears to play a critical role in suppressing fat breakdown,[3262] which explains why lower-glycemic foods can have less of an effect.[3263] Lentils were identified as a promising option for maintaining athletic endurance,[3264] which can take a hit on an empty stomach,[3265] while maintaining more of the fat dissolution. They are "unlikely to be consumed by the general population," though, wrote one research team, "due to low palatability."[3266] (They obviously haven't tried my mom's lentil soup.)

A systematic review and meta-analysis on exercise timing for fat metabolism found that exercising in a completely fasted state may work best.[3267] The Japanese team who published some of the seminal work in this area went as far as asserting: "If exercise were a pill to burn body fat, it would be effective only when taken before breakfast."[3268] Surveys show few people exercise before breakfast, though.[3269] Before asking people to make the switch, we need to make sure that these tantalizing, twenty-four-hour results translate into weight loss over the long term. There's a solid theoretical basis, but you don't know until you put it to the test.

In a study of experimental weight gain, volunteers were fed up to 4,500 calories a day for six weeks while vigorously exercising a total of three hundred minutes a week, always either after an overnight fast or after a meal. A control group who didn't exercise at all but consumed the same extra calories gained about six and a half pounds, compared to three pounds gained in the exercise-after-a-meal group. The premeal exercise group worked out the same amount and ate the same amount, but they only gained half as much, one and a half pounds.[3270] What about weight *loss*, though?

Twenty young women on calorie-restricted diets were randomized to exercise for three hours a week either before or after a meal. Same diets, same amount of exercise, and, disappointingly, about the same amount of weight loss. The premeal exercise group did lose about an extra pound of body fat (total weight loss of three and a half pounds versus two and one-fifth pounds), but this did not reach statistical significance, meaning such a small difference could very well have been due to chance.[3271] Similarly, a study of six weeks of low-volume, high-intensity interval training before or after meals also failed to show a difference.[3272]

One explanation that's been offered for this failure is that the increased fat loss during premeal exercise might be "neutralized" by the lesser diet-induced thermogenesis.[3273] It costs our bodies fewer calories to process food if we eat after physical activity compared to eating before. When we exercise after a meal, our bodies get mixed signals. Exercise is all about mobilizing energy stores for fuel, whereas eating is more about assimilation and storage. So the metabolic challenge presented by the ensuing hormonal "tug-of-war"[3274] might be responsible for the 15–40 percent greater calorie cost.[3275] This has led some to recommend exercising *after* meals to facilitate weight loss.[3276] If you do the math, though, diet-induced thermogenesis makes such a small contribution that this might only come out to be three to twelve calories.[3277] Such a slight difference would be easily overwhelmed by the big disparity in fat loss, as confirmed by the twenty-four-hour fat-balance studies.

I would suggest a more reasonable explanation might be that the clear body-fat deficit on premeal exercise days is made up for by extra fat storage on nonexercise days. Our bodies like to hold on to body fat if they can, so, on days you aren't driving it down, it may try to even things out. Both of the failed weight-loss studies had people exercising only three days a week, so their bodies had most of the week to compensate. The study I'd love to see is pre- versus post-meal exercise on all or at least most of the days of the week to see if we can continue to drive down fat stores.

Blood Sugar Taming Through Timing

You can imagine how that siphoning effect muscles have on excess blood sugar during exercise might be great for those suffering from elevated blood sugars. Indeed, exercising after a meal can bring down blood sugars as well as some blood sugar–lowering drugs.[3278] Randomize type 2 diabetics to a leisurely twenty-minute stroll (about 2 mph) before dinner or after dinner, and you can show that after-dinner walking can

(continued)

comparatively blunt blood sugar spikes by 30 percent.[3279] Same meal, same amount of exercise, same intensity of exercise, but with a significant bonus effect on blood sugar control, thanks to a little tactical timing. Even just a ten-minute walk after a meal may make a difference.[3280] So for those with blood sugar problems, it's better to exercise after meals than before them.

Blood sugar from a meal starts appearing in the bloodstream fifteen to twenty minutes after the first bite. It ramps up after thirty minutes to peak around the one-hour mark before declining to premeal levels within a few hours.[3281] For optimal blood sugar control, prediabetics and diabetics should start exercising thirty minutes after the start of a meal and ideally go for an hour to completely straddle the blood sugar peak.[3282] If you had to choose a single meal to exercise after, it would be dinner,[3283] due to the circadian rhythm of blood sugar control that wanes throughout the day. Ideally, though, breakfast would be the largest meal of the day, and you'd exercise after that—or, even better, after every meal.[3284]

A Walk in the Park

Exercise recommendations for obesity have been referred to as the "mysterious case of the public health guideline that is (almost) entirely ignored." Governmental, scientific, and professional organizations call for at least an hour of exercise a day for weight management, but almost no obese adults meet this target.[3285] Surveys suggest Americans watch TV about ten times more than they exercise, and for obese Americans, it may be even worse.[3286] Only 2 percent even reach thirty minutes of exercise a day,[3287] and the percentage exceeding an hour a day is expected to be close to zero.[3288]

Why don't obese individuals exercise more? Rather than speculate, why don't we just ask? When questioned, obese adults typically describe exercise as being "unpleasant, uncomfortable and unenjoyable."[3289] So how can we break this vicious cycle, where inactivity can lead to weight gain, which can lead to further inactivity and even more weight gain? The first thing to recognize is that it is normal and natural to be physically lazy.[3290]

Laziness is in our genes. We evolved to instinctually avoid unnecessary exertion to conserve energy for survival and reproduction. These days, there's no shortage of available fuel, yet the hardwired inertia remains. Our ancient ancestors are presumed to have exercised only when it was necessary or when it was fun, as a form of play.[3291] The only way exercise is going to work long term for weight control is if it becomes a stable, lifelong habit,[3292] so you need to restructure your surroundings to require more physical activity (like working at a treadmill desk) and figure out how to make exercise more enjoyable.[3293]

Here's a piece of wise advice from a 1925 medical journal entry: "The best prescription to be written for a walk is to take a dog . . . and a friend."[3294] Listening to your favorite music might also help. Music has been described as a "legal method"[3295] for improving peak performance and, more importantly, the enjoyment of high-intensity interval training.[3296] During exercise, listening to a preferred playlist can significantly reduce our "rate of perceived exertion," which is how hard you feel your body is working.[3297] Put severely obese youth on a treadmill and have them go until exhaustion with or without music, and those listening to their favorite tunes tended to make it about 5 percent longer. This was chalked up to "attentional distraction"—the music may have helped keep their minds off feelings of fatigue.[3298] If that's the case, listening to a podcast or audiobook may have a similar effect.

Spin Class

The recommendation to exercise sixty to ninety minutes for weight control has been dismissed as "too ambitious,"[3299] "too daunting,"[3300] and "too much, too soon," fearing people will feel overwhelmed and not exercise at all.[3301] In short, America, you can't handle the truth.[3302]

Maybe we should just tell it like it is. In a paper titled "Effects of Threatening Communications . . . on Weight Change in Obese Children," mothers of obese kids were randomized to receive one of two messages from their pediatrician's clinic. In the "low-threat" group, the message was gentler and more "generic":

> There are health problems related to obesity, most of which take years to develop. Being obese can interfere with things that people want to do . . . All in all, obese people are more likely to have health problems.

The "high-threat" group got a more blunt, "threatening" message:

The overweight child is likely to become an obese adult . . . Heart attacks, strokes, high blood pressure, and diabetes happen a lot more often to obese people—add it all up and you get a shorter life expectancy.

Whose kids do you think consistently lost more weight? Did the stronger message overwhelm the moms into paralysis? No. Their kids lost nearly twice as much weight as the children whose mothers got the milder message.[3303] Ignorance is less blissful when lives are on the line.

Some of the most influential voices in exercise promotion don't think we should focus on health at all. After all, Big Business is smart enough to keep its true goal of profit hidden from consumers, shrouding its advertising in promises of success and happiness. We should learn from the drug companies, they say. Pharmaceutical ads are less educational than aspirational.[3304] If we took a page from Big Pharma's playbook and listened to those exercise-promoting influencers, we would appeal to emotions, rather than "logical benefits such as better health" to promote exercise and instead prescribe "pleasure and meaning." We would need to "shift from a medical to a marketing paradigm."[3305]

I bristle at the marketing talk, but the nice thing about exercise is that it really can deliver on all those fronts—fostering elixir-of-life feelings of joy and vitality while helping people physically fulfill their goals in life. Frame a walk as exercise, and people report feeling more fatigued and in a worse mood than after going the same distance on a walk framed as fun.[3306] And it really can be fun. When sedentary individuals are started on an exercise regimen, they report enjoying it significantly more than they had expected.[3307]

FOOD FOR THOUGHT

The bottom line with exercise is that any amount is good[3308] and the more the better.[3309] If, however, you are a man over forty-five, are a woman over fifty-five, have diabetes, or experience symptoms such as chest pain, dizziness, or shortness of breath, I would recommend checking with your health professional before starting a new exercise regimen.[3310]

The evidence for the health benefits of exercise in general is overwhelming. Obesity can exacerbate disabling, painful conditions, such as osteoarthritis of the knees, making exercise more difficult but all the more essential. Losing weight doesn't just ease pain in the overloaded joints in the lower back, hips, knees, and ankles. The anti-inflammatory effects of exercise can also alleviate headaches and more diffuse, chronic, musculoskeletal aches and pains that disproportionately affect overweight individuals.[3311] However, the efficacy for weight loss is underwhelming for all but the most voluminous regimens. I did offer some suggestions to maximize fat loss, but on the whole, the limitations just make the calories-in side of the equation—that is, the dietary tweaks—all the more important. But overall, exercise is win-win: adding years to your life and life to your years.

FAT BLOCKERS

Eat Your Thylakoids

Turn Over a New Leaf

What on earth is a thylakoid? No big deal, just the source of nearly all known life and the oxygen we breathe. Thylakoids are where photosynthesis, the process by which plants turn light into food, takes place. Microscopic saclike structures composed of chlorophyll-rich membranes concentrated in the leaves of plants, thylakoids are the green engine of life.

When we eat them, when we bite into a leaf of spinach, for instance, the thylakoid membranes are able to resist our digestive enzymes. They can last for hours in our intestines before finally getting broken down,[3312] and it is in those hours when they work their magic. Thylakoid membranes bind to lipase, the enzyme our bodies make to digest fat, thereby helping to block fat absorption.[3313] This mechanism is like a natural version of the fat-blocking drug orlistat, but without the anal leakage.[3314] Unlike the drug, the thylakoids do finally break down, eventually freeing the lipase enzyme to do its job before fat comes spilling out your other end.[3315] Ultimately, fat absorption is not so much blocked by thylakoids as it is delayed.

If all the fat is eventually absorbed, what's the benefit? Location, location, location. Remember that ileal brake effect I described in the High in Fiber-Rich Foods section? By delaying calorie absorption until that tail end of the small intestine, strong satiety signals are sent to our brains saying, in effect, that you are full from stem to stern, thus dialing down your appetite.[3316] If you feed someone a meal with added thylakoids (by slipping in some powdered spinach, for instance) and measure the level of hormone release into their bloodstreams over the next six hours, you see a significant rise in a satiety hormone called CCK, as well as a drop in the hunger hormone ghrelin.[3317] Does this then translate into a drop in appetite? Researchers were eager to find out.

Spinach extracts were disguised in jam[3318] and juice[3319] to sneak thylakoids into meals, and those unwittingly eating the equivalent of about a half cup of cooked spinach felt significantly less hungry and more satiated over the next few hours. Give someone the equivalent of a shot of wheatgrass juice or what they might get in a "green drink" or green smoothie, and not only do they feel more satiated, but their cravings for sweet, salty, and fatty snacks, such as potato chips, chocolate, and cinnamon buns, drop by about a third. Feed them candy anyway, and those who unknowingly had been snuck some spinach report liking the sweets significantly less.[3320] The satiating power of greens has been attributed to their high fiber and water contents and low-calorie density,[3321] but the thylakoids may be their secret weapon.

The majority of thylakoid trials to date have shown improvements in satiety,[3322] but what about weight loss? Researchers in Sweden randomized overweight women to blended blueberry drinks every morning with or without "green-plant membranes" (powdered spinach). Within twelve weeks, the women who had been slipped spinach lost three pounds more than the control group. The spinach group's cravings for sweets diminished, and as a bonus, their bad LDL cholesterol dropped, too, even before the weight loss started kicking in.[3323] If you instead fix their caloric intakes to force the same weight loss, those randomized to the spinach group appeared to have an easier time with eating less. They experienced less hunger after a test meal after weeks of eating green.[3324]

Extracts of spinach were used in these studies so the researchers could create convincing placebos, but you can get just as many thylakoids eating about a half cup of cooked greens. Which greens have the most? You can tell just by looking at them.[3325] Because thylakoids are where the chlorophyll is, the greener the leaves, the more potent the effect.[3326] So go for the darkest-green greens you can find. In the store where I shop, that's the Lacinato (or dinosaur) kale.

What happens when you cook greens? Blanched for fifteen seconds or so in steaming or boiling water, they actually get even brighter green, but if you cook them too long, they eventually turn a drab olive brown. When greens are overcooked, the thylakoids physically degrade, along with their ability to inhibit lipase. Within that first minute when the green gets even more vibrant, though, there's a slight boost in fat-blocking ability.[3327] So you can gauge thylakoid activity in both the grocery store and the kitchen with your own two eyes.

Which are the best greens, and what is the best cooking method? The best green vegetable and the best way to cook it is whichever, and however, you'll end up eating the most. We've been chewing on leaves for millions of years,[3328] but today, the greenest thing about some people's diets may be a St. Patrick's Day pint. Americans average fewer than two grams of spinach a day, not even half a teaspoon.[3329] Our bodies were designed to have thylakoids passing through our systems on a daily basis, so the delay in fat absorption can be thought of as the default, normal state.[3330] It's only when we eat greens-deficient diets that the accelerated fat digestion undercuts our natural satiety mechanisms. In the *Journal of the Society of Chemical Industry,* a group of food technologists argued that given their fat-blocking benefits, "thylakoid membranes could be incorporated in functional foods as a new promising appetite-reducing ingredient"[3331]—or you can just get them in the way Mother Nature intended.

Choose Low-Oxalate Greens

Kidney stones affect as many as one in ten people in their lifetime and can cause excruciating pain.[3332] I instinctively cross my legs just thinking about them. Oxalate stones are the most common type,[3333] forming when the oxalate concentration gets so high in our urine it basically crystallizes out of

(continued)

solution like rock candy. Some foods, like spinach, have lots of oxalates in them. Should we try to reduce our intakes of oxalates to lower our risk? It turns out that people who get stones don't appear to eat any more oxalates on average than people who don't get stones.[3334] It's less what you eat and more what you absorb. People who are predisposed to kidney stones just appear to be born with a higher intestinal oxalate absorption.[3335] Their guts just really soak it up. So-called super absorbers assimilate up to 50 percent more oxalate than non-stone-formers.[3336]

Overall, the impact of typical dietary oxalate on urine levels appears to be small.[3337] Feed people a "massive"[3338] dose of dietary oxalates, and most only experience a relatively mild increase in the amount that makes it into their urine.[3339] Still, until you get your first stone, how do you know if you're a super absorber or not? Is it safer to just generally avoid higher oxalate fruits and vegetables? Well, people who eat more fruits and veggies actually tend to get *fewer* kidney stones.[3340] In fact, when researchers put it to the test and removed produce from people's diets, their kidney stone risk went up.[3341]

Removing fruits and vegetables can make our dietary oxalate intakes go down, but it also impairs our bodies' ability to get rid of the oxalate we produce on our own. Oxalate is formed internally as a waste product, and our bodies have more difficulty getting rid of it without the alkalizing effects of fruits and vegetables on our urine's pH.[3342] This may help explain why those eating plant-based diets get fewer kidney stones, though it also may be due to their reduction in meat intake, as meat consumption can have an acid-forming effect in the kidneys.[3343] A single can of tuna a day can increase our risk of forming stones by 250 percent,[3344] for example, and just cutting back on animal protein can help cut kidney stone risk in half.[3345]

Surely, there must be some level of oxalate intake that could put people at risk regardless. The study that showed a "massive" load of dietary oxalate didn't have much of an effect on urine levels used 250 mg of oxalates.[3346] That's a massive dose if we were talking about most greens—for example, 25 cups of collard greens, 60 cups of mustard greens, 125 cups of kale, or 250 cups of bok choy—but it's less than a half cup of spinach.[3347] Spinach really is an outlier. Even though there are small amounts of oxalates found throughout the food supply, spinach alone may account for 40 percent of oxalate intake in the United States.[3348] The Harvard cohorts found that men and older (but not younger) women who ate spinach eight or more times a month had about 30 percent higher risk of developing kidney stones.[3349]

Oxalates are water-soluble, so blanching collard greens, for example, can reduce oxalate levels by up to a third.[3350] (In that case, the oxalate load of those twenty-five cups of raw collards could be bumped up to thirty-three cups of blanched collards!) Steaming spinach reduces oxalate levels by 30 percent, and boiling cuts them by more than half. Boil the three high-oxalate greens—spinach, beet greens, and swiss chard—and up to 60 percent of the oxalates are leached into the cooking water.[3351] They start out so high, though, that they would still contain hundreds of times more oxalates than low-oxalate greens like kale.

Who may benefit from avoiding the big three high-oxalate greens? Anyone who has a history of kidney stones, is otherwise at high risk (for example, those who take megadoses of vitamin C,[3352] have a history of long-term broad-spectrum antibiotic use,[3353] or had Roux-en-Y gastric bypass surgery[3354]), or who eats cups of greens a day. (I personally try to eat at least a pound of greens a day, which is about three cups cooked or a dozen raw.) This is especially important for those who juice or blend their greens, as oxalates appear to be absorbed more rapidly in liquid than solid form.[3355]

Other high-oxalate foods that have been associated with kidney problems at high enough doses include chaga mushroom powder (four to five teaspoons a day),[3356] rhubarb (four cups a day),[3357] almonds[3358] or cashews (more than a cup a day),[3359] and star fruit (a single dose of one and a quarter cup juice[3360] or four to six fruit).[3361] Excessive tea consumption can also be a problem, especially of instant tea powder, which boosts urine oxalate nearly four times higher than brewed tea.[3362] Two cases of kidney damage attributed to drinking sixteen daily glasses of iced tea have been reported.[3363,3364]

The Calcium Effect

Another reason to give preference to low-oxalate greens is that they are less stingy with their calcium. While less than a third of the calcium in milks (whether from cow[3365] or plant[3366]) may be bioavailable, most of the calcium in low-oxalate greens is absorbed.[3367] The bioavailability of some greens is twice that of milks, but the oxalates in spinach, swiss chard, and beet greens bind to the calcium, preventing the absorption. It works both ways, though.[3368] The calcium binds to the oxalate too. That's why some gastric bypass surgeries result in enhanced oxalate absorption.[3369] The procedures can cause fat malabsorption. The fat steals away the calcium bound to the oxalate to form a type of soap in our intestines,[3370] and the oxalate is then freed to be absorbed.

Wait a second. If calcium is so good at grabbing onto fat in the gut, might calcium-rich foods act as fat blockers too? The problem with fat-blocking drugs is that the undigested fat comes out the other end, resulting in fecal leakage. But if calcium turns the fat into a semisolid soap, there's no oily discharge,[3371] and when we poop out the fat-calcium soap, we poop out all those fat calories contained therein.

The dairy industry was excited to put it to the test. When 1,200 mg or so of calcium in the form of cheese was added to people's diets, instead of losing about four grams of fat in their stool each day, they excreted closer to six grams of fat.[3372] The extra calcium caused the body to absorb two fewer grams of fat. Of course, that much cheese has more than fifty grams of fat,[3373] so it makes no sense to add fifty grams so you can get rid of two. You can imagine, though, how adding a fat-free source of calcium—skim milk, or even healthier, low-oxalate greens—could result in a small, negative fat balance every day. Orlistat can block about sixteen grams of fat a day,[3374] whereas a meta-analysis of the calcium fat-blocking studies confirmed only the two-gram difference.[3375] But if you absorbed two fewer grams of fat a day, that's eighteen calories you won't be holding on to, which, if not compensated for, could add up to a pound of fat loss.[3376] (Of course, another way to prevent two grams of fat from being absorbed is just to consume a half-teaspoon less oil every day.)

Nondairy sources of calcium appear to work just as well as dairy sources,[3377] and the small fat-blocking effect does not appear to diminish with time.[3378] Does this translate into weight loss? When people were randomized to take 1,000 mg of calcium supplements a day, all the extra little bits of daily fat loss added up to about two pounds of body fat lost over six months compared to placebo.[3379] Interventions using dairy didn't show any significant body fat loss,[3380] presumably because the added calories from the dairy itself counteracted any fat-blocking effects.[3381]

Caloric-restriction trials in which dairy calories were swapped in rather than added, though, did show an average of about two pounds of fat loss over an average of five months, helping to confirm the calcium effect. Unfortunately, none of the dairy studies lasting a year or longer showed a significant benefit, but they were mostly nonsubstitution trials, so presumably people just weren't able to compensate for the added dairy calories.[3382] Even dairy industry–funded scientists have been forced to conclude that dairy consumption has "no clinically meaningful effect" when it comes to promoting weight loss.[3383] We know the calcium fat-blocking effect *is* real, though. If only it could be provided in a safe, satiating form. It can. That's why greens—high in fiber, low in calories—may be the perfect delivery vehicle, combining the effects of thylakoids and calcium into one package deal.

Calcium Supplement Safety

In twelve short years, expert panels went from suggesting widespread calcium supplementation to prevent osteoporosis[3384] to "do not supplement,"[3385] the recommendation that remains for most people to this day.[3386] What happened? It all started with a 2008 study in New Zealand.[3387]

Researchers were hoping to prevent heart attacks by giving people calcium supplements. Short-term studies have shown that calcium supplementation may drop blood pressures by about a point.[3388] Though the effect appears to be transient, disappearing after a few months, it's better than nothing.[3389] Further, the fat-blocking effect of calcium could theoretically lower cholesterol levels by preventing a bit of saturated fat from getting into the system.[3390] To the researchers' surprise, however, instead of fewer heart attacks, there appeared to be *more* heart attacks in the calcium-supplement group.[3391] Was this just a fluke?

All eyes turned to the Women's Health Initiative, the largest and longest randomized controlled trial of calcium supplementation. If that name sounds familiar, it's because that's the very study that uncovered how dangerous hormone replacement therapy was. Would it uncover the same for calcium supplements?

The Women's Health Initiative reported no adverse effects. However, the majority of the participants were already taking calcium

(continued)

supplements before the study started. So, effectively, the study was just comparing higher versus lower doses of calcium supplementation rather than supplementation versus no supplementation. What if you go back and see what happened to the women who started out not taking supplements and then were randomized to the supplement group? Those who started calcium supplements suffered significantly more heart attacks or strokes.[3392] Thus, whether high dose or low dose, any calcium supplementation seemed to increase cardiovascular disease risk.

Researchers went back, digging through other trial data for heart attack and stroke rates in people randomized to calcium supplements, and they confirmed the danger.[3393] Most of the population studies also agreed: Users of calcium supplements tended to have increased rates of heart disease, stroke, and death.[3394]

The supplement industry was not happy, accusing researchers of relying in part on self-reported data—that is, simply asking if people had had a heart attack or not, rather than verifying it.[3395] That's not as much of a stretch as it may sound. Long-term calcium supplementation can cause all sorts of gastrointestinal distress, including twice the risk of being hospitalized with acute symptoms that may have been confused with a heart attack.[3396] However, the increased cardiovascular risk was seen consistently across the trials, regardless of whether the heart attacks were verified or not.[3397]

The calcium supplementation and heightened cardiovascular risk link continues to be a rising concern.[3398] Thankfully, supplementation rates dropped when the news came out, though some doctors continue to prescribe calcium for prevention.[3399] This inertia has been attributed to a complex web of industry ties with advocacy organizations and academia to protect the $6 billion business.[3400]

Why might calcium supplements increase heart attack risk, whereas the same calcium you get in foods does not? When you take calcium pills, you get an unnaturally large, rapid, and sustained spike of calcium in your bloodstream that can last as long as eight hours. This can cause your blood to clot more easily, which could increase the risk of forming clots in the heart or brain.[3401] Of course, if you're worried about heart attacks, there are risky food sources of calcium too. (I'm looking at you, cheese.)

The best sources of calcium are Green Light foods like leafy greens. In

How Not to Die, I defined my Green Light category as foods of plant origin to which nothing bad has been added and from which nothing good has been taken away. Green Light whole plant foods, unlike dairy, package calcium with lots of fiber, folate, iron, antioxidants, and thylakoids, instead of the baggage that too often accompanies milk products, such as sodium, cholesterol, and saturated butterfat. Despite the global dairy industry's campaign to "neutralise the negative image of milkfat among regulators and health professionals as related to heart disease," the American Heart Association is explicit about our need to cut down on dairy fat (and coconut oil and meat) to reduce the risk of our number one killer.[3402,3403] The American Heart Association put out a special Presidential Advisory in 2017 to clearly "set the record straight on why well-conducted scientific research overwhelmingly supports limiting saturated fat in the diet."[3404]

Drink Hibiscus Tea

Flower Power

Hibiscus tea, also known as *roselle* or *Jamaica,* is enjoyed around the world, hot or cold, for its bright red color and tart cranberry-like flavor. It's the "zing" in Red Zinger tea. I talk about its benefits in the chapter on high blood pressure in *How Not to Die,* working as well as,[3405] or even beating out; some antihypertensive medications in head-to-head tests.[3406]

Within three hours of drinking hibiscus tea, one hundred different metabolites can be detected in the human bloodstream.[3407] Alterations in gene expression at the three-hour mark suggest an improvement in metabolism and a downregulation of cholesterol synthesis, but randomized controlled trials have failed to consistently find cholesterol-lowering benefits.[3408] An interesting side effect did pop up, though: weight loss.[3409]

In Mexico, hibiscus tea has been used traditionally for the treatment of obesity, sparking lots of research interest.[3410] Computer modeling studies have suggested that certain hibiscus compounds might bind to the fat-digesting enzyme lipase like a key in a lock.[3411] (Uncreative names of compounds found from the flower include *hibiscin, hibiscitrin, hibiscetin,* and *hibiscus acid.*[3412]) Test-tube studies screening a variety of medicinal plants did indeed find that hibiscus inhibited lipase more than the others,[3413] and hibiscus has been found to reduce body fat in hamsters,[3414] mice,[3415] and rats, increasing fecal fat excretion.[3416] However it wasn't tested in people until recently.

To design a randomized double-blind trial, instead of trying to create an artificially colored and flavored placebo tea, the researchers dried the hibiscus tea into a powder and put it into capsules. After twelve weeks, there was a greater reduction in waistlines and body-fat percentage in the hibiscus group compared to those who got placebo capsules,[3417] but the dose they used was the equivalent of nine cups of hibiscus tea a day.[3418] I recommend people stick to no more than a quart a day on a regular basis due to the high manganese content. (Manganese is an essential trace mineral, but nine cups a day might result in too much of a good thing.[3419])

Finally, in 2018, a study was published using a reasonable dose—the equivalent of about a single twelve-ounce glass of tea a day. The complicating factor is that the researchers also added lemon verbena to the mix. That's another herbal tea, better known for improving recovery after intense bouts of strength training,[3420] but there were some promising in vitro data on effects of lemon verbena on fat cells in a petri dish,[3421] so they tried a combination. The dose came out to be about a cup and a half of hibiscus tea[3422] and a quarter cup of lemon verbena tea[3423] once a day for two months.[3424]

Both the tea and placebo groups were prescribed diets containing the same number of calories, yet those randomized to the tea group lost significantly more weight—eight pounds compared to five. That's only an extra pound a month, but an extra pound a month on a same-calorie diet.[3425] That's the advantage of fat-blocking interventions that actually cause you to lose more calories: Beyond reducing hunger, they can make you feel fuller for longer in hopes that you'll subsequently eat fewer calories.

Why not just pop pills instead of brewing tea? There are all sorts of herbal extract supplements on the market, but do we know enough to extract out the right active ingredients? For example, it does not appear to be the red anthocyanin pigments in hibiscus, since white varieties seemed to have similar effects.[3426] When the various compounds in hibiscus tea are isolated out and tested in various combinations, synergistic effects are found, meaning the whole may be greater than the sum of its parts.[3427]

Other than my manganese caveat, the only potential downside of hibiscus tea is the effect it can have on our tooth enamel if we're not careful. As with any sour food or beverage, like after eating citrus, it's important to wash the natural acids off your teeth by rinsing out your mouth with water to protect your teeth.[3428] You also want to wait at least an hour before brushing so as not to erode your enamel when it's in a softened state.[3429]

FOOD FOR THOUGHT

The best source of the fat-blocking agents thylakoids and calcium is low-oxalate, dark green leafy vegetables, meaning essentially all greens except spinach, beet greens, and swiss chard. To be clear, I encourage everyone to eat huge amounts of dark leafy greens every day, the healthiest food on the planet. Greens answer the question: *What if the food with the lowest calorie content also had the highest nutrient content?* But if you follow this advice (and you should!), then just choose any of the other wonderful greens. If you eat mere-mortal amounts of greens (like a serving a day), then it doesn't matter which type of dark green leafy you choose. I continue to enjoy spinach, beet greens, and chard all the time. It's just that you can overdo those three. To make sure I don't end up consuming more than a serving or two a day of the high-oxalate ones when I'm trying to hit my pound-a-day green leafy quota, I personally do mostly kale, collards, and arugula, which also happen to have the added benefit of being *cruciferocious*. And you can enjoy it with a cup of hibiscus tea for added zing.

FAT BURNERS

Up to BAT

Fat in the Fire

Even if the majority of fat absorption was blocked, we could still accumulate excess body fat in the context of excess calories due to burning less of our own fat stores. Is there any way to ramp up the burn? Let's take a look.

During World War I, it was discovered that some of the ingredients used to make the new explosives had toxic or even lethal effects on the workers in the munitions factories. Chemicals such as dinitrophenol (DNP) can boost metabolism so much that workers were found wandering along the road after work, soaked in sweat with fevers up to 109°F. Then they died. Even after deaths, their temperatures kept going up as if they were having a total-body meltdown. At lower doses of DNP, workers claimed to have grown thin after several months working with the chemical.[3430] That got some Stanford pharmacologists excited about DNP's "promising metabolic applications."[3431]

DNP became the first bona fide fat-burning supplement, boosting resting metabolic rate by 30 percent after a single dose. People started losing weight with no apparent side effects. They felt great.[3432] Then thousands of people started going blind, and users started dropping dead from hyperpyrexia (fatal fever) due to the heat created by the burning fat.[3433] Of course, it continued to be sold. The ad copy read:

> Here, at last, is a [weight] reducing remedy that will bring you a figure men admire and women envy, without danger to your health or change in your regular mode of living. . . . No diet, no exercise!

DNP works, but its therapeutic index—the difference between the effective dose and the deadly dose—is razor thin. It was not until thousands suffered irreparable harm that it got pulled from the market.[3434] Until, that is, its availability was brought back by the internet.[3435] DNP deaths continue to be reported among those dying to be thin.[3436]

There is, however, a way our bodies naturally burn fat to create heat. When we're born, we go from a balmy, tropical 98.6°F in our mothers' wombs straight out into room temperature, when we're still all wet and slimy. As an adaptive mechanism to maintain warmth, the appearance of a unique organ around 150 million years ago allowed us warm-blooded mammals to maintain our high body temperatures.[3437] That unique organ is called brown adipose tissue, or BAT for short, and its role is to consume fat calories by generating heat in response to cold exposure.

The white fat in our bellies stores fat, but the brown fat, located high in our chests, burns fat. In newborns, BAT is essential for thermogenesis—the creation of heat—but was considered unnecessary in adults since we have the muscle mass to warm ourselves by shivering. We used to think BAT just shrank away when we grew up, but then an exciting discovery was made.[3438]

When PET scans were invented to detect metabolically active tissues like cancer, oncologists kept finding hot symmetrical spots in the neck and shoulder regions[3439] that were initially dismissed as muscle tension.[3440] Then, some observant radiologists noticed they appeared in patients mostly during the cold winter months.[3441] When they looked closer at tissue samples taken from people who had undergone neck surgery, they found it: brown fat in adults.[3442]

Go to BAT Against Fat

By the time a baby is born, brown fat may make up 5 percent of an infant's body weight.[3443] As we get older, our brown fat deposits start withering away.[3444] Some adults are left with more than others, and that may help determine how heavy we may become. The amount of body fat we accumulate as we age is correlated with how much brown fat we lose.[3445] The more BAT you have and the more active it is, the thinner you tend to be.[3446] Those who have active BAT have less than half the visceral belly fat[3447]—but which came first: the BAT or the lack of fat? It's possible that underactive brown fat leads to obesity, but maybe obesity leads to underactive brown fat. With all the extra body fat acting as insulation, perhaps our bodies are just able to turn down their internal heaters.[3448] There is, however, reason to believe that brown fat does play a causal role in regulating our weights.

A hibernoma is a rare, benign tumor of brown fat, so named because it resembled the "hibernating gland" of animals like bears, who utilize brown fat to keep them warm through the winter. This condition allows us the opportunity to see if growing extra brown fat can cause weight loss, and indeed, people with hibernomas can lose as much as thirty-five pounds but then may gain it right back after surgical removal of the tumor.[3449] Brown fat transplantation studies showing you can reverse obesity in lab animals have even led scientists to suggest that perhaps we should start harvesting brown fat cells from cadavers.[3450]

Could this explain why some people gain more weight while others seem to be able to overeat and remain slim? Might that just be a consequence of how much brown fat they retained as they grew up? Is it all because of BAT?[3451]

Initially, scans of thousands of people revealed active brown fat deposits in fewer than one in ten, raising doubts about BAT's public health significance. But when they were put in a cool room in their undies for an hour or two *before* the scan, more than half of the people started lighting up when they were scanned. Of those who didn't, however, when they were dunked in cold water or made to sit with their bare feet on a slab of ice, their detection rate shot up to 100 percent.[3452] Given these findings, instead of just a lucky few, it seems nearly everyone retains brown fat, and much more than we used to think.

Initial estimates posited as few as two ounces of brown fat survived into adulthood,[3453] but advanced mapping techniques have revealed it's more like a full cup.[3454] That's still only about 1 percent of our total body mass, though. Is that enough to make a difference? Maximally stimulated, that much brown fat could produce as much heat as a sixty-watt incandescent light bulb.[3455] Developmentally, brown fat cells may derive from the same precursors that go on to form muscle cells.[3456] BAT cells are little fat-burning machines. Theoretically, just our BAT alone could burn off fifty pounds of fat a year without us lifting a finger.[3457] The potential is there, but in most people, their brown fat is just lying dormant. So how can we wake it up?

Turning Up the Heat

Brown fat can be activated rapidly by exposure to cold. There are temperature-sensitive thermoreceptors in our skin connected to nerves that send signals to a special region in our brains that then triggers brown fat activation.[3458] If you focus an infrared thermography camera on someone's upper chest as they stick their hand into a bowl of ice water, you can see areas above their collarbones light up within minutes,[3459] indicating the presence of BAT.

Even mild cold exposure, like a few hours spent in a chilly room, can boost our metabolic rates up to 90 percent, thanks in part to brown fat activation.[3460] Even if that means hundreds more calories burned every day, it only translates into weight loss if there isn't any compensatory increase in appetite.[3461] In the short term, there doesn't seem to be any change in hunger or food intake after a mild cold exposure,[3462] but you can't know about longer-term impacts until you put it to the test.

In a famous study entitled "Recruited Brown Adipose Tissue as an Anti-obesity Agent in Humans," people were randomized to spend two hours a day at 63°F. By the end of six weeks, the cold-exposed group was burning

180 more calories a day and lost significantly more body fat than the control group. At first, only about half the study subjects had detectable brown fat activation in response to the cooler temperatures, but as the weeks went by, BAT hot spots started to ignite.[3463]

Beige Can Be Slimming

Once cells become specialized, they tend to stay that way. A muscle cell can't just decide one day to turn into a skin cell or a nerve cell. Fat cells, though, are different. They're flexible. In the breast, for example, mature fat cells can morph into gland cells and start producing milk. Imagine if there were a way to reprogram a white fat cell into a brown fat cell, turning it from fat-*storing* to fat-*burning*.

Brown fat is brown because the cells are packed with mitochondria, the little power plants in our cells that burn fat using iron-containing enzymes that give them a deep reddish color.[3464] Brown fat is also riddled with a dense network of blood vessels to pump in oxygen and distribute the heat. White fat, on the other hand, is just the regular body fat you can see in a cut of meat. The latest entry in the new color code of fat is beige fat, also known as *brite* (a contraction of *brown in white*).[3465] Apparently, when we're exposed to cold, not only do we make new brown cells from scratch, but some of our white fat cells also transform into brown fat cells, offering a dual benefit.[3466] The fat around our middles can become speckled with brown fat cells to start burning off the fat of their neighboring cells. (In fact, that's one of the ways the FTO "fat gene" may work. It was the first obesity-related gene discovered and may increase risk of obesity by decreasing the formation and activity of this beige fat.[3467])

So the next time you get chilly, look on the "brite" side.

Lose Weight by Chilling Out

Thomas Jefferson purportedly used a cold footbath every morning for most of his life to "maintain his good health."[3468] Was he on to something? Cold exposure is the most powerful known stimulus for BAT activation.[3469] Just twenty minutes at cool temperatures can boost metabolism for hours.[3470] The colder the better, but putting people in a room chilled down into the 50s Fahrenheit is "often not appreciated by [research] subjects."[3471] It's not called a "thermal *comfort* zone" for nothing.

Exposure to cold (or lack thereof) might even help explain the rise in obesity rates. Wintertime bedroom temperatures have been slowly creeping up over the last few decades.[3472] The U.S. standard for winter comfort evidently increased from 64°F in 1923 to 76°F by 1986. All other things equal, spending just 10 percent of one's life at 72°F instead of 82°F could theoretically result in an eighteen-pound weight loss over a decade.[3473]

In an extreme example, lumberjacks in Finland who incidentally died in the dead of winter were found to be replete with brown fat on autopsy, but one need not live Beyond the Wall to reap some BAT benefits.[3474] You burn 164 more calories a day living at 62°F instead of 72°F, about sixteen calories per degree.[3475] If not otherwise compensated for, this could translate into a pound of fat a year per degree.[3476] A climate of 62°F is pretty chilly, but simply moving within the range of climate-controlled buildings from 75°F down to 66°F has been proven to boost BAT activation. This resulted in a 5 percent boost in metabolic rate, so about one hundred more calories burned every day or an annual calorie-deficit equivalent of approximately twenty days of fasting.[3477] So just a slight thermostat shift to a cool-but-not-too-cold ambient temperature may have a significant effect.[3478]

Former NASA scientist Ray Cronise, recognized for helping Penn Jillette lose one hundred pounds,[3479] advises people to twist their faucet handle to incorporate some twenty-second cold-water blasts while showering. The purported benefits of cold-water immersion remain largely anecdotal, though.[3480] (Our founding father's footbaths might have worked even better had Jefferson laid off the opium and mercury.[3481]) Since BAT burns both fat and sugar to make heat,[3482] brown fat activation could help with blood sugar control,[3483] but as far as I'm aware, there has only been a single study published on the effects of regular cold-water showering on health. Those randomized to even just thirty seconds a day of a cold-water blast ended up taking off fewer sick days from work.[3484]

Foods That Turn On BAT

Metabolic Magic Bullet

Mild cold exposure by "slightly" decreasing home temperatures has been suggested as a "cure for obesity,"[3485] but the insulating layer of fat worn by obese individuals makes BAT activation harder[3486]—though not impossible.[3487] Even without cold exposure, however, those who carry active BAT deposits appear to burn off about an extra fifty calories a day without even trying.[3488] This has led to brown fat being regarded as a "magic metabolic bullet,"[3489] with drug companies scrambling to design pills to activate it.[3490]

Fat-burning drugs have a sordid history. When DNP was banned in 1938, amphetamines (speed) took up the slack until they were declared a controlled substance in the 1970s. Then came fenfluramine, followed by dexfenfluramine, and then sibutramine—all of which were later pulled from the market.[3491] Supplements like ephedra also seemed to work, until people started suffering from seizures, strokes, and sudden death, that is.[3492,3493] Thankfully, there are safer options that don't involve phrases like *cold shower* or *ice vest*. Brown fat can be activated by certain foods, herbs, spices, and beverages.

Those same thermoreceptors in our skin are also found in our intestines.[3494] No, you don't have to eat a brain-freezing Slurpee. There are dietary, as well as temperature, triggers. Unfortunately, most of the studies on food components that can activate brown fat or turn white fat beige were only performed in petri dishes or lab animals. These include studies involving beets,[3495] broccoli,[3496] grapes,[3497] greens,[3498] olives,[3499] omega-3s,[3500] onions,[3501] raspberries,[3502] rose hips,[3503] soybeans,[3504] and turmeric, but so far, none of these has been shown to activate BAT in humans.[3505] In ironic contrast to the cold, one of the first foods to pass the test was hot peppers.

Chili Peppers

Capsaicin, the pungent compound in chili peppers that gives them their heat, fits like a lock-and-key into the thermoreceptors that lead to the activation of brown fat.[3506] Studies have investigated the "antiobesity effects" of "Tabasco hot sauce in rats,"[3507] and according to some population studies, those who eat spicier foods tend to gain less weight. This has led researchers to conclude that "regular and higher chilli consumption may provide a low cost and simple strategy to reduce the incidence of overweight and obesity."[3508] But you don't *really* know until you start feeding people some peppers.

Remember how you can point a thermography camera at someone and see the area above their collarbones light up when you plunge their extremities into ice water as their brown fat revs up? The same happens if you skip the ice and just feed people a chili pepper extract.[3509] If you give people 2 mg of purified capsaicin, which is about what you'd find in a jalapeño pepper[3510] or a half teaspoon of red pepper powder,[3511] you can potentially increase the rate at which they burn calories by up to 150 calories a day.[3512]

The reason we know this metabolic boost is from the ignition of brown fat is because capsaicin-like compounds only seem to work in people with active BAT deposits.[3513] Even if yours are lying dormant, cold can not only light up the brown fat you have but also recruit its formation in the first place—and chili peppers appear to do the same thing.[3514] Eight weeks of consuming chili pepper extracts boosted both BAT activity and density by almost 50 percent.[3515] Even just six weeks of taking in chili pepper compounds can so bulk up our BAT that we can get a tenfold increase in cold-induced heat generation.[3516] The researchers concluded that their findings could contribute to "developing practical, easy, and effective antiobesity regimens."[3517] These studies used straight capsaicin or purified extracts so they could hide it in a pill to pit them head-to-head against sugar pill placebos. What about using the whole pepper?

Normally, diet-induced thermogenesis—the extra calories you burn after a meal to digest it—just bumps up your metabolic rate by about 10 percent. Add some red pepper powder to that meal, however, and you can bump up the rate at which you burn calories immediately afterward by more like 30 percent.[3518] The original pepper powder studies were done in Japan, though, where men[3519] and women[3520] happily sprinkled two tablespoons of red pepper powder onto a meal, so people with less affinity for spice might not find it as nice.

Some Like It Hot

Chili pepper may be one of the world's most popular spices, but it's enjoyed more in some places than others.[3521] In Mexico, for example, studies consider anyone eating less than the equivalent of three jalapeño peppers per day as "low-level consumers," whereas high consumers averaged nine to twenty-five jalapeño peppers' worth of capsaicin daily.[3522] In contrast, in the United States, only about one in ten individuals eats peppers of any kind on a daily basis.[3523] So researchers in Indiana sought to determine if a red pepper dose "hedonically acceptable" to Americans would still have an effect.

Instead of two tablespoons, the researchers tried ten times less—about a half teaspoon of cayenne pepper—and mixed it into tomato soup. Over the next four and a half hours, those who had eaten the spicy tomato soup burned about ten more calories than those who had had the unspiced soup.[3524] Since cayenne has essentially zero calories, the spicy group ended up with a relative calorie debt, but ten measly calories is hardly anything to write home about. But that's not the end of the story.

Two years later, a study was published in the Netherlands that reignited interest in the use of chili peppers for weight loss. The researchers started by cutting everyone's caloric intake by 20 percent, which is typical for those on portion-controlled diets. It's the equivalent of removing 500 calories out of a 2,500-calorie day. Your body doesn't like that and tries to compensate, for example, by slowing your sleeping metabolic rate. So, in reality, cutting 20 percent of calories only results in a 16 percent calorie deficit. You may have cut out 500 calories, but since your body is able to make some of that up by slowing your metabolism enough to burn 100 fewer calories, you end up only being down 400 calories by the next morning. The study subjects then were randomized into one of two groups: those who got capsules containing one-half teaspoon of cayenne pepper with each meal or those who got placebos.[3525]

Both groups had 20 percent of calories cut from their diets, but while the bodies of those in the placebo group successfully compensated that reduction down to only a 16 percent deficit, those who had unknowingly ingested the cayenne experienced the full 20 percent drop. The red pepper powder counteracted the body's attempts to ratchet down the metabolism to slow the weight loss. Indeed, the cayenne group woke up the next morning with nineteen fewer grams of body fat, whereas the placebo group had only lost fourteen.[3526] That's about a thick pat of butter's worth of difference, which may not seem like much on any given day, but could add up over time. A study where researchers openly sprinkled red pepper onto people's meals—in tomato juice for breakfast and then in pâté and pizza—experienced a similar benefit.[3527]

Fire in the Belly

A meta-analysis of studies on capsaicin, whether in extract or pepper form, found that overweight individuals burned, on average, about an extra seventy calories a day compared to those in the control groups.[3528] At the same time, taking capsaicin-like compounds before a meal may actually decrease caloric intake, so it may help from both sides of the energy-balance equation.[3529] No wonder capsaicin has been referred to in the medical literature as an "anti-obesity drug,"[3530] a "spicy solution to the management of obesity."[3531] But does it work long term?

The supplement data are mixed. Some randomized, double-blind, placebo-controlled trials using pepper extracts found a benefit in terms of significantly enhanced loss of abdominal fat over time,[3532] but others did not.[3533] Even if the extracts the researchers used contained the right mixture of active ingredients, it's possible some of the effect is mediated by nerve signals coming off our tongues or stomachs.[3534] This would explain why capsaicin supplements that do not dissolve and open up until they're well into the intestine don't appear to work as well.[3535] However, findings from the whole pepper powder studies are inconsistent too.

In an Australian study, where participants were switched between bland and spicy diets, the subjects didn't lose any relative weight in the month they had been adding chili powder to their meals.[3536] A subsequent study in Korea, however, did find a benefit. CT scans revealed significant reductions in visceral fat among those randomized to use Korean chili paste (*kochujang*, a signature component of bibimbap) compared to a placebo paste that evidently looked, tasted, and smelled the same, but had no actual peppers. To accomplish this, however, the researchers had to manipulate the ratios of some of the other ingredients in the placebo paste, such as the salt and soybeans, so other factors may have crept in. Study duration may have also played a role. The twelve-week Korean study lasted three times longer than the Australian study, perhaps allowing time for BAT levels to ramp up sufficiently.[3537]

A nice thing about studies on healthy foods is that even if there are conflicting data about the specific benefits for a particular malady, these foods are by definition healthful. So, with no downsides, I figure you might as well give them a try. But is that the case for chili peppers? Capsaicin has been put to the test as an ergogenic (performance-enhancing) aid and appears to help both with running performance[3538] and strength training,[3539] but what about effects on chronic disease? Do people who eat red hot chili peppers live longer?

Apparently so. The diets of more than sixteen thousand people across the United States were tracked for nearly twenty years. Over that time, one in three passed away—but they were among those who reported they did *not* eat chili peppers. Over that same period, only one in five chili-pepper eaters died.[3540] That's significantly lower overall mortality, but it doesn't necessarily mean the peppers had anything to do with it.

Remember the Hispanic paradox[3541] I discussed in the Rich in Legumes section, where despite having on average less education, a higher poverty rate, and worse access to health care,[3542] Hispanics and Latinos in the United States have a 24 percent lower risk of premature death compared to Caucasians?[3543] That translates into Hispanic men and women living about seven years longer than non-Hispanic black Americans and three years longer than non-Hispanic white Americans.[3544] Latino longevity has been chalked up to their eating up to four to five times more beans,[3545] which have been a staple among all the longest-living populations in the world[3546] and have been called "the most important dietary predictor of survival."[3547] Is it possible that chilis are just being added more often to beans than burgers, and that explains the apparent pepper protection?

Apparently not. The chili pepper longevity study controlled for race and ethnicity, and adjusted for other dietary factors, such as fruit, vegetable, and meat intake, as well as income, education, alcohol, and exercise.[3548] A similar study in China that followed hundreds of thousands of individuals confirmed that those who eat spicy food more frequently do appear to lower their risk of premature death, attributed to the "anti-obesity, antioxidant, anti-inflammatory, and antihypertensive effects of spicy foods."[3549]

As the saying goes, *good peppers burn twice,* but are burning our butts or freezing our bodies our only two options for boosting brown fat? Thankfully, there are a variety of structurally similar flavor molecules in other foods that can go to BAT for us.

Ginger

Ginger has been used in India and China to treat disease for thousands of years,[3550] but both the Chinese and Indian systems of medicine also prescribed mercury,[3551] so there's only so much that "traditional use" can tell us. That's why we have science.

Randomized, double-blind, placebo-controlled trials have found ginger to be effective for treating morning sickness[3552] and migraine headaches,[3553] as well as reducing cholesterol, triglycerides,[3554] blood sugars,[3555] and signs of inflammation.[3556] What about fat burning? There are weight-loss reviews in the medical literature with titles like "Beneficial Effects of Ginger . . . on

Obesity . . ." that sound promising. It's only after you hand over the thirty-eight dollars to buy access to the paper that you may realize disappointedly they're mostly talking about the effects on fat rats. The authors suggest the lack of clinical studies is due to factors such as "ethical issues [and] limited commercial support."[3557] The limited commercial support I can see. Ginger is dirt cheap, so who's going to pay for such studies? But ethical issues? We're just talking about feeding people some ginger. Maybe they think it would be unethical to deprive the people in the control group of ginger yumminess.

Cross-sectional studies, where you take a snapshot in time of ginger consumption and body weight within a population, are relatively inexpensive to conduct. One such study in China found that those who are obese do seem to eat less ginger, which the investigators felt "demonstrated that the use of ginger could have relevance for weight management." But maybe ginger consumption is just a marker of a more traditional, less Westernized diet.[3558]

A randomized controlled trial was performed to assess the effects of having a "hot ginger beverage"—two grams of ginger powder stirred into a cup of hot water—with breakfast. That's about a teaspoon of ground ginger, around five cents' worth. Over the next few hours, those in the ginger group reported feeling significantly less hungry than those who had been given plain hot water instead.[3559] Obviously, the study subjects knew which group they were in, so part of the response may have just been the placebo effect, but not all the effects described were subjective. Four hours after breakfast, the metabolic rate in the ginger group was elevated compared to control.[3560]

What happens when subjects don't know if they're getting a placebo or the real deal? When hidden inside capsules, a half teaspoon's worth of powdered ginger can increase the rate at which our bodies burn fat by about 10 percent two hours after consumption compared to placebo capsules. This only seemed to work in the morning, though. The same amount of ginger given in the afternoon did not appear to have the same effect.[3561] Surprisingly, dried ginger may work better than fresh.[3562] When ginger is dried, some of the gingerol compounds turn into shogaols (from the Japanese word for *ginger*), which may be even more effective at activating brown fat.[3563] Indeed, fresh ginger at breakfast did not appear to affect metabolism at all.[3564]

Human trials with grains of paradise, an African plant in the ginger family, demonstrate that the boost in metabolism is indeed through brown fat activation,[3565] which can then lead to a drop in visceral body fat.[3566] We don't have to search for grains of paradise, though, because plain old ginger spice will do.

Bottom line: Putting together all the randomized controlled trials of ginger powder, two to twelve weeks of a quarter teaspoon to one and a half teaspoons a day of ground ginger significantly decreased body weight for just pennies a day.[3567] And the side effects?

I searched in vain for downsides to ginger consumption and didn't find any, other than "ginger paralysis."[3568] What?! That doesn't sound good. In 1930, thousands of Americans were poisoned by purportedly drinking ginger extract. First of all, who drinks ginger extract? Well, it was 1930, during Prohibition, so ginger extract was a way to sneak a little alcohol. Little did folks realize that the bootleggers had been taking advantage of the demand by swapping in a ginger substitute, a varnish chemical called *triorthocresyl phosphate,* in order to make greater profits.[3569] So actual ginger is fine. The moral of the story is don't drink varnish.

Cinnamon

Cinnamon is another spice with some heat that can cause browning of white fat cells in a petri dish and the slimming of mice in a lab,[3570] but what about in people? Is it all cinnamon bark and no cinnamon bite?

A number of studies have put cinnamon to the test for a variety of maladies. Did the study subjects happen to lose weight in the process? Eight weeks of about a half teaspoon of cinnamon a day (stuffed into capsules) caused about a pound of weight loss in a group of women suffering from polycystic ovary syndrome.[3571] In a group of type 2 diabetics, just about a third of a teaspoon a day for twelve weeks caused four pounds of weight loss over placebo, and, as a bonus, their blood sugar control and cholesterol also improved.[3572] Another study on diabetics using triple the dose, however, failed to find a weight-loss benefit.[3573] A longer study—sixteen weeks with subjects getting about a teaspoon of cinnamon a day—resulted in about seven pounds of weight loss and a two-inch-slimmer waist, with improvements in blood sugars and pressures, cholesterol, and triglycerides.[3574] However, at least a half dozen other studies failed to show any significant change in weight with cinnamon supplementation.[3575,3576,3577,3578,3579,3580]

It's not clear why some studies found a weight-loss benefit and others didn't, but it can't hurt to sprinkle some cinnamon on your oatmeal every morning. Just make sure to choose *real* cinnamon (also known as *Ceylon cinnamon*), not cassia cinnamon (also known as *Chinese cinnamon*). In the United States, if it doesn't specify *Ceylon* on the label, it's probably cassia, which, as I described in *How Not to Die,* has too much coumarin for comfort. A single daily teaspoon of cassia cinnamon could exceed the safety limit for liver toxicity risk in an adult, and even a quarter teaspoon may be too much for a small child.[3581] So make sure it says *Ceylon* on the label, and then sprinkle to your heart's desire.

Peppermint

What about a cooling compound like the menthol in mint? The same receptor in the body that is activated by cold temperatures is also activated by menthol.[3582] Studies on fat biopsies taken from people during surgery discovered that these cold receptors are found on our fat cells. What's more, when they are activated by menthol, they can be "browned" into burning fat in a petri dish.[3583] This discovery led to the 2016 proposition that chronic, menthol-induced browning "could provide a promising novel therapeutic approach for increasing energy expenditure, regulating body weight, and preventing obesity."[3584]

It works in mice.[3585] Mimicking long-term cold exposure with dietary menthol can prevent obesity in rodents. What about in us? While giving people more than ten cups of peppermint tea's worth of menthol a day didn't appear to significantly raise their metabolic rate, rubbing the same amount on their skin did.[3586] Our livers rapidly modify the menthol we eat to remove it from the body. The tobacco industry found a not-so-Kool way to skirt the liver by selling menthol cigarettes to provide a purported edge in weight control,[3587] but topical application may have a similar effect, allowing more menthol to circulate throughout the body before getting metabolized. Research subjects who applied a gel that contained about a half teaspoon of peppermint essential oil's worth of menthol got a significant rise in resting metabolic rate within hours.[3588]

Menthol had been used for medicinal purposes for thousands of years before the menthol receptors in our bodies were discovered.[3589] The reason sports injuries are often iced is to reduce the swelling by reducing blood flow to the area. When our skin is exposed to cold, our bodies clamp down on blood flow to prevent heat loss, and the same happens when we apply menthol. Researchers found that applying about three-quarters of a teaspoon of a 3.5 percent menthol gel on someone's forearm can reduce blood flow as much as applying a cold pack of crushed ice. Not only was the menthol less uncomfortable than the ice pack,[3590] it has also been shown to work better in reducing muscle soreness after a tough workout.[3591]

Topical menthol has also been found to work for chronic pain (carpal tunnel syndrome in slaughterhouse workers[3592]) and migraine sufferers (rubbed on the forehead and temple of the affected side[3593]), but what about weight loss? It works in rats.[3594] Rub rodents with menthol, and their metabolic rates go up and they gain less weight. Unfortunately, it has never been tested in people. If you want to give it a try, menthol concentrations up to 16 percent are considered safe for topical application.[3595] Since peppermint essential oil is comprised of one-third to one-half pure menthol,[3596] you could safely add a tablespoon to a quarter cup to your favorite hand lotion or massage oil. Allergic reactions or skin irritation to menthol is rare,[3597] and no serious adverse effects have been filed with the FDA.[3598] However, that is not the case with other "cooling" chemicals such as methyl salicylate (oil of wintergreen) or camphor (found in products like Bengay and Tiger Balm), which can cause serious, even life-threatening, reactions when used improperly.[3599] So I advise you to stick to menthol-only preparations.

Any other herbs out there with potential?

Cannabis

Pop culture often depicts marijuana users as a "sluggish, lethargic, and unproductive subculture of compulsive snackers,"[3600] but the majority of large population studies have found that pot smokers actually tend to be thinner.[3601] You might be thinking, *But what about the munchies?* Even a single dose of marijuana has been found to increase food intake.[3602] In fact, the first documented medical use of cannabis, dating back over a thousand years, was as a treatment for loss of appetite.[3603] Today, THC, the main psychoactive component of cannabis, is FDA-approved as an appetite stimulant and has been shown to help slow the wasting syndrome associated with AIDS.[3604]

When young, healthy individuals were put in a live-in laboratory setting with all-you-can-eat cake, cookies, Doritos, and other snacks, they gained as much as six pounds over six days smoking joints four times a day. They then lost that weight after they were switched to placebo joints made with cannabis that had had the THC removed.[3605] If cannabinoids like THC can cause weight gain, Big Pharma figured cannabinoid-blocking drugs might be able to cause weight loss.

In 1973, scientists discovered that we have specific receptors in our brains for opioid drugs like heroin and morphine.[3606] Since we didn't evolve shooting up dope, it stood to reason there were natural compounds produced by our bodies that fit into those receptors. Scientists went looking and discovered we did indeed make endogenous morphines, or *endorphins* for short. In 1990, scientists discovered that we also have specific receptors in our brains for marijuana compounds, cannabinoids like THC.[3607] Since we didn't evolve toking up either, it stood to reason there were natural compounds produced by our bodies that fit into *those* receptors. This led to a similar discovery: Our brains make endogenous cannabinoids, or endocannabinoids.

Drug giant Sanofi-Aventis designed a drug called *rimonabant,* which was sold as Acomplia, to block these endocannabinoid receptors to suppress appetite, and it worked. People lost about ten more pounds on the drug compared to placebo over a six- to twelve-month period.[3608] However, the drug also made some people want to kill themselves, which led to its hasty removal from the market for its serious psychiatric side effects.[3609] Our bodies make their own endocannabinoids for a reason.

If cannabis is so good at stoking our appetites, why do regular users tend to be skinnier on average? It does not appear to be due just to concurrent tobacco use.[3610] The boost in appetite may be outweighed by the boost in metabolism.[3611] We've known for more than forty years that our metabolic rates shoot up by about 25 percent within fifteen minutes of lighting up a joint and stay there for at least an hour.[3612] This may be due in part to the activation of endocannabinoid receptors found on brown fat cells.[3613] Unfortunately, there have yet to be any formal weight-loss trials to put cannabis to the test.

Those considering cannabis for weight loss should familiarize themselves with the balance of risks and benefits. On NutritionFacts.org, I have a twenty-part video series that takes a deep dive into the topic. In short, while there is little evidence to support an association between cannabis use and the two main concerns linked to smoking tobacco—lung cancer and emphysema[3614]—

using cannabis can result in addiction, chronic bronchitis, and altered brain development, and may increase the risk of schizophrenia.[3615]

Marijuana liberalization has also led to an increase in the incidence of a rare condition known as *cannabinoid hyperemesis syndrome*,[3616] which is believed to be caused by long-term heavy use of high-potency cannabis.[3617] Characterized by intractable vomiting relieved by hot-water immersion, resulting in some sufferers ending up in the shower for hours a day, it's thought to be caused by a numbing of the same thermoreceptors we've been talking about due to an overload of cannabis stimulation.[3618] This realization has led to the successful topical use of a capsaicin cream—in effect, treating fire with fire—to help mediate the debilitating disease. Bottom line? There are safer ways to boost brown fat. If cannabis is not your cup of tea, then next up to BAT? You guessed it: a cup of tea.

Tea

Brewing Evidence

Simply drink a cup of tea, and, within an hour, you may be burning up to 10 percent more calories.[3619] Drink four cups of tea in the twenty-four hours before a thirty-minute walk, and you burn an extra gram of fat during your half-hour stroll.[3620] Take about ten cups' worth in the form of green tea extract supplements the day before thirty minutes of cycling, and burn an extra two grams of fat.[3621] So is this just from the caffeine naturally found in tea, or is something else at work?

Researchers randomized people to one of three groups: getting either the equivalent of a cup of tea with every meal, just the amount of caffeine in the tea, or a placebo with neither tea nor caffeine. The caffeine alone didn't seem to have any effect, but having tea three times a day raised the number of calories burned in that twenty-four-hour period from about 2,280 to 2,360, around 80 calories more.[3622] And tea without anything added has practically zero calories, so based on these findings, tea may be thought to have "negative" calories. In effect, each cup of tea swept away about 25 calories.

Interventional studies putting around three to six cups' worth of daily green or oolong tea to the test showed an average metabolic boost of about one hundred calories a day, shaving off three butter pats' worth of extra fat every day.[3623] Tea only seems to work half as well as ephedra,[3624] but unlike the drug, tea hasn't chalked up eighteen thousand cases of adverse events or killed any professional baseball players.[3625]

Although more than two thousand compounds have been identified in tea leaves, most attention has been paid to a family of antioxidants called *catechins*, such as *EGCG*.[3626] This is because even straight EGCG has been shown to boost metabolism and the rate at which fat is burned at rest.[3627] That is one reason most of the spotlight has been on green, white, and oolong teas, as they have about five times more EGCG than black tea.[3628]

Originally, we thought this stimulant effect was due to tea compounds keying up our metabolisms by inhibiting an enzyme that degrades adrenaline in the body.[3629] This was based largely on test-tube studies, though, using EGCG concentrations higher than what you might expect to reach in your bloodstream.[3630] Green tea can boost metabolism without raising heart rate[3631] and, if anything, reduces blood pressure a bit—both of which are inconsistent with an adrenaline rush.[3632] Indeed, when put to the test in people, the adrenaline-eating enzyme wasn't suppressed after all,[3633] calling the whole theory into question.[3634] More likely, what's causing this reaction is the BAT signal.

A brown fat effect could help explain the variability in weight-loss responses. In one study, for example, overweight women randomized to about a half teaspoon of green tea powder a day lost an average of twelve pounds more than the placebo group over eight weeks. But, even the twelve-pound difference didn't reach statistical significance because there was such a wide range of responses.[3635] Could it be that some individuals started out with more brown fat than others? In a petri dish, tea compounds like EGCG can induce the browning of white fat cells to beige[3636] and green tea extracts have been shown to reduce shivering under cold conditions,[3637] but BAT activation from tea wasn't proven until 2016.

Like cold and capsaicin, tea only acutely boosted metabolism in those with active BAT deposits,[3638] and furthermore, could recruit the formation[3639] and activation of additional brown fat over time.[3640] It didn't work as well as some of the cold experiments, but drinking tea, the researchers concluded, may be an "easier and more convenient treatment than chronic cold exposure."[3641] But does it get us to lose weight?

Choose Unleaded

China burns about half of the world's coal, spewing toxic heavy metals such as mercury and lead into the atmosphere. Even if you don't live in China or eat any food produced there, you could still be exposed to mercury that settles in the oceans if you eat fish and other seafood, or be exposed to lead if you drink something from China: tea.[3642]

Beyond the mercury from its coal plants to its tea plants, China didn't ban leaded gasoline until the year 2000, which is reflected in the fact that lead levels on Chinese tea plantations are highest closest to highways.[3643] How can you limit your exposure? Just as longer-living fish accumulate more mercury, longer-living leaves accumulate more lead.[3644]

Young tea leaves appear to have two to six times less lead than mature leaves,[3645] so the younger leaves that are used to make green tea and white tea have significantly less lead than the older leaves used to make black and oolong teas. Furthermore, the lead in black and oolong teas appears to be released much more readily into tea water when brewed. Only 7 percent of the lead in green tea leaves leaches into hot water, compared to more than half in the darker varieties. Combining all these factors, the health risk from heavy metals is approximately one hundred times lower for green tea compared to oolong and black.[3646]

Since certain fungicides may have heavy metal impurities, one might assume organic teas would be less contaminated,[3647] but in a study of thirty common teas off North American store shelves, there did not seem to be less toxic element contamination in organic versus conventional tea.[3648] In terms of lead, the country of origin may be the most important factor. Based on the most stringent safety limits in the world,[3649] such as California's Proposition 65 parameters, and the largest studies of tea leaf contamination in two of the largest tea-exporting countries, this is what I was able to come up with:[3650]

(continued)

Safe Level of Tea Consumption

	Chinese Green Tea		Chinese Black Tea		Japanese Green Tea	
	Drinking (cups/day)	Eating (teaspoons/day)	Drinking (cups/day)	Eating (teaspoons/day)	Drinking (cups/day)	Eating (teaspoons/day)
Non-Pregnant Adult	>10	3	3	2	>10	(8)
70-Pound Child	(4)	1	1	0	(4)	(2)
During Pregnancy	1	0	0	0	(4)	0

If you're not pregnant and just *drinking* green tea, from a lead standpoint, it doesn't matter where you source your tea. Given the average levels of lead in Chinese black tea samples, however, more than three cups a day would exceed the most conservative daily safety limits for lead. That's if you're just drinking brewed tea and throwing away the tea leaves or tea bag. If you're actually eating the leaves, like drinking powdered green (matcha) tea or throwing tea leaves into your smoothie like I do, I wouldn't use more than two or three heaping teaspoons a day unless your tea is sourced from Japan. The parenthetical numbers in the chart indicate caution only from a standpoint of caffeine limit, rather than that of any sort of contamination.

If you're the weight of an average ten-year-old, lead still isn't a problem when drinking green tea, but the safe caffeine intake for children is more restrictive. I wouldn't add more than two spoonfuls of Japanese green tea to a child's smoothie due to the caffeine or more than one spoonful of Chinese green tea because of the lead. Similarly, I wouldn't like to see children drinking more than one cup of black tea a day and wouldn't want them eating the leaves at all.

Pregnant women should be able to drink a cup a day of green tea throughout pregnancy, regardless of source, based on average tea lead levels. The cap for Japanese green tea is really just the suggested American College of Obstetrics and Gynecology's 200 mg per day caffeine limit.[3651]

> I wouldn't recommend drinking black tea during pregnancy at all, though, or eating any kind of tea leaves unless you know you're getting tea from a low-lead source.

Weak Tea

A shallow survey of the medical literature might leave one with the impression that tea is more effective at inducing weight loss than it actually is. Case in point: a study published in the journal *Clinical Nutrition* in 2016. Researchers reported in the abstract that the green tea preparation they used "resulted in significant weight loss" and "reduced waist circumference."[3652] The abstract of a scientific paper is a concise summary listing all the important findings, and it's often the only part of a study people read since the rest of the paper can be concealed behind a paywall, as it was in this case. Only after shelling out $35.95 to read the paper in its entirety would you learn the truth: Technically, the green tea supplements did result in significant weight loss and a slimmer waist, but the placebo pills did *better*. Those taking capsules filled with cellulose (essentially purified sawdust) instead of green tea lost more weight and waistline than the green tea group.[3653] That's why you always have to read the entire study (or just have me do it for you).

There certainly are studies showing impressive results, like fifteen pounds of weight loss over placebo for about three cups' worth of green tea a day for three months.[3654] Part of that may be the metabolic boost on the calories-out side of the equation, but improved satiety after a meal with green tea, compared to plain hot water, may also be helping out on the calories-in side.[3655] If you feed two groups of people the exact same diets, but one gets tea and the other does not, would you still see a benefit? Researchers randomized obese sedentary individuals to two thousand calories a day with either a green tea extract supplement equivalent to about a half cup of tea at each meal or an indistinguishable placebo. Within eight weeks, those in the green tea group were down an average of ten pounds compared to about four pounds in the placebo group. Given the identical diets and no significant change in exercise, this suggests the primary green tea benefit is from burning more calories, which was confirmed by calorimetry. The green tea resulted in a significantly higher resting metabolic rate.[3656]

However, after putting all the weight-loss studies together, meta-analyses seem split between statistically insignificant weight loss[3657] or clinically insignificant weight loss, an average of about three pounds over twelve weeks.[3658] Green tea seems less magic bullet and more BB gun pellet, but a pound a month may be worth it for something that's healthy anyway. After nearly five thousand years of tea drinking,[3659] science has finally caught up and shown green tea can lower cholesterol[3660] and prevent colon polyps.[3661] You can even gargle with it to help prevent the flu.[3662] And a meta-analysis of observational studies where tea-drinking populations were followed over time shows consumption of green or black tea is associated with living a significantly longer life.[3663]

What About Green Tea Extract Supplements?

A head-to-head comparison between brewed green tea and green tea extract supplements found a similar amount of weight loss over the control group over an eight-week period.[3664] Those randomized to drink the tea lost six pounds, while those randomized to take the supplements lost four pounds, so why not just take the pills? First of all, because the supplement industry is so poorly regulated, you never know what you're getting. There are supplements on the market that list green tea as an ingredient on the label, but when tested, didn't appear to contain any at all.[3665] Even if supplements are labeled accurately, the fillers may bind to the active components and reduce bioavailability,[3666] or the capsule shell may not disintegrate properly.[3667] This may help explain why, in cholesterol-lowering trials, for example, green tea in beverage form worked, but green tea in supplement form did not.[3668] More concerning, though, are the side effects.

Twelve years ago, when I first started producing videos about cases of liver toxicity tied to green tea extract supplements, it was thought to be rare, on the order of one in one hundred thousand.[3669] Now that we have large studies like the Minnesota Green Tea Trial, we realize it may be more like one in twenty. In contrast, not a single liver problem has been reported in any of the trials that used green tea in regular beverage form.[3670] Even in Japan, where nine cups a day is not uncommon,[3671] adverse effects have not been reported.[3672] An incredible five billion kilos of tea are produced worldwide annually, enough for more than two trillion cups of tea a year.[3673] I think we'd know if just drinking tea could cause liver issues.

Another problem with supplements may be the dose.[3674] Some studies used extract supplement regimens equivalent to drinking more than forty cups of tea a day.[3675] To be on the safe side, I recommend enjoying tea in beverage—not pill—form. I encourage people to stay away from green tea extract supplements, but if you do take them, please stick to less than 300 mg EGCG a day[3676] and stop immediately if you develop symptoms of liver trouble, such as abdominal pain, dark urine, or yellowing of the skin or whites of the eyes (jaundice).[3677]

Not Milk?

Both green and black teas have been shown to improve artery function within hours of consumption.[3678] Why then in population studies is green tea consumption associated with lower heart disease risk than black tea?[3679] In two British studies, in fact, tea consumption was associated with an *increased* risk of coronary artery disease.[3680,3681] Is it because Brits tend to drink their tea with milk, whereas green tea is typically taken straight? If only there were a country that drank black tea, but without milk. There is—the Netherlands. And in those studies, black tea was associated with the same drop in risk as the green tea studies.[3682,3683] So maybe it has something to do with the milk.

Researchers found the addition of milk "completely prevents the biological activity of tea."[3684] Both the artery function benefits and the thermogenic calorie-burning effects were inhibited by casein, a protein in milk that apparently wraps itself about the catechins and blocks their function.[3685] (Interestingly, this is presumably the same mechanism by which adding milk to tea can reduce teeth staining.[3686]) Milk protein also undercuts the benefits of berries,[3687] chocolate,[3688] and coffee.[3689]

What about soy milk? In a test tube, coffee phytonutrients bind not only to dairy proteins but also to egg and soy proteins.[3690] Eggs haven't been put to the test in people, so we don't know yet if having an omelet with black coffee would impair absorption, but soy has been given the all-clear.[3691] Soy proteins do initially bind up the coffee compounds in the small intestine, but then our good bacteria release them so they can be absorbed down in the lower intestine.[3692] Almond-, rice-, oat-, and coconut-based milks have so little protein that I'd assume binding would not be a problem, but they have yet to be directly tested.

When the original milk-blocking study on tea was published, the European Society of Cardiology suggested people consider skipping the creamer, noting the protective cardiovascular effects are "totally wiped out by adding milk."[3693] This advice did not go over well. "As doctors," read one letter to the medical journal editor, "we would not prescribe a new drug to patients if it was studied only in one small study. In analogy, milk abstinence should not be recommended to tea drinkers on the basis of evidence of similar strength."[3694] The researchers replied that the effect was so great—milk didn't just reduce the benefit but "completely blunted the effects of tea"—that they didn't need to do a large study.[3695] As far as I'm concerned, the reason we don't prescribe drugs without overwhelming evidence is that drugs can kill. In fact, prescription drugs kill an estimated 106,000 Americans every year,[3696] so the benefits better outweigh the risks. But what's the downside of a little milk abstinence?

Coffee

In the Black

What About Green Coffee Extract

Green coffee extract is a supplement made from green (unroasted) coffee beans.[3697] Advertised as a miracle weight-loss cure, it was hyped by Starbucks and TV doctors citing a study that found remarkable results[3698]—a randomized, double-blind, placebo-controlled, crossover trial that reported an average of eighteen pounds of weight loss over placebo within six weeks.[3699] Sadly, the too-good-to-be-true study turned out to be too good to be true. It was a disgraceful fraud. Though the lead "researchers" claimed no conflicts of interest, it seems they were glorified ghostwriters handed falsified data, bought and paid for by the supplement manufacturer.[3700]

The company was fined millions by the Federal Trade Commission for making false claims,[3701] and the study has since been retracted.[3702] There have been a few other studies on different green coffee extracts that suggest modest weight-loss benefits,[3703,3704,3705] but the field has been so tarnished by the scandal that green coffee may forever remain branded a cautionary tale on the corrupting power of commercial influence in medicine.

We've known for more than a century that caffeine can boost our metabolisms.[3706] But what about that tea study where a cup with every meal raised the metabolic rate, yet the same amount of caffeine alone did not? That's probably because even black tea usually has less than 50 mg of caffeine per cup, and it typically takes at least 100 mg of caffeine, about the amount found in a typical cup of coffee,[3707] to have a thermogenic effect.[3708] In fact, that's where caffeine got its name—from the German word for coffee, *kaffee*.[3709]

Give people about four cups of coffee's worth of caffeine and they burn about two extra spoonfuls of fat from an hour of cycling.[3710] Is that just because they pedaled harder, though? Caffeine can make exercise seem less difficult and more enjoyable.[3711] Runners randomized to drink coffee shaved about six seconds off their mile,[3712] for example, and weightlifters randomized to coffee were able to squat more weight, worth about six hundred more pounds of reps.[3713] The cycling workout was standardized, however, so the extra fat loss wasn't just because the caffeine group pedaled faster.[3714]

The metabolic boost also occurs at rest. Drink two cups of coffee, and over the next few hours, your resting metabolic rate goes up about 10 percent.[3715] In fact, you can tell whether someone had just consumed coffee by measuring the heat coming off their skin. Two hours after drinking two cups of coffee, our skin temperatures rise by about half a degree.[3716]

On average, every cup of coffee may cause you to end up burning seventeen extra calories.[3717] Since a cup of black coffee only has about two calories,[3718] that leaves a net deficit of fifteen calories per cup. But only a third of U.S. coffee consumers drink their coffee without cream or sugar.[3719] While drinking coffee black could push your calorie ledger into the red, added creamer or caloric sweeteners could easily wipe out any benefit.[3720] There are some Dunkin' Donuts coffee drinks with more than a thousand calories.[3721]

Drinking coffee throughout the day has been shown to burn in excess of one hundred calories,[3722] but might we compensate by eating more? One study found that when overweight individuals were given coffee with about 500 mg of caffeine for breakfast, they didn't eat more throughout the day. In fact, they ate less—550 calories less.[3723] A more typical appetite suppression from coffee seems to be on the order of 55 calories over the course of a day,[3724] but with fewer calories going in and more calories going out, one might expect significant weight loss over time.

Sixteen weeks of five cups of coffee a day did lead to statistically significant decreases in body weight, but it was hardly clinically significant with less than an inch off the waist.[3725] What about combining coffee and capsaicin? Canadian researchers tried giving people cups of coffee with meals sprinkled with about a tablespoon of red pepper powder. Appetites were suppressed and metabolisms were boosted, leaving people nearly a whopping one thousand calories down by the end of the day.[3726] Now if they just would have eaten their meals while sitting on an ice block out in the snow . . .

No trial has ever put the cayenne-and-caffeine combination to the test for weight loss, however, so we're just left with the underwhelming coffee data. So again, it comes down to whether it's healthy for you anyway. Nine out of ten North Americans consume caffeine on a daily basis,[3727] with three billion pounds of coffee consumed annually in the United States alone.[3728] Are there any grounds for concern?

In my chapters on liver disease, depression, and Parkinson's disease in *How Not to Die*, I discussed the benefits of coffee for the liver, mind, and brain. Coffee drinkers do seem to live longer and have lower cancer rates overall,[3729] but coffee may worsen acid reflux disease,[3730] bone loss,[3731] glaucoma,[3732] urinary issues,[3733] and sleep.[3734]

We used to think as long as you didn't drink caffeine in the evening, it wouldn't affect sleep, but having the equivalent of four cups of coffee up to even six hours before bedtime can reduce total sleep time by more than an hour.[3735] Even just two cups at 7:00 a.m. can change what our brain waves look like on EEG later that night,[3736] indicative of shallower sleep.[3737] It's not clear, however, if this has any clinical relevance beyond delaying the onset of sleep by an average of ten minutes.[3738] On balance and on average, coffee consumption is more often associated with benefits than harms.[3739]

What About Energy Drinks?

If caffeine can help burn fat, what about energy drinks? The first energy drink—Dr. Enuf—dates back more than a half century, launched in 1949. Today, there are more than one hundred different brands[3740] fueling a $50 billion industry.[3741] Some military leaders have questioned their safety,[3742] based in part on the skyrocketing number of energy drink–related visits to the ER over recent years.[3743] To be fair, though, if you look at some of the reports, you'll see cases like this: A 24-year-old male didn't feel well after drinking a can of energy drink . . . and "3 bottles of vodka."[3744] Because energy drinks are often co-consumed with other substances like alcohol, it's hard to specify the culprit.[3745] That's why you have to put them to the test.

One concern that has been raised by public health advocates is increased blood pressure.[3746] If you have people chug a can of Red Bull, there's no significant change in blood pressure thirty minutes later.[3747] Okay, but that was just the little eight-ounce can. What about the big sixteen-ounce cans of Red Bull? Forty minutes after drinking one of those, there was still no significant change, so concerns about energy drinks raising blood pressure were dismissed as overblown[3748] . . . until the bomb dropped in 2014.

Red Bull did indeed significantly raise blood pressure after all. The reason the earlier studies missed it is because the spike doesn't start peaking until about an hour after consumption. And the big shocker was that blood flow in the brain took a dive. These energy drinks are promoted as having beneficial effects, but this instead suggests they're potentially harmful because of the extra workload they force on the heart and the decreased cerebral blood flow.[3749]

(continued)

Other adverse effects of Red Bull have been found, such an increased inflammation,[3750] and that goes for other brands like Rockstar[3751] and Monster energy drinks too.[3752] Is it possible it's just the caffeine? Is downing an energy drink any different from having a cup of coffee? To figure that out, a study was conducted in 2017 that compared the effects of an energy drink with a plain drink with the exact same amount of caffeine.

Young, healthy volunteers were randomized to drink two large cans of either an energy drink or a control drink that had the same amount of sugar and caffeine but none of the other proprietary blend ingredients common in energy drinks, such as taurine, carnitine, ginseng, and guarana. It turns out it was *not* just the caffeine. Significantly higher blood pressures were noted on the energy drink, along with a longer "QT interval," which is an EKG finding corresponding to the time it takes for the heart to contract and then refill with blood before beginning its next beat. QT prolongation—which is what the energy drink did, but not the caffeine alone—is a recognized marker of increased risk for developing a sudden fatal heart rhythm.[3753]

Prolongation of the QT interval by more than sixty milliseconds is a marker for life-threatening arrhythmias. Though the energy drink only prolonged it by about ten milliseconds, there have been drugs pulled from the market—profitable drugs bringing in billions of dollars—because of a five- to ten-millisecond prolongation. The researchers suggested we need to start investigating some of these other ingredients in energy drinks.[3754] Case in point: Authorities once found cocaine in Red Bull, though the manufacturers insisted that they were just adding the coca leaf for "flavor."[3755]

Food for Thought

Everything we eat and drink can be grouped into one of four categories:

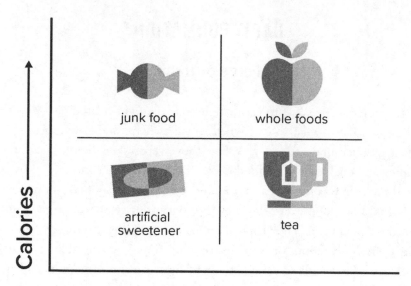

Most of what we consume fits into the upper-right corner, foods that provide both nutrition and calories, but some offer calories without any nutrition, like candy. Others, like artificial sweeteners, offer neither nutrition nor calories. Then there's a fourth category: nutrition without calories. That's where tea comes in, along with many spices. So imagine making a spicy chai with green tea, ginger, and cinnamon. You'd be nailing three fat burners in just one cup.

Note that premenopausal women or anyone at risk for iron-deficiency anemia ideally should not drink tea within an hour of meals to minimize tea's impact on reducing iron absorption.[3756]

Another option is to try feeling *hot! hot! hot!* by spicing up your meals with chili peppers or hot sauces. (You can even add red pepper flakes to your favorite chai tea.) Then you can cool yourself down by lowering your thermostat in the winter for a money-saving, carbon-friendly way to try to burn off some extra fat. A peppermint lotion foot rub may or may not help, too, but it'll feel good either way.

HABIT FORMATION

Force of Habit

When people were asked to estimate how many food-related decisions they make every day—what to eat, when to eat, where, and how much—most pick a number under twenty. When they were asked to carry around a counter and click each such food choice made over the course of a day, the actual number was more than two hundred.[3757] We may make hundreds of decisions about food every day, yet the vast majority appear to pass under our conscious radars. They happen almost automatically, without cognizant reflection, deliberation, or even awareness.[3758] We may be able to take advantage of this mindless eating, though, by harnessing the power of habit formation.

It's been said that "most of the time what we do is what we do most of the time."[3759] Many of our eating habits are indeed just that—habitual. And the busier we are and the more distracted we are, the more likely we are to fall back on habits.[3760] That's what they're there for. Habits are like reflexive subroutines our brains use as mechanisms to free up our mental resources. That can work against us, in the case of bad habits, or for us, in the case of good ones. Imagine if you had to add "buckle seat belt" to your to-do list every day. Maybe put a sticky-note reminder on your dashboard or tie a string around your car keys? If you're in the habit of buckling up, though, your hand will start reaching for the seat belt without you even knowing.

Once you do something long enough, your brain commits the actions to memory and can whip them out at will to automate away some of your cognitive workload—and the automation happens automatically. The mere repetition of a simple action in a consistent context ultimately leads to the action being activated upon exposure to that same situation.[3761] Do it enough times, and getting into a car (contextual cue) can automatically lead to reaching for the seat belt (action).[3762]

Habits are defined as "learned behavioral responses to situational cues,"[3763] so there are two parts—the cue and the action. The cue can be in any context—for example, an event (such as arriving at work), a time (after breakfast), a location (in the car), or even a mood (anxious).[3764] It just has to be something salient that is frequently and consistently encountered in daily life.[3765] Do something over and over again in the same context—whether intentionally or unintentionally—and a habit can form.[3766]

How long does it take? You may have heard that habits take twenty-one days to form. That's a myth that evidently originated from anecdotal evidence of how long it takes plastic surgery patients to psychologically adjust to their new appearance.[3767] When it was actually put to the test, the average time to reach automaticity was sixty-six days. Study volunteers were asked to choose an eating, drinking, or activity behavior to carry out each day in the same context. Examples chosen included "eating a piece of fruit with lunch," "drinking a bottle of water with lunch," and "running for 15 minutes before dinner." There was considerable variation in the time it took for these actions to become automatic, from 18 days to 284 days, but the average was 66.[3768] That might seem like a long time, but be reassured that it does get progressively easier with time, and you only have to maintain your motivation until the habit forms. After that, you're golden. It's like uploading a new piece of software into your brain for a built-in, lifelong body hack.

The magic of habits lies in their persistence even after losing conscious motivation or interest. They just become second nature. You don't have to worry about them anymore. Health can happen effortlessly.

Breaking Bad . . . Habits

Of course, bad habits can also form. The first time you snacked in front of the TV at night, you may have been genuinely hungry, but over time, the two activities can become indelibly linked such that your prime-time shows trigger snack cravings even if you're not really in the mood to eat. It can become something you can't help—in other words, a bad habit.[3769] In one oft-cited study, people in the habit of eating popcorn in the movie theater were asked why.[3770] Most gave some variation of the answer "it tastes good." Seems reasonable, but then why did they end up eating the same amount when they were given stale, week-old popcorn they "decidedly disliked"? Put people who aren't habituated in the same scenario, and they eat more of the fresh popcorn and less of the stale,[3771] but strong habits can perpetuate independently of the intentions or consequences of your behavior.[3772]

There are two ways to break a bad habit: change the cue, or change the action. The most straightforward approach is to try to avoid the situational triggers.[3773] Recovering alcoholics and drug addicts know all too well the power of social or environmental cues to prompt cravings and re-lapses. That may be the reason some people find it easier to quit smoking when they're traveling or otherwise removed from their typical everyday circumstances.[3774] So anytime we can remove ourselves from triggering situations—by walking a different route to work to avoid the donut shop, for instance—we can capitalize on contextual changes to avoid the habitual call-and-response.[3775]

In the popcorn study, when the habituated eaters were moved out of the cinema to instead watch videos in a conference room, the spell was broken. Without the same contextual cues, their actions were released from habitual control, and they, too, pushed away the stale popcorn. That's the first way to break a habit: Block its activation. The other way is to block its execution. In the popcorn study, this was accomplished by surreptitiously forcing the habituated eaters to eat with their nondominant hand.[3776]

There they were, seated in the theater with a bucket of popcorn, so their reflexive response to mindlessly eat even stale popcorn was triggered. Just by having to eat it with their other hand, however, was enough to disrupt the subroutine and regain intentional control.[3777] Change the cue, or change the action. We can block either a habit's initiation or its fluid implementation.

The researchers went as far as to suggest that dieters "actively disrupt the execution of the activated eating sequence by simple manipulations such as eating with the nondominant hand and, in so doing, bring their eating under their personal control."[3778] But do that manipulation long enough and it, too, will become a habit. Junk from the left is just as fattening as junk from the right. A better strategy would be to form new habits of healthy eating.

Change the Cue

Health-wise, it matters little what we eat on birthdays, holidays, or special occasions (unless for you every day is National Hot Dog Day). It's the day-to-day that adds up, which is why our eating habits are so important, for good or for ill.[3779] Our food choices may start out planned and purposeful but can morph into well-worn tracks over time, and we can become stuck in the rut. There is a tendency for habits to continue regardless of our intentions.[3780] This may be why just knowing the right thing to do often isn't enough.

Knowledge is power, but it may not be powerful enough on its own to break a habit. Historically, anti-smoking campaigns have been successful in making people aware of the dangers of cigarettes, but they were not very effective in and of themselves in getting people to quit. Media interventions to reduce youth substance abuse may have even backfired. A meta-analysis of more than one hundred papers showed knowledge and attitudes improved, but the information campaigns appeared to actually increase youth drug use.[3781]

Habits are propensities to repeat behaviors given the recurring circumstances.[3782] As habits form, deliberate decision-making recedes by design and is replaced by these reflexive circuits within our brains. The strength of habits, however, is also its weakness. The dependence of habits on contextual triggers renders them vulnerable to modification.[3783]

Just like smokers trying to quit can remove from sight all their ashtrays, we can try to get rid of all the junk from our pantries.[3784] If you're used to having a cookie every time you see the cookie jar, it might be better to replace it with a fruit bowl. Strategies like packing healthy snacks to go can help shift our immediate surroundings to become more conducive to healthy choices. To change all our habits at once, though, we can try exploiting major life events, such as a change in living arrangements.

Public health campaigners try to take advantage of this by targeting those experiencing natural shifts in their lives, like when they start a new job.[3785] A study of personal accounts of successful versus failed attempts at major life changes found that altering one's immediate environment or moving to an entirely different location appeared to help.[3786] When our existing habits are disrupted, this offers an opportunity to start anew, but you don't have to relocate to start fresh. You can change your existing bad habits to good ones, or establish new good habits from scratch, using a technique known as *implementation intentions.*

How to Get Teenagers to Change

Millions of taxpayer dollars were spent on the D.A.R.E. (Drug Abuse Resistance Education) program to get teens to *just say no* to drugs[3787] until the U.S. General Accounting Office publicized the fact that all the studies that had been done to evaluate its impact showed it had "no statistically significant long-term effect on preventing youth illicit drug use."[3788]

(continued)

It's hard enough to get adults already beset with chronic disease to live healthier. How can we possibly motivate teenagers, who feel invincible and for whom concepts like lung cancer and heart disease are nebulous notions better fit for a grandparental purview?

The classic challenge facing public health efforts is to figure out how to counter the temptation of the immediate reward with the hope of distant future health benefits. This is particularly difficult in the adolescent age group, so much so that leading experts in teen development have said things such as, "Classroom-based health education is an uphill battle against evolution and endocrinology, and it is not a fight we are likely to win."[3789] A landmark study published in the *Proceedings of the National Academy of Sciences* entitled "Harnessing Adolescent Values to Motivate Healthier Eating" broke through the defeatist pessimism by first starting with a question: *What motivates teens?*[3790]

If you were going to design educational materials to get teens to freely choose baby carrots over Cheetos, what would you do? One of the reasons it's so difficult to convince teenagers to take better care of themselves is that they are extremely sensitive to perceived encroachments on their autonomy. They seek independence from parents and other authority figures telling them what to do—so the researchers sought to turn this obstacle into an asset. They developed a healthy eating message framed as an exposé of manipulative food industry marketing practices designed to deceive. They talked about how Big Food scientists use sophisticated, industrial techniques to maximize product craveability using salt, sugar, fat, and other flavor additives. The goal was to portray healthy eating as a way to rebel and "stick it to the man."[3791]

The other commonly shared value they tapped into was a concern about injustice. Teens are often stereotyped as self-centered, but anyone who's worked with them can attest to their sensitivity to unfairness and inequity. So the researchers talked about how the food industry disproportionately targets poor communities and young children with ads for some of their unhealthiest products. Avoiding junk food was presented as a way to take a stand for social justice.

In theory, these two avenues eliminate the need to think about long-term consequences, instead offering immediate symbolic benefit in terms of stoking their rebellious spirits and acting in accordance with their deeply held beliefs. Or at least that's the theory. To test it, researchers set up a double-blind, randomized, placebo-controlled experiment with more than five hundred eighth graders. They were allocated randomly to one of three groups: the new approach, traditional nutrition education, or a nonfood-related control group. Then hidden observers spied on them surreptitiously at a later date in an unrelated context. The students had access to unhealthy choices, such as Coke, Sprite, Oreos, Doritos, and Cheetos, as well as healthy options, such as sparkling water, fruit cups, trail mix, and baby carrots. What happened? It worked! Compared to the other groups, those given the healthy eating message framed to teen values independently chose to forgo some of the fattening snacks and drinks in favor of the healthier options.[3792]

Change the Action

Fancied as asphalt for the highway to hell, good intentions have a bad reputation. Oscar Wilde wrote, "Their origin is pure vanity. Their result is absolutely *nil*."[3793] Many who have failed to stick to their New Year's resolutions can relate.

To help secure our goals, we can call on our built-in cognitive capacity to create habits to automate our actions.[3794] This starts with implementation intentions.[3795] Instead of vague self-promises to "do our best," implementation intentions are specific if-then plans to perform a particular behavior in a specific context. They take the form of *When situation* X *arises, I will perform response* Y.[3796] For example, *If I get hungry after dinner, I will eat an apple*. If the triggering circumstance is a regular, daily occurrence, implementation intentions can be the beginning of a beautiful habit.[3797]

Note that to break a bad habit or create a new one, we have to select a new action (eat an apple) rather than just give up an existing behavior (don't eat potato chips).[3798] To activate the habit-forming mechanism, you likely need a new alternative response, rather than a nonresponse.[3799] Evidently, you can't form a habit of not doing something.[3800] Then, to lock it in, you have to purposefully repeat it day after day, week after week, and maybe even month after month before it takes on a mind of its own. It may be a lot of work up front, but once it's ingrained in our brains, then the need for willpower is replaced by an eerie compulsion to just do the right thing.

During the process of habit formation, it gets easier as we go along. This is particularly the case with dietary interventions because our palates change along the way. For example, ever since I stopped regularly drinking coffee,[3801] I've been having a really strong chai tea in the morning. At first, I was using one of the less harmful, low-calorie sweeteners to cut the bitterness. Preliminary data suggest sweeteners like monk fruit,[3802] erythritol,[3803] and allulose[3804] are relatively benign in small doses, but low-calorie sweeteners tend to have a bad track record when it comes to safety. Given that I'm always trying to expand the percentage of Green Light foods in my diet, I could have tried a more nutritive sweetener like date syrup, but I decided to try to cut down altogether. Every day, I vowed to use less sweetener than the day before. Now, not only do I take my morning tea unsweetened, I *prefer* it that way. As a "treat" to myself one day, I decided to add a little sweetener, and it just tasted gross. So now I'm in the best of both worlds where taste and health preferences unite.

Implementation Intentions Put to the Test

Given their simplicity, implementation intentions appear to be surprisingly effective.[3805] Imagine you're a dentist who wants your patients to floss their teeth daily. You give them a complimentary pack of dental floss with a handout telling them how important flossing is and encourage them to floss every day. Having read this book, though, you recall the supposed power of implementation intentions. You're skeptical, so you randomize half your patients to get the same free floss and identical handout except their version contains one additional message:

> You are more likely to carry out your intention to perform dental flossing every day if you make a decision about when and where. Most people perform dental flossing in the bathroom immediately after they brush their teeth at night. Others prefer to do it in the morning after breakfast. Write down where and when you intend to floss your teeth every day for the next 4 weeks.

Just such an experiment was carried out, and that one additional tweak, that one additional message, *doubled* flossing frequency, from eight days of flossing out of the following month to nineteen days.[3806] That's the power of implementation intentions. (Note that all randomized, controlled, crossover trials to date show that flossing *before* brushing gets rid of significantly more plaque.[3807,3808])

Does what works for flossing work with eating? When researchers interviewed maintainers of significant weight loss, action planning to develop healthy habits arose as a consistent theme. The successful losers often decided in advance what they were going to eat, when, and where. Many consciously planned their meals for the day or week, often getting into the habit of eating similar meals for breakfast and lunch every day. They meal-prepped and kept healthy snacks like carrots and fruits in plain sight. Some made double portions of wholesome meals to refrigerate or freeze in case they got busy.[3809] Several brought home only healthy foods from the store. (As one put it, "You cannot eat what you don't buy.")

Those all sound like good ideas, but just because those successful at weight loss tended to use lots of implementation intentions doesn't necessarily mean the intentions had anything to do with it. You can only prove cause and effect with interventional trials where you randomize people to an intervention—or not—and put it to the test. So that's just what researchers did.

Hundreds of middle-aged women were randomized into one of two groups. Both groups were told about the health benefits of fruits and vegetables, and both groups were encouraged to boost their intakes, but one group got additional instructions to form implementation intentions. They were told to think of all the barriers to healthy eating they encounter on a daily basis and come up with three implementation intentions to overcome them. Typical examples included *If I have no fruits at work, then I will buy an apple in the canteen at lunch* or *If I am eating out for lunch, then I order a salad*.[3810]

In the first couple of months, both groups succeeded in eating more fruits and veggies, but by month four, the implementation-intention group pulled ahead. Two years later, the fruit and vegetable consumption in the information-only group had, unsurprisingly, fallen back toward baseline, but the implementation-intention group was still going strong. After just that single meeting with the experimenters years before, they were still eating significantly more fruits and vegetables, presumably because it had become so routine as to become habit.[3811] All because of that simple psychological trick.

Other studies have found intention formation to be a useful tool for solidifying healthy eating and exercise interventions,[3812] but what about weight loss? Randomized controlled studies show forming new habits or breaking old ones can not only produce significant weight loss but, more importantly, help keep it off.[3813] For example, in one twelve-week study, participants randomized to try to turn the "Top Ten Tips" for weight loss into daily habits lost about seven pounds (compared to no significant weight loss in the control group). The tips were just your run-of-the-mill good advice, such as "Make water your first choice," "Try reaching ten thousand steps each day," "Pack healthy snacks," and "Eat more fruits, vegetables, and pulses (beans, split peas, chickpeas, and lentils) and less fast food and high-fat dairy and meats."[3814] Losing seven pounds is nothing to sneeze at, but the excitement came from what happened after the study ended.

A year later, not only did the participants randomized to try to habituate the weight-loss tips not gain back the weight, they continued to lose another five pounds on average.[3815] Participants described that healthy eating and activity just became "pretty much second nature."[3816] They "just worm their way into your brain," one person remarked. "Now I actually feel quite strange if I haven't [eaten a salad]." Overall, 65 percent achieved clinically significant, sustained weight loss by automating healthy behaviors into habits.[3817]

Avoiding a Snowball's Chance

In the study that determined it took an average of sixty-six days of repetition to form a habit, the researchers found that sporadically missing a day resulted in a tiny dip in automaticity the next day but had no longer-term consequences.[3818] So if you stumble or forget one day, just pick it back up the next. A series of experiments dating back to the 1970s did uncover a curious quirk of human psychology you should be aware of, though, so you don't fall into the trap.

Imagine enrolling dieters in a study ostensibly to "investigate the effects of prior taste on subsequent taste perception" by having them "taste test" different flavors of ice cream after drinking a milkshake. Half were told the preload milkshake was "very high calorie," and the other half were told it was "very low calorie"—though, in truth, all shakes were identical. All the subjects were then instructed to taste and rate three bowls of ice cream, eating as much or as little as they wanted and feeling free to finish them all off if they so wished. What do you think happened?

The rational thing to do if you're trying to watch your weight is to eat less ice cream after you've just had a high-calorie milkshake, right? Well, the exact opposite happened. Those told they were drinking the high-calorie shake went on to eat 43 percent more ice cream than those who had drank what they thought was the low-calorie shake.[3819] How does that make any sense? Instead of telling themselves they'd overeaten and shouldn't make it worse, their attitude appeared to be, "It's too late now, so I might as well enjoy myself."

As I mentioned on page 85, this irrational reaction to overindulge after overeating because now the "day is lost" has a name in the scientific psychology literature. It's been coined the "what-the-hell effect."[3820,3821]

Though proximal subgoals, like promising yourself no more than one treat a day, can help keep you on track, they can be counterproductive if they cause you to lose sight of the end goal—that is, losing weight. Slipups can feel like you've let yourself down and demotivate you into all-or-nothing thinking.[3822] Two cookies can lead you to binge-eat the whole bag.

There are a few ways to counter the what-the-hell effect. You can try extending the time period of the subgoal. So instead of committing to no more than one treat a day, if you swore to yourself that you wouldn't have more than seven treats in a week, having two cookies in one day might no longer feel like such a face-stuffing failure. You can just make it up tomorrow.[3823]

Another way identified by researchers to fight the what-the-hell effect is to choose acquisitional, rather than inhibitional, goals. People seem to be better able to deal with coming up short on positive goals than negative ones. So framing your subgoals as things you want to accomplish, rather than avoid, can help you escape the fatalistic, black-and-white thinking that can subvert your longer-term goals. For example, if you aim to drink a large glass of water before every meal but miss one time, there isn't the same defeatist feeling. *Well, I messed up and didn't drink water before lunch, so forget it. I might as well not drink water before dinner either* doesn't tend to race through your mind. When we have positive subgoals, we're more likely to think positively— *Thankfully, I remembered at breakfast and now dinner, so at least I'm making progress*—whereas violating a negative, don't-do-something goal, like vowing not to touch soda, appears more likely to make what-the-hell break loose.[3824]

Finally, you can recognize the feeling when what-the-hell arises, realize how ridiculous it is, and try to laugh it off. I had to chuckle at myself the other day when my writing was interrupted by an urgent media call that forced me to delve into a few hours of research unrelated to this book. Afterward, I remember thinking, *Well, my day's shot, so I might as well just stop now and watch a movie or something and start fresh tomorrow.* I had just what-the-hell'd myself! I missed a few hours of writing time, so therefore I should miss *more* time? Realizing how silly that was, I got back to work.

Avoiding the Self-Licensing Trap

The flip side of subgoal setbacks blowing your end goal is when subgoal successes do the same thing. Remember self-licensing, the other irrational phenomenon where dietary supplements led smokers to light up more and dieters to eat more junk? It's when movement toward our goals can justify indulgences that set us further back. Excuses like *I worked hard this week so I deserve it* fall into this category.[3825] There's a reason it's the catchphrase for marketers the world over. (Who can forget, *You deserve a break today at McDonald's?*)

Would you guess that smokers of "light" cigarettes would be more or less likely to quit compared to those who smoke regular cigarettes? You might reason that those choosing to find lower-tar varieties are already acknowledging and trying to cut down on the risks, so they would probably be more ripe to quit, right? But no. They are more than 50 percent *less* likely to kick the habit. This failure is presumed to be a licensing effect, where their imagined progress toward their goal of not dying from lung cancer is subconscious justification to indulge their addictions that may end up killing them. (The cruel irony of light cigarettes is that smokers tend to use more of them or instinctively hold the smoke in longer such that the same amount of tar ends up being deposited in their lungs.[3826])

Check out how this manifests in the world of weight loss. The best predictor of future performance is past performance, right? Haven't we all heard past-as-prelude aphorisms? Well, if you follow dieters over time, it turns out the opposite can be true. Weight loss in one week appears to have a strong negative impact on weight loss in the subsequent week.[3827] Naïvely, you might think that progress begets progress, with good news on the bathroom scale inspiring further motivation to stick with it. But instead of taking a victory lap (burning even more calories!), people tend to use the occasion of their progress as a pretext to indulge. After all, they figure, they deserve it.

This counterintuitive consequence draws from a larger literature on "moral licensing." Researchers have found a prior good deed can lead people to act questionably later on. Virtue can lead to veritable villainy. You'd think people would take pride in the integrity of moral consistency, but instead, being good appears to liberate us to be bad.[3828]

Consider this disturbing study out of the University of Toronto: People were randomly assigned to purchase items from one of two online shopping sites, identical except the products were described as environmentally friendly on one of the sites. Then, in a supposedly unrelated task, they played a computer game and were told to pay themselves out of a provided envelope of money for each correct answer. They were told no one was watching and it was all on the honor system. Who do you think acted more honorably? In actuality, the experimenters really *were* watching them, tallying up the actual number of correct answers, how many the subjects claimed they had gotten correct, and how much money they subsequently took. Shockingly, those randomized to purchase the green products were significantly more likely to then lie, cheat, and steal.[3829] Ethical acts may license unethical behaviors, and it may only take a molehill of virtue to create a mountain of immorality.[3830]

Self-licensing can also involve self-delusion. The effect is so powerful that when people are presented with a temptation, they tend to exaggerate in their minds how well they've been eating in order to justify the indulgence. So not only may progress toward a goal rationalize lapses, but even misremembered distortions of progress can cause us to slide.[3831] This is why it's so important to be aware of the psychological tricks our minds can play on us so we can counter them.

Even visions of *future* progress can trigger licensing and undercut our goals. How many times have you been tempted to slip "just this once," resolving to make up for it tomorrow? But "tomorrow" may never come. If you offer people watching their weight the choice of a "large Mrs. Field's cookie" or a snack they perceive as healthy (plain fat-free yogurt) around 50–60 percent choose the cookie. If, however, as you offer them the choice, you tell them they'll be given the same choice the following week, the number choosing the cookie jumps up to 70 or 80 percent. Do you see what happened? People told themselves they'll choose the healthier option the next week, thereby justifying their choice to jump at the cookie this week.

What happens if you tell people they can choose between the cookie or the yogurt this week, but only the healthier option will be offered the following week? Those choosing the cookie shoots up to 90 percent! Sadly, our brains don't work the other way around. Telling people they're just going to get the cookie next time doesn't increase their odds of making healthier choices in the present.[3832] Our minds are always reaching for the rationalization.

Ironically, those with the greatest self-control are the most vulnerable to this kind of behavior.[3833] They're so sure they're going to be able to resist the temptation—*next* time—they feel licensed to indulge now. To neutralize this effect, try to make each decision on its own merits in the here and now. In that present moment, regardless of what you did before or plan on doing later, consider the best choice to fulfill your long-term goals.

Does that mean you should never splurge, never veer off the path? Self-licensing is dysfunctional if it's your mind tricking you into stumbling too easily or too often, but it can be useful if it supports long-term dietary adherence. If cheating every once in a while helps you sustain a healthier lifestyle, then it could be beneficial in the long run.[3834] The difference is in the design. Cheating isn't cheating if it's baked into the plan. Those who prearrange to give themselves a certain number of passes every month to skip the gym or eat whatever they want can do so without deceiving themselves or inviting the wrath of the what-the-hell effect. Because it's all just part of the plan.

FOOD FOR THOUGHT

The business world knows all about how to make things easy. It's the reason Amazon has a 1-Click Buy button.[3835] This is why the term *habit-forming* can be a good thing when you consciously turn it to your advantage. It can turn healthy decisions into an impulse buy.

Using implementation intentions, we can begin the process of automating healthy urges away from conscious control. Then we can relax and let the habitual subroutines do all the work. There's no need for willpower when you have chill power.

Those who've seen my "blender burpees" cooking video know a bit about how I style implementation intentions in my own life. A typical if-*X*-then-*Y* for me is *As I fill up my water bottle, I'm going to try to fit in ten squats.* Better that than just standing there getting nothing else done as I get my water, right? That's actually where my

Daily Dozen checklist sprang from, a set of acquisitional goals to remind me to fit in more of the healthiest of healthy foods.

For example, burdened with the knowledge that dark green leafy vegetables are the healthiest foods on the planet, I'm always trying to intentionally implement ways to fit more into my diet. Every time I shop for groceries, for instance, I make myself buy at least two bunches of greens for every day of the week. (But if I run out, I know I always have an emergency stash of bags of frozen greens in my freezer.) I also changed a snacking habit to *If I get hungry, I'll snack on roasted nori.* For me, it was less about the calories (though nori does only have about five to ten calories a sheet), and more about the marvel of enjoying dark green leafy vegetables as a snack. I even sip on matcha tea, so I can drink my dark green leafies too.

To maintain healthy habits, I described the pitfalls—the two psychological glitches that can threaten your goals from both directions. Say you're trying to get into the habit of drinking water instead of soda. On the one hand, if you slip, your morning Mountain Dew can turn into a what-the-hell chugfest. If, on the other hand, you succeed, the licensed self-indulgence side could rationalize one or two "live a little" liters. I know it can be seductive to rationalize. Sometimes when I'm on the road for a weeks-long stretch, jet-lagged after some hectic four-hour book-signing, the junky snacks in the late-night hotel minibar start looking pretty enticing. I've found for me it helps to turn those feelings of entitlement around. *No,* I tell myself. *You know what you* really *deserve? To be healthy.*

HYDRATION

Just Add Water?

According to a national survey, "Drink plenty of water" was one of the weight-control practices most associated with successful weight loss. The strategy was also associated with *unsuccessful* attempts at losing weight, however.[3836] In other words, it's one of the most popular weight-loss tips across the board, heralded in the mainstream media and commonly recommended by physicians to their patients.[3837] But does it work?

About a dozen studies have been published on the matter, and overall, there does appear to be a weight-reducing benefit to increased water consumption.[3838] What's the obvious confounder, though? Confounding factors, sometimes called *lurking variables,*[3839] are those third elements that may end up being the true explanation for a supposed link between two things. For example, there may be a tight correlation between ice cream sales and drowning deaths, but that doesn't mean ice cream causes drowning. A more likely explanation is that there is a lurking third variable—like hot weather or summertime—that explains why drowning deaths are highest when ice cream consumption is at its peak. So what might be a confounding factor that can offer an alternate explanation as to why those who drink more water tend to lose more weight? The most obvious might be that those who drink more water tend to drink less soda.[3840]

The primary reason that the Centers for Disease Control and Prevention, U.S. Department of Agriculture, American Medical Association, American Diabetes Association, American Heart Association, and American Academy of Pediatrics all recommend drinking water for weight management is as a replacement for sugary beverages.[3841] Swapping just one sweetened beverage or beer a day with water is associated with a lower incidence of obesity over time.[3842] American children and adolescents drink so much soda that replacing all sugary beverages with water could result in an average reduction of 235 calories a day.[3843] So does that explain it? Not quite. Even if you take the consumption of calorie-containing beverages into account, water consumption is *still* associated with better weight control, so there has to be something else going on.[3844]

What about exercise? That's another obvious confounder candidate. After all, who drinks a lot of water? Those who spend hours working out. No wonder heavy water drinkers might be slimmer. However, a study of dieting overweight women that took both soda intake and exercise habit into account still found a benefit associated with increased water consumption. Over a year, those who drank at least a liter of water a day lost about five more pounds on average than those who didn't.[3845] Okay, the researchers were able to account for other beverages and physical activity, but what about other foods? It turns out those who drink more water also tend to eat more fruits and vegetables, greens and beans, and whole grains,[3846] as well as less fast food[3847] and total sugars.[3848] No wonder they're a healthier weight.

To control for dietary factors, the scientific world brought out the big guns: Harvard's massive cohort studies that followed the diets and health of more than one hundred thousand doctors and nurses for decades. The researchers were able to control not only for other beverages and lifestyle factors like exercise, smoking, sleeping, and TV watching but also a wide range of healthy and unhealthy food intakes, from fruits and vegetables to meat and candy. They were the first to show that "increasing water intake per se was independently and significantly associated with less weight gain" over the long term.[3849]

Consumption patterns in these studies were by self-report, though. Participants were asked to fill out detailed questionnaires about their diets. For more objective measure, researchers directly assessed people's hydration status by measuring their blood and urine concentrations. In both children[3850] and adults,[3851] the more hydrated they were, the less likely they were to be obese. Spot-checking urine from nearly ten thousand men and women, researchers found that nearly half the obese individuals were walking around underhydrated compared to fewer than one in three individuals who were normal weight or lighter.[3852]

The problem with snapshot-in-time studies is you don't know which came first: Did underhydration lead to obesity, or did obesity lead to underhydration? At a heavier weight, you actually need more water. The daily water requirement of a man of average height weighing 210 pounds may be four cups more than if he weighed 160 pounds.[3853] And who's more hydrated? Those who eat more water-rich foods like fruits and vegetables.[3854] There's that specter of confounding again. The only way to prove cause and effect is to put it to the test.

Milked Dry

Overweight adolescents were randomized into one of two groups, either advised to drink eight cups of water a day or not. What happened after six months? Before you look at the results of any interventional study, the first question you always have to ask is: *Did the participants actually comply with the intervention?* In this case, both groups started out drinking around two cups of water a day, so the study was designed to see if there was a weight-loss benefit to consuming six extra cups of water. Unfortunately, in the end, the difference in water intake between the groups came out to be less than a cup and a half, which evidently wasn't enough to show any benefit. Only a tiny percentage of teens in the water group reported reaching the target intake.[3855]

To improve compliance, another set of researchers asked kids to keep an eye on their pee. The group of overweight nine- to twelve-year-olds randomized to the water intervention was told to increase their water intakes to the point their urine became straw-colored (pale yellow). Once again, not every kid complied, but those who did lost significantly more weight.[3856]

Inspired by these small pilot studies and early successes with school-based interventions in Europe,[3857] researchers launched the most ambitious study yet, involving more than a million students in New York City public schools. They compared obesity rates and weight gain in schools that installed cooled, filtered water dispensers compared to control schools that hadn't, and the increased water access appeared to translate into less weight gain and lower likelihood of overweight kids.[3858]

The accompanying editorial in the American Medical Association's pediatrics journal was entitled "The Power of a Simple Intervention to Improve Student Health: Just Add Water."[3859] But was it the addition of water per se that caused this, or could it have been the subtraction of something like soft drinks? Isn't it possible the students with greater water access just grabbed fewer sodas and that's why they had less weight gain?

The study had been performed a decade *after* NYC schools removed soda from all their vending machines, but they still sold low-fat milk. The corresponding drop in milk purchases is in fact what the researchers suspect may have accounted for the weight-loss benefit in the water group.[3860] Intake of milk, like soda, can result in weight gain.[3861] This is true for skim milk or even just straight dairy protein, pure whey or casein added to beverages even without the naturally occurring milk sugars.[3862] The increased fat mass from drinking milk[3863] may be in part from the elevation in insulin levels caused by milk protein.[3864] Even dairy industry–funded studies have found that drinking less than a cup of milk with a low-glycemic-index meal can exaggerate the insulin spike as much as if you just had eaten high-glycemic white bread.[3865]

Burn Fat, Preserve Muscle

While milk can impair fat burning,[3866] water may have the opposite effect. To get to the bottom of the water-and-weight-loss question, tightly controlled metabolic experiments were performed in which whole-body protein and fat breakdown were measured under different degrees of hydration. Well-hydrated individuals experienced the best of both worlds: increased fat burning and decreased protein breakdown.[3867] The way the body responds to high water intake is similar to how it responds to acute fasting—by switching toward fat as a fuel source while trying to spare the muscle.

These were proof-of-principle experiments with limited real-world relevance, though. The high fluid states were induced not only by having the participants drink ten cups of water over a twelve-hour period but also by dripping extra free water straight into their veins and even giving them an antidiuretic hormone to cause them to retain even more water. However, there are mechanisms by which our day-to-day hydration status can affect our metabolisms.

When we get dehydrated, our blood volume actually shrinks. This drop is detected by our kidneys, which then release an enzyme into our bloodstreams that triggers the cascade that results in the formation of a hormone called *angiotensin,* which, in turn, causes us to become thirsty and constricts our blood vessels to raise our blood pressures to compensate for the diminished blood volume. (This is how a popular class of blood pressure–lowering medications works. The *ACE* in *ACE inhibitors*—like captopril—stands for *angiotensin-converting enzyme*.)

That isn't all that angiotensin does, though. Drip the hormone onto human fat cells in a petri dish, and they start piling on more fat.[3868] This may help explain why those with higher angiotensin levels in their bloodstreams tend to be heavier.[3869] The thought is that those who don't drink enough end up with chronically elevated angiotensin levels, which can lead to weight gain.[3870] The most convincing evidence comes from genetic studies showing that those born predisposed to higher angiotensin levels are significantly more likely to become obese.[3871] We can keep our levels down in the normal range, though, by staying adequately hydrated.

What Kind of Water Should You Drink?

Though many distrust the safety of tap water,[3872] bottled water may be no safer, no cleaner, or of no higher quality than water straight out of the faucet.[3873] How much is that saying, though? Two studies published back in the 1970s forever changed our perception that drinking water safety was just about waterborne diseases.[3874] In fact, it was our fight against microbial contaminants that led to a new kind of contamination in the form of disinfection by-products.

The two landmark papers from 1974 solved the mystery of the source of chloroform in drinking water: We have met the enemy, and he is us. The chlorination of drinking water—crucial for maintaining microbiological safety—was interacting with natural organic matter from the water's source and creating chlorinated compounds that can not only result in off flavors and smells but may also pose a potential public health risk.[3875] More than six hundred disinfection by-products have been identified so far.[3876]

After decades of research into the matter, it appears that the lifelong ingestion of chlorinated drinking water results in "clear excess risk" for bladder cancer.[3877] There is also some evidence of increased risk of birth defect rates,[3878] but most of the concern has focused on the bladder cancer link.[3879] Forty years of exposure may increase your odds of bladder cancer by approximately 25 percent.[3880] Environmental Protection Agency scientists estimated that between 2 and 17 percent of bladder cancer cases in the United States are due to these disinfection by-products in drinking water.[3881] However, this is assuming the link is cause and effect, which has yet to be firmly established.[3882]

The best way to reduce risk is to treat the cause. Countries could prevent the formation of disinfection by-products in the first place through better initial removal of the source water's natural organic matter[3883] (or *schmutz,* as my grandmother would say). Some countries in Europe such as Switzerland have newer, well-maintained drinking-water systems that can distribute tap water free from residual disinfectants, but the cost to upgrade the infrastructure of even a small city in the United States could run in the tens of millions.[3884] As the tragedy in Flint, Michigan, has revealed, we seem to have trouble keeping even undeniable toxins out of the tap.

Nearly 40 percent of Americans use some sort of water purification device.[3885] Two of the most common approaches—pour-through pitchers and refrigerator filters—were tested head-to-head against Tucson tap water. Both of the fridge filters (GE and Whirlpool) did similarly well, removing more than 96 percent of trace organic contaminants, edging out the three pitcher filters, which ended up catching 93 percent (ZeroWater), 84 percent (PUR), and only 50 percent (Brita).[3886] A similar discrepancy was found between PUR and Brita brand filters tested specifically against disinfection by-products.[3887] Reverse osmosis systems can work even better, but their cost, water waste, and loss of trace minerals[3888] make them seem unworthwhile.

The annual cost for purifying your water with a pour-through pitcher or fridge filter was calculated to be about the same, at only around a penny per cup (with the exception of the ZeroWater brand, which is up to four times more expensive).[3889] I figured the "change by" dates on the filters were just company scams to get you to buy more, but I was wrong. Since I drink filtered water mostly just for taste, I used to wait until the water started tasting funky before I changed the filter. Bad idea. Not only do the filters eventually lose much of their removal capacity, but bacterial growth can build up inside them, resulting in your filtered water having higher bacterial counts than the water straight out of the tap.[3890]

FOOD FOR THOUGHT

You can check your hydration situation by monitoring the color of your urine. Originally validated as a way to detect acute dehydration in athletes,[3891] it's now used more broadly in studies of the general population to track hydration status[3892] (including pregnant and lactating women).[3893] The gold standard (or rather, the *pale* gold standard) is the color of straw. For those of you who didn't grow up playing on bales in barns like I did, that means a light yellow. Note that if you take B vitamins or eat riboflavin-rich foods, that can throw off the results.[3894] Riboflavin (also known as vitamin B2) gets its name from the Latin word *flavus,* for *yellow.*[3895] So if you dust your air-popped popcorn with nutritional yeast, a vitamin-packed cheesy topping (spritzing the popcorn first with apple cider vinegar to get it to stick, of course), your urine stream can light up neon yellow like a light saber. This can give the false impression that your urine is more concentrated than it is and, hence, that you're more dehydrated than you actually are.

Is there any danger in drinking too much water? Absolutely, yes. Even healthy kidneys can only handle about three cups of water an hour.[3896] Beyond that, we risk washing the electrolytes out of our brains with potentially lethal consequences. Can you just replenish with a sports drink? No. In fact, there is a high-profile case of a high school athlete who died after drinking two gallons of Gatorade.[3897] Drinking too much of anything can be dangerous.

So how much water should you drink every day? Unless you have a condition like heart or kidney failure or your physician otherwise advises you to restrict your fluid intake, here is how much water I recommend you drink every day to help your weight (based on the Institute of Medicine's adequate intakes and assuming moderate physical activity at moderate ambient temperatures):[3898]

Recommended Daily Cups of Water

Ages	Female	Male
9–13	7	8
14–18	8	11
19+	9	13

Note that for adults, that comes out to nearly one cup every waking hour, so you could set your watch or phone to ping you if you find yourself forgetting. I always travel with a water bottle wherever I go.

There are shatter-resistant glass bottles with silicone sleeves, but I find I drink more when my water's cold, so I use a vacuum-insulated stainless steel bottle. It's really remarkable. I can still hear the tinkle of ice cubes when I land after a transoceanic flight.

INFLAMMATION QUENCHERS

Down in Flames

In the Dietary Inflammatory Index scoring system I discussed in the Anti-Inflammatory section, the single most pro-inflammatory food component is saturated fat. The single most *anti*-inflammatory food component? Fiber.[3899] Since saturated fat is found mostly in meat, dairy, and junk food, whereas fiber is abundant in whole grains, beans, vegetables, and fruit, that information alone is enough to get a general sense of what an anti-inflammatory diet might look like: one centered around whole plant foods.[3900] Indeed, in dozens of interventional trials where different diets were put to the test in thousands of individuals, the more plant-based diets won the day in terms of bringing down markers of systemic inflammation, such as C-reactive protein.[3901]

What about fish? The purported benefits of the omega-3 fats in seafood are often ascribed to their anti-inflammatory nature, but that's not actually what the medical literature shows. When healthy people were given fish oil supplements equivalent to eating about a serving of salmon, a can of tuna, or ten fillets of tilapia every day[3902] for weeks or months, overall there was no benefit in terms of reducing key inflammatory markers.[3903] No surprise, then, that a compilation of more than twenty randomized placebo-controlled trials of fish oil supplements found no demonstrable effect on weight loss.[3904]

A completely plant-based diet, however, can help drop C-reactive protein levels by 30–40 percent within just a few weeks in both adults[3905] and children, but it need not be all or nothing.[3906] Yes, those randomized to a no-meat diet dropped the inflammatory potential of their diets more than those placed on a low-meat diet,[3907] but even swapping out just a few servings of meat for beans, split peas, chickpeas, or lentils a few days a week can lower measures of inflammation in the body by about a third within only two months.[3908] Adding plant foods alone can help too. Five servings of fruits and veggies a day don't appear to be sufficient, but eight daily servings significantly drop C-reactive protein levels compared to those randomized to eat close to the American average,[3909] a paltry two servings a day.[3910] That's one of the reasons my Daily Dozen recommendation includes a minimum of nine daily servings.

In 2018, researchers at the University of Nebraska published a paper pitting whole grains against fruits and vegetables head-to-head for their anti-inflammatory properties. Which won? Both! Both groups experienced anti-inflammatory benefits, but in distinct ways, affecting different markers of inflammation. This implies that whole grains, fruits, and vegetables lower inflammation through different mechanisms, suggesting consuming them all together could have a synergistic effect.[3911] So our best bet may be to eat a variety of foods as grown. Have any plants been shown to be particularly potent?

Crying Wolf(berry)

Obesity is associated with elevated levels of oxidative stress,[3912] which can result in free radical damage to proteins within the body that can trigger inflammation.[3913] Might an antioxidant-rich fruit be able to help break this vicious cycle? Goji berries, also known as wolfberries, have at least four times the antioxidant activity compared to other dried fruits like raisins or dried cranberries that you might sprinkle on your oatmeal or add to your trail mix.[3914] Beyond its rich antioxidant content, a number of anti-inflammatory compounds have also been specifically identified in the fruit.[3915] In the lab, goji berries do have anti-inflammatory effects on cells from umbilical cords, one of the most convenient sources of human tissue, but what about in whole humans outside the lab?[3916]

Petri dish studies on goji berries have concluded they "could be developed as a new anti-inflammatory therapeutic herbal medicine,"[3917] but you don't know until you put it to the test. Randomized, double-blind, placebo-controlled trials have shown anti-inflammatory effects[3918] while otherwise potentially improving immune function (boosting vaccination response among elderly individuals),[3919] but does that translate into weight loss?

Goji berry juice doesn't seem to work for weight loss, or at least the Go-

Chi beverage sold by a multilevel marketing company[3920] accused of making such false and misleading claims didn't.[3921] What about just giving people actual berries? (What a concept!) Brazilian researchers split people into two groups.[3922] Both were given identical instructions to follow a healthier diet, but one group was also given fourteen grams of dried goji berries a day, which is about two tablespoons.[3923] Forty-five days later, the goji group appeared to cut two and a half inches off their waistlines compared to no change in the control group. This presumed drop in abdominal fat was accompanied by significant drops of about 20 percent in both LDL cholesterol and triglycerides.[3924] Of course, it would have been better if the researchers had given the control group something like raisins (which haven't shown a slimming effect)[3925] to help discount the placebo effect, but what's the downside of giving gojis a go?

Anti-Inflammatory from My Head To-ma-toes

How about a weight-reducing, anti-inflammatory vegetable? There's no need to look for an exotic goji equivalent. If you don't count french fries and other potato products, tomatoes are America's most popular vegetable[3926] and have been shown to have anti-inflammatory effects in both petri dishes[3927] and people.[3928] Randomize overweight individuals to a little less than a can of tomato juice a day (330 ml), and see a drop in inflammation within three weeks.[3929] Low-sodium V8 juice may also help.[3930]

Give people about a quarter cup a day of tomato paste, and get an improvement in artery function within fifteen days, an effect attributed to both anti-inflammatory and antioxidant effects.[3931] Anti-inflammatory benefits can even be realized at a single meal. Men and women were randomized to a pro-inflammatory meal (containing saturated fat in the form of cream cheese and coconut milk) with or without about a third of a cup of tomato paste. The tomato paste significantly blunted the rise of an inflammatory mediator that occurred within hours of consumption.[3932]

Tomatoes are so anti-inflammatory that tomato extracts have been investigated as a potential replacement for aspirin as a blood thinner.[3933] The effects have been attributed to lycopene, the red pigment[3934] in tomatoes, watermelon, and other such hued fruits and vegetables, but we now know that tomatoes contain a large number of diverse anti-inflammatory compounds.[3935] That may be why giving people Lyc-O-Mato lycopene supplements alone appears to have no effect.[3936] The question is: *Can tomatoes help you lose weight?*

Perimenopausal women asked to drink nearly a cup of tomato juice twice a day had an improvement in menopausal symptoms, but no weight loss—though they did appear to get about a 150-calorie-per-day boost in their resting metabolic rates.[3937] That may help explain why a study of younger normal-weight women drinking about a cup of tomato juice a day experienced a reduction in weight, body fat, and waist circumference. The changes were minuscule, though, with only about a pound of weight and a half inch off the waist, and more importantly, there was no control group.[3938] As we know, just being in a study under observation can get people to lose weight. There was a controlled study, however, that did suggest there may be something special about tomatoes.

UK researchers fed people sandwiches made out of white bread, tomato-enriched white bread that was 40 percent tomatoes by weight, or carrot-enriched white bread that was 40 percent carrots by weight. The tomato bread was significantly more filling, but apparently not only because it was replacing some of the white flour, since the 40 percent carrot-enriched bread failed to cause the same dip in hunger.[3939] Where can you find tomato bread, though? Can't you just eat a tomato? Good idea!

Women who were asked to eat a ripe tomato before lunch every day for one month dropped two pounds with improvements in blood sugars, cholesterol, and triglycerides.[3940] Again, this study had no control group, but you can imagine how such a result could be possible. A tomato is 95 percent water, so you'd effectively be filling up a fist-sized portion of your stomach with only about fifteen calories right before a meal.[3941] This reminds me of the pears-and-apples study that found a similar effect interspersing meals with fruit.[3942]

Turmeric and Nutritional Yeast—Good as Gold?

If you recall, the spice turmeric is scored as the most anti-inflammatory food in the Dietary Inflammatory Index.[3943] In vitro, curcumin—the pigment in turmeric responsible for its bright yellow color—has a stronger and broader anti-inflammatory profile than the powerful anti-inflammatory corticosteroid drug prednisolone.[3944] Various turmeric preparations have been shown to offer benefit for inflammatory diseases of the joints,[3945] lungs,[3946] skin,[3947] and gut.[3948] This includes turmeric extracts, purified curcumin, and just about a half teaspoon a day of the plain spice you can find at the store.[3949] Though curcumin from turmeric doesn't appear to blunt the acute, pro-inflammatory effects of a milkshake,[3950] randomized controlled trials clearly show a drop in a variety of inflammatory markers when it is taken over time.[3951,3952]

Turmeric is one of the few foods that have actually been put to the test in people. A turmeric-based spice mix was found to suppress hunger after a meal,[3953] but what about weight loss?

Turmeric curcumin "blocks obesity" in mice fed a high-fat diet,[3954] but the human data are disappointing. Out of eight randomized controlled trials, only three showed any kind of significant weight-loss benefit.[3955] A different golden-colored seasoning—nutritional yeast—shows more promise.

A special type of fiber called *beta-glucan* in brewer's, baker's, and nutritional yeasts displays anti-inflammatory effects[3956] sufficient to improve wound healing[3957] and alleviate symptoms in ragweed sufferers.[3958] Randomized, double-blind, placebo-controlled clinical trials of about two teaspoons of nutritional yeast's worth of beta-glucans have resulted in about an inch off the waist within six weeks[3959] or up to a five-pound weight benefit compared to controls in twelve weeks, along with an improvement in blood pressure.[3960] Both of these studies were funded by companies trying to sell supplements, but I figure what are the side effects—tastier popcorn? I would, however, caution against the use of nutritional yeast for those with Crohn's disease[3961] or a skin condition known as *hidradenitis suppurativa*[3962] due to immune reactivity. (Further details can be found on NutritionFacts.org.)

FOOD FOR THOUGHT

The evidence base for weight loss from specific anti-inflammatory foods is pretty weak, but one would only expect benefits from swapping in goji berries for raisins, nailing my Daily Dozen recommendation for at least a quarter teaspoon of turmeric every day, seasoning with nutritional yeast instead of parmesan, for example, or trying my nutritional yeast–based Savory Spice Blend instead of salt (from my *How Not to Die Cookbook,* recipe online at www.nutritionfacts .org/recipe/savory-spice-blend/). Brewer's yeast has the same inflammation-modifying beta-glucan fiber as nutritional yeast, but it also has a bitter flavor that I remember all too well from my childhood. My mom used to mix a spoonful into orange juice to make what she used to call Yeast Juice (and yes, it tastes as bad as it sounds).

You can also try eating a tomato salad as an appetizer. What I like to do is quarter a ripe tomato, grind on some freshly cracked pepper, and add a drizzle of balsamic vinegar and some shreds of fresh basil. Delish!

INTERMITTENT FASTING

Caloric Restriction

The 3,500-Calorie Rule Is Wrong

Fasting is the practice of abstaining from all food for a period of time, while caloric restriction is a dietary regimen that simply reduces caloric intake. Anyone who's seen *The Biggest Loser* television shows knows that hundreds of pounds can be lost with enough exercise and caloric restriction.[3963]

Similarly, there are cases in the medical literature of what some doctors refer to as *super obesity,* defined as a BMI of 50 or more,[3964] in which individuals lost up to 374 pounds largely on their own without professional help and kept it off for years.[3965] In the case of the 374-pound loss, the guy lost about 20 pounds a month cycling two hours a day and reducing intake to eight hundred calories a day, which is down around what some were getting in World War II prisoner camps.[3966]

Perhaps America's most celebrated TV weight loss was when Oprah pulled out a wagonful of fat, representing the sixty-seven pounds she had lost on a very-low-calorie diet, onto the set of her talk show.[3967] How many calories did she have to cut to achieve that weight loss in four months? If you consult leading nutrition textbooks,[3968] read prestigious medical journals,[3969] refer to trusted authorities like the Mayo Clinic,[3970] or listen to the U.S. Surgeon General,[3971] you'll learn the simple weight-loss rule: One pound of fat is equal to 3,500 calories. Quoting from *The Journal of the American Medical Association,* "This means if you decrease (or increase) your intake by 500 calories daily, you will lose (or gain) 1 pound per week. (500 calories per day × 7 days = 3,500 calories.)"[3972]

Simple, but not true.

The 3,500-calorie rule can be traced back to a paper published in 1958 that simply noted that since fatty tissue in the human body is 87 percent fat, a pound of body fat would have about 395 grams of pure fat. Multiplying that by 9 calories per gram of fat gives us that 3,500-calories-per-pound approximation.[3973] The fatal flaw that leads to "dramatically exaggerated" weight-loss predictions is that the 3,500 rule fails to take into account the fact that changes in the calories-in side of the energy-balance equation automatically lead to changes in the calories-out side—the slowing of metabolic rate that accompanies weight loss known as *metabolic adaptation*, for example.[3974] That's one of the reasons weight-loss plateaus.

Imagine a thirty-year-old sedentary woman of average height who weighs 150 pounds. According to the 3,500-calorie rule, by cutting 500 calories from her daily diet, she'd lose a pound a week or 52 pounds a year. In three years, then, she would apparently vanish. She'd go from 150 pounds to -6. Obviously, that doesn't happen. What *would* happen is that, in the first year, instead of losing 52 pounds, she'd likely only lose 32 pounds and then, after a total of three years, stabilize at about 100 pounds.[3975] This is because it takes fewer calories to exist as a thin person.

Part of it is simple physics in the same way a Hummer requires more fuel than a compact car.[3976] Think how much more effort it would take just to get out of a chair, walk across the room, or climb a few stairs while carrying a fifty-pound backpack. That's no lighter than carrying fifty pounds in the front in your belly. Even when lying at rest, sound asleep, there's simply less of our bodies to maintain as we lose weight. Every pound of fat tissue lost may mean one less mile of blood vessels our bodies have to pump blood through every minute.[3977] Since the basic upkeep and movement of thinner bodies take fewer calories, as you lose weight by eating less, you end up needing less. That's what the 3,500-calorie rule doesn't take into account.

Imagine it another way. A 200-pound man starts eating 500 more calories a day. That's like two donuts. According to the 3,500-calorie rule, in ten years, he'd weigh more than 700 pounds. That doesn't happen because the heavier he is, the more calories he burns simply existing.

If you're one hundred pounds overweight, that's like the skinny person inside you trying to walk around balancing thirteen gallons of oil at all times or lugging around a sack containing four hundred sticks of butter wherever you go. It takes about two donuts' worth of extra energy just to live at 250 pounds compared to 200, so that's where he'd plateau if he kept eating those extra 500 daily calories.[3978] So weight gain or weight loss, given a certain calorie excess or deficit, is a curve that flattens out over time rather than a straight line going up or down.

Nevertheless, the 3,500-calorie rule continues to crop up—even in obesity journals.[3979] That may be a consequence of the well-described innumeracy—mathematical illiteracy—that pervades the medical profession.[3980] Public health researchers used it to calculate how many excess pounds children might avoid gaining each year if, for example, fast-food kids' meals included apple slices instead of french fries.[3981] They figured two meals a week could add up to four pounds a year.[3982] The actual difference, National Restaurant Association–funded researchers were no doubt delighted to point out, would probably add under half a pound—ten times less than the 3,500-calorie rule would predict.[3983]

The original article was subsequently retracted.[3984]

A Slow Burn

Other players in the weight-loss game are all the compensatory survival mechanisms our bodies use to defend against weight loss. Because of our millions of years of evolution hardwiring us to survive scarcity,[3985] when we start losing weight, we may unconsciously start moving less as a behavioral adaptation to conserve energy.[3986] There are metabolic adaptations as well. Our metabolisms slow down.[3987] Every pound of weight loss may reduce our resting metabolic rates by seven calories a day.[3988] This may only translate to a difference of a few percentage points for most,[3989] but it can rapidly snowball for those who achieve massive weight loss.

During one season, some of *The Biggest Loser* contestants famously had their metabolic rates tracked. Above and beyond the hundreds of fewer calories it takes just to exist more than one hundred pounds lighter, by the end of filming for that season, their metabolic rates had slowed by an extra five hundred calories a day.[3990] The mindblower was that when they were retested six years later, they still had the five-hundred-calorie-a-day handicap.[3991] So the contestants had to cut five hundred calories *more* than anyone else their size to maintain the same weight loss. No wonder the bulk of their weight was regained. Most did remain at least 10 percent lower than their starting weight, and even a 7 percent drop may cut diabetes rates by more than half,[3992] but still—the metabolic slowing means they have to work that much harder than everyone else just to stay in place.

Analyzing four seasons of *The Biggest Loser* minute by minute, researchers noted that 85 percent of the focus was on exercise rather than diet,[3993] though the exercise component accounted for less than half of the weight loss.[3994] Even six years after their season ended, the contestants had been maintaining the hour of daily, vigorous exercise, yet still regained most of the weight. Why? They started eating more. They could have cut their exercise from sixty to just twenty minutes a day and still maintained 100 percent of their initial weight loss if they would have just kept their intakes under three thousand calories a day.[3995] That may not sound like much of a challenge, but weight loss doesn't just slow our metabolisms—it boosts our appetites.

Appetite for Destruction

If it were merely a matter of our weight settling at the point at which our reduced caloric intakes match our reduced caloric outputs, it would take years for our weight loss to plateau. Instead, the plateau often occurs within six to eight months.[3996] You probably know the drill: Start the diet, stick to the diet, and then weight loss stalls six months later. What happened? Don't blame your metabolism—that only plays a small part. What likely happened is you actually stopped sticking to your diet because your appetite went on a rampage.

If you cut eight hundred calories out of your daily diet and your weight loss stalls after six months, what happened is that despite thinking you're still down eight hundred calories a day, you may actually only be down six hundred daily calories at the end of the first month. By month two, you're only down about five hundred calories, down three hundred by month three, and by month six, you're only eating two hundred fewer calories than before you had started the diet. In other words, you inadvertently suffered an exponential increase in caloric intake over those six months without even realizing it, because, by that time, your body may have ramped up your appetite by six hundred calories. So it still *feels* as if you are eating eight hundred fewer calories, but you're actually only down two hundred. By then, your metabolism and physical activity also may have slowed by two hundred calories a day, so with no difference between calories in and calories out, that's how your weight loss grinds to a complete halt.[3997]

The slow, upward drift in caloric intake on a new diet is not because you got lazy. Once your appetite is boosted by six hundred calories after you've been dieting for a while, eating two hundred fewer calories is as hard as eating eight hundred fewer calories had been at the beginning. So you can maintain the same disciplined level of willpower and self-control, yet still end up stagnating.[3998] To prevent this from happening, we need to maintain the calorie deficit. How is that possible in the face of a ravenous appetite?

Hunger is a biological drive. Asking someone to eat smaller portions is like asking them to take fewer breaths. You can white-knuckle it for a bit, but eventually nature wins out. That's what this book is for. Remember how I discussed in the Eating Rate section that you can cut more than a thousand calories out of people's daily diets without them even noticing? Sustainable weight loss is not about eating *less* food—it's about eating *better* food.

The Ten-Calorie Rule

If you are able to take advantage of some of the techniques in this book and dutifully maintain a calorie deficit, what weight loss could you expect? If the 3,500-calorie rule is bunk, what's the alternative? There are validated mathematical models that take into account the dynamic changes that occur when you cut calories, such as the metabolic slowdown. They've been turned into free online calculators you can use to make personalized estimates. There's the Body Weight Planner from the National Institutes of Health (NIH) and the Pennington Biomedical Research Center's Weight Loss Predictor out of Louisiana State University (LSU).

- NIH Body Weight Planner: www.bit.ly/NIHcalculator
- LSU Weight Loss Predictor: www.bit.ly/LSUcalculator

The NIH Body Weight Planner has been found to be more accurate, as the LSU model appears to overestimate the drop in physical activity,[3999] but they each have their pluses and minuses. The Body Weight Planner tells you how many calories you need to restrict and/or how much more you need to do to achieve a specific weight-loss goal by a specific date. Clicking on the Switch to Expert Mode button gives you a graph and exportable chart showing your day-by-day weight-loss trajectory. The LSU Weight Loss Predictor, on the other hand, doesn't allow you to adjust physical activity, but its advantage is that you don't have to choose a goal or time frame. Just put in different calorie changes, and it graphs out your expected course.

Is there any easy rule of thumb you can use? Yes—the Ten-Calorie Rule. Every permanent, ten-calorie drop in daily intake will eventually lead to about one pound of weight loss.[4000] It takes about a year to achieve half the total weight change and about three years to completely settle into the new weight. So cutting five hundred calories a day can cause the fifty-pound weight loss predicted by the 3,500-calorie rule, but that's the total weight loss at which you plateau, not an annual drop, and it takes about three years to get there. A five-hundred-calorie deficit would be expected to cause about a twenty-five-pound weight loss the first year and then an additional twenty-five pounds over years two and three, but that's only if you can *maintain* the five-hundred-calorie deficit.

If you're eating the same diet that led to the original weight problem but just in smaller servings, you should expect your appetite to rev up about forty-five calories for each pound you lose.[4001] So if you were cutting five hundred calories a day through portion control alone, before you were down even a dozen pounds, you'd feel so famished that you'd be driven to eat *more* than five hundred calories a day and your weight loss could vanish. That's why if you're dead set on eating the same diet with the same foods only in smaller quantities, you have to cut down more than forty-five calories per pound of desired weight loss to offset your hunger drive.

So to get that one pound off, instead of eating just ten fewer calories a day using the Ten-Calorie Rule, you'd have to eat ten fewer calories *on top of* the forty-five fewer calories to account for the revving of your appetite, so that's a total of fifty-five fewer daily calories. Indeed, just changing diet *quantity* and not *quality* requires you to take in fifty-five fewer calories per day to lose a single pound. That five-hundred-calorie daily deficit would only net you about a nine-pound weight loss (500 ÷ 55) three years later instead of fifty pounds.[4002] That's why portion-control methods can be such a frustrating failure for so many people.

The Flame That Burns Twice as Bright
Burns Half as Long

Though a bane for dieters, a slower metabolism may actually be a good thing. We've known for more than a century that caloric restriction can increase the life spans of animals,[4003] and the metabolic slowdown may be the mechanism.[4004] That could be why the tortoise lives ten times longer than the hare.[4005] (Harriet, a tortoise evidently collected from the Galapagos by Charles Darwin in the 1830s, lived until 2006.[4006]) Slow and steady may indeed win the race.

One of the ways our bodies lower our resting metabolic rates is by creating cleaner-burning, more efficient mitochondria, the power plants that fuel our cells.[4007] It's like our bodies pass their own fuel-efficiency standards. These new mitochondria appear to create the same energy with less oxygen and produce less free-radical "exhaust." After all, our bodies are afraid famine is afoot, so they try to conserve as much energy as they can.

Indeed, the largest caloric-restriction trial to date found both metabolic slowing and a reduction in free radical–induced oxidative stress, both of which may slow the rate of aging.[4008] Whether this will translate into greater human longevity is an unanswered question. Caloric restriction is said to extend the life span of "every species studied,"[4009] but this isn't even true of all strains within a single species.[4010] Some scientists don't think caloric restriction will improve human longevity at all, while others suggest a 20 percent caloric restriction starting at age twenty-five and sustained for fifty-two years could add five years onto our life spans.[4011] Either way, the reduced oxidative stress would be expected to improve our *health* spans.[4012]

Members of the CR Society International, self-styled CRONies (for *calorie restriction with optimal nutrition*), appear to be in excellent health, but they're a rather unique, self-selected bunch of individuals.[4013] As always, you don't really know until you put it to the test. Enter CALERIE, the Comprehensive Assessment of Long-term Effects of Reducing Intake of Energy, the first clinical trial to test the effects of caloric restriction.[4014]

Hundreds of nonobese men and women were randomized to two years of 25 percent caloric restriction. Though they only ended up achieving half of that, they still lost about eighteen pounds and three inches off their waists, wiping out more than half their visceral abdominal fat.[4015] That translated into significant improvements in blood pressure, insulin sensitivity, triglycerides, and cholesterol levels.[4016] Eighty percent of those who were overweight when they started were normal weight by the end, compared to a 27 percent increase in those who became overweight in the control group.[4017]

In the famous Minnesota Starvation Experiment that used conscientious objectors as human guinea pigs during World War II, the study subjects suffered both physically and psychologically, experiencing depression, irritability, and loss of libido.[4018] The subjects started out lean, though, and had their caloric intakes cut in half. The CALERIE study ended up being four times less restrictive, at only about 12 percent below baseline caloric intake, and enrolled normal-weight individuals, which in the United States these days means overweight on average. As such, the CALERIE subjects experienced nothing but positive quality-of-life benefits with significant improvements in mood, general health, sex drive, and sleep.[4019] During the final year, they were eating only about three hundred fewer calories than they had been at baseline,[4020] so they got all those benefits after cutting only about a snack-sized bag of chips' worth of calories from their daily diets.

What happened at the end of the trial, though? In both the Minnesota Starvation Experiment[4021] and experiments on U.S. Army Rangers,[4022] as soon as subjects were released from restriction, they tended to rapidly regain the weight—and sometimes more. The leaner they started out, the more their bodies seemed to drive them to overeat to pack back on extra body fat.[4023] In contrast, after the completion of the CALERIE study, even though their metabolisms were slowed, they retained about 50 percent of the weight loss two years later.[4024] They must have acquired new eating attitudes and behaviors that allowed them to keep their weight down. Indeed, after extended caloric restriction, cravings for sugary and fatty foods do go down.[4025]

Potential Pitfalls of Caloric Restriction

One of the most consistent benefits of caloric restriction is improvement in blood pressure in as short as one or two weeks.[4026] Unfortunately, this can work a little too well and cause orthostatic intolerance,[4027] manifesting as light-headedness or dizziness upon standing, which, in severe cases, can cause fainting. Staying hydrated can help, though,[4028] as I discuss in more detail in the Metabolic Boosters section.

What about loss of muscle mass? In the CALERIE trial, 70 percent of the lost body weight was fat and 30 percent was lean body mass,[4029] so the subjects ended up with an improved body composition, from 67 percent lean and 33 percent fat to 72 percent lean and 28 percent fat.[4030] Though leg muscle mass and strength declined in absolute terms, relative to their new body size, they generally got stronger.[4031] Is there any way to preserve more lean mass, particularly among older individuals who naturally tend to lose muscle mass with age?

Increased protein intakes are commonly suggested, but most studies fail to show a beneficial effect on preserving muscle strength or function, whether young or old, active or sedentary.[4032] For example, researchers randomized overweight older men and women to either a normal-protein diet of four grams for every ten pounds of body weight or a high-protein diet with about eight grams per ten pounds, during a 25 percent caloric restriction. A doubling of protein intake had no discernible effect on lean body mass, muscle strength, or physical performance.[4033] Most such studies have found the same lack of benefit,[4034] but after putting them all together, one can tease out a "very small" advantage.[4035] Unfortunately, high-protein intake during weight loss has been found to have "profound" negative metabolic effects, undermining the benefits of weight loss on insulin sensitivity.[4036]

Though you can always bulk back up after weight loss, the best way to preserve muscle mass during weight loss is exercise. The CALERIE study had no structured exercise component, and, just like after bariatric surgery, about 30 percent of the weight loss was lean mass. In contrast, that proportion was only about 16 percent in *The Biggest Loser* contestants, chalked up to their vigorous exercise programs.[4037] Resistance training even just three times a week can prevent more than 90 percent of lean body mass loss during caloric restriction.[4038]

The same may be true of bone loss. Lose weight through caloric restriction alone, and you experience a decline in bone mineral density in fracture-risk sites like the hip and spine. However, in the same study, those randomized to lose weight with exercise didn't suffer any bone loss. The researchers concluded: "Our results suggest that regular EX [exercise] should be included as part of a comprehensive weight loss program to offset the adverse effects of CR [caloric restriction] on bone."[4039]

You can never argue with calls for increased physical activity, but even without an exercise regimen, the "very small" drop in bone mineral density in the CALERIE study might only increase ten-year risk of osteoporotic fracture by about 0.2 percent.[4040] The benefits of caloric restriction revealed by the CALERIE trial—improved blood pressure, cholesterol, mood, libido, and sleep—would seem to far outweigh any potential risks. The fact that a reduction in calories seemed to have such wide-ranging positive effects led commentators in the American Medical Association's internal medicine journal to write: "The findings of this well-designed study suggest that intake of excess calories is not only a burden to our physical homeostasis but also on our psychological well-being."[4041]

Fasting

The Fast Track to Weight Loss

The greatest caloric restriction is no calories at all. Fasting has been branded the "next big weight loss fad" but has a long history throughout various spiritual traditions, practiced by Moses, Jesus, Muhammad, and Buddha.[4042] In 1732, a noted physician wrote, "He that eats till he is sick must fast till he is well."[4043] Today, about one in seven American adults reports using some sort of fasting as a means to control body weight.[4044]

Case reports of the treatment of obesity through fasting date back more than a century in the medical literature. In 1915, Harvard doctors described "two extraordinarily fat women" whose weight-loss success led the physicians to conclude that "moderate periods of starvation constitute a perfectly safe, harmless, and effective method for reducing the weight of those suffering from obesity."[4045]

The longest recorded fast, published in 1973, made it into the *Guinness Book of World Records*. To reach his ideal body weight, a twenty-seven-year-old man fasted for 382 days straight, losing 276 pounds, and managed to keep nearly all of it off.[4046] He was given vitamin and mineral supplements, but no calories for more than a year. In their acknowledgments, the researchers thanked him for "cheerful cooperation and steadfast application to the task of achieving a normal physique."[4047]

In a U.S. Air Force study of twenty-five individuals, the majority of whom were at least one hundred pounds overweight and "unable to lose weight on previous diets," the subjects were fasted for as long as eighty-four days. Nine people dropped out of the study, but the sixteen who remained were "unequivocally successful" at losing between forty and one hundred pounds. According to the researchers, such subjects lose as much as four pounds a day in the first few days. That is mostly water weight, shed as the body starts to adapt to the fast, but after a few weeks, they can be steadily losing about a pound of mostly straight fat per day. The investigator described their "starvation program" as a "dramatic and exciting treatment for obesity."[4048]

Of course, this single *most* successful diet for weight loss—namely, no diet at all—is also the single *least* sustainable. What other diet can cure morbid obesity in a matter of months but be practically guaranteed to kill you within a year if you stick with it?

The reason diets don't work almost by definition is that people go on them, and then they go off them. Permanent weight loss is only achieved through permanent lifestyle change. So what's the point of fasting if you're just going to go back to your regular diet and gain all the weight right back?

Fasting proponents cite the psychological benefit of realigning people's perceptions and motivation.[4049] Some individuals have resigned themselves to the belief that weight loss is somehow impossible for them. They may think they're made differently in some way, and the pounds just won't come off no matter what they do.[4050] The rapid, unequivocal weight loss during fasting demonstrates to them that, with a large enough change in eating habits, it's not just possible but also inevitable. This morale boost from reasserting control may then embolden them to make better food choices once they resume eating.[4051]

The break from food may allow some an opportunity to pause and reflect on the role food is playing in their lives—not only the power it has over them but the power they then have over it.[4052] In a fasting study entitled "Correction and Control of Intractable Obesity," a subject's personality was described as changing "from one of desperation, with abandonment of hope, to that of an eager extrovert full of plans for a promising future." She realized that her weight was within her own power to control.[4053] The researchers reported: "This highly intellectual social worker has been returned to a full degree of exceptional usefulness."

After a fast, newfound commitments to more healthful eating may be facilitated by a reduction in overall appetite reported post-fast compared to pre-fast.[4054] Even during a fast, hunger may start to dissipate within thirty-six hours.[4055] As such, challenging people's delusions about their exceptionality to the laws of physics with a period of total fasting may "seem barbaric," wrote a group of researchers in the journal of the American Medical Association, but "in reality, this method of reduction is remarkably well tolerated by obese patients."[4056] This seems to be a recurring theme in these published series of cases. In an influential paper entitled "Treatment of Obesity by Total Fasting for Up to 249 Days," the researchers remarked, "The most surprising aspect of this study was the ease with which the prolonged fast was tolerated." Evidently, all their patients spontaneously commented on their increased sense of well-being throughout the process. The researchers concluded: "We are convinced that it is the treatment of choice, certainly in cases of gross obesity."[4057]

Fasting for a day can make people moody, irritable,[4058] and distracted,[4059] but a few days into a fast, many report feeling clear, elated, and alert—even euphoric.[4060] This may be due in part to the significant rise in endorphins that accompanies fasting.[4061] Mood enhancement during fasting is thought perhaps to represent an adaptive survival mechanism to motivate the search for food. This positive outlook toward the future may then facilitate the behavioral change necessary to lock in some of the weight-loss benefits.[4062]

Is Fasting Effective?

How do fasted patients do long term? (As we've said, in obesity research, *long term* typically means only one or two years, which itself says much about the field.) Some research groups reported "extremely disappointing" results. At around the one-year follow-up after an average weight loss of twenty-seven pounds in twenty-five days of "inpatient starvation," one study of twenty-three subjects found they had gained back an average of twenty-nine pounds.[4063] In another study with follow-ups ranging up to fifty months, only four out of twenty-five "superobese" patients achieved even partial sustained success.[4064] Based on these kinds of data, some investigators concluded that "complete starvation is of no value in the long-term treatment of obese patients."[4065]

Other research teams have reported better outcomes. One series of more than one hundred individuals found that 60 percent either retained at least some weight loss at follow-up (43 percent) or even continued losing weight (17 percent).[4066] The follow-up periods varied from one to thirty-two months with no breakdown as to who lasted how long, though, making the data hard to interpret.[4067] In another study, one year after fasting sixty-two patients down sixteen pounds in ten days, 40 percent retained at least seven pounds of that weight loss.[4068]

Putting six such studies together, hundreds of obese subjects who fasted for an average of forty-nine days lost an average of fifty-two pounds, and around one or two years later, 40 percent had retained at least some of the weight loss.[4069] So although most gained back all their weight, 40 percent keeping off at least some weight is extraordinary for a weight-loss study. By comparison, researchers followed one hundred obese individuals on a standard low-calorie diet while getting treatment at a weight-loss clinic and found only one out of one hundred had lost more than forty pounds, and only about one in ten had lost even twenty pounds, with the overall successful weight maintenance at only 2 percent over two years.[4070] That's why having a control group is so important. What may look like a general failure in the fasting trials may actually be a relative success compared to more traditional weight-loss techniques.

Researchers new to the field may find the results reported in a seventy-five-subject "long-term follow-up of therapeutic starvation" to be "clearly disappointing."[4071] One year later, two-thirds were "failures" with more than one-third regaining all the weight they had initially lost. But 12 percent were labeled successes, maintaining sixty pounds of weight loss two years later.[4072] In a direct comparison of different weight-loss approaches at another clinic, five years after initiating a conventional low-calorie approach, only about one in five was down twenty pounds compared to nearly half in the group who instead had undergone a few weeks of a fasting program years previously. By year seven, most of those instructed on daily caloric restriction were back to, or had exceeded, their original weight, but that was true of only about one in ten of the fasted group.[4073] In an influential paper published in *The New England Journal of Medicine* on seven myths about obesity, fallacy number three was that "large, rapid weight loss is associated with poorer long-term weight-loss outcomes, as compared with slow, gradual weight loss."[4074] In reality, the opposite is true. The hare may end up skinnier than the tortoise.

Researchers set up a study comparing the sustainability of weight loss at three different speeds: six days of fasting, three weeks of a very-low-calorie diet of six hundred daily calories, or six weeks of a low-calorie diet of twelve hundred daily calories. A year later, the fasting group was the only one who had sustained a significant loss of weight.[4075] That was just after one year, though. How about nine years later? "Therapeutic Fasting in Morbid Obesity" is the largest, longest follow-up study I could find.[4076] At least some of the fast-induced weight losses sustained a year later were maintained by the "great majority" (90 percent) of the 121 patients. Nine years later, however, that number dropped to fewer than one in ten. Almost everyone had regained the weight they had fasted away. Many patients reported they thought the temporary loss was worth it, though. As a group, they had lost an average of about sixty pounds. They described improved health and quality of life, claiming reemployment was facilitated and earnings increased during that period of time, but the fasting didn't appear to result in any permanent change in eating habits for the vast majority. The small minority for whom fasting led to sustainable weight loss "all admit to a radical change in previous eating habits."[4077]

Fasting only works long term if it can act as a jump-start to a more healthful diet.

In a retrospective, long-term comparison of weight reduction after an inpatient stay at a naturopathic center, those who were fasted lost more weight at the time but were back to the same weight around seven years later. No surprise, since most returned to the same diet they had eaten before. Those who were placed instead on a more healthful, whole-food, plant-based diet were more likely to make persistent changes in their eating patterns and, seven years later, were on average lighter than when they had started.[4078]

Can't we have it both ways? Why not use fasting to kick-start a big drop in weight and *then* start a healthy diet? The problem is that initial big drop is largely illusory.

Fasting for a week or two can cause more weight loss than caloric restriction, but, paradoxically, it may actually lead to *less* loss of body fat. Eating more calories can lead to more fat loss? Yes. During fasting, the body starts cannibalizing itself and burning more of our protein for fuel.[4079] Emperor penguins, elephant seals, and hibernating bears can survive just burning fat without dipping into their muscles, but our voracious, big brains appear to need at least a trickle of blood sugar, and if we're not eating any carbohydrates, our bodies are forced to start turning our protein into sugar to burn.[4080] Even just a few grams of carbs, like those consumed by people who add honey to their water when they fast, for example, can cut protein loss up to 50 percent.[4081] What about adding exercise to prevent loss of lean tissues during a fast? That may make it even worse![4082] At rest, most of our heart and muscle energy needs can be met with fat, but if we start exercising, some of the blood sugar meant for our brains is used and our bodies may have to break down even more protein.[4083]

Less than half the weight lost during the first few weeks of fasting comes from our fat stores.[4084] So even if we double our daily weight loss on a fast, we may actually be losing less *fat*. An NIH-funded study placed obese individuals on an eight-hundred-calorie-a-day diet for two weeks, and they steadily lost about a pound of body fat a day. They then switched to about two weeks of zero calories and started losing more protein and water, but, on average, only lost a few ounces of fat a day. When the subjects were subsequently switched back to the initial eight-hundred-calorie-a-day diet for a week, they rapidly replaced the protein and water they had lost, so the scale registered that their weight went up, but their body fat loss accelerated back to the approximate pound lost a day.[4085] The scale made it look as though they were doing better when they were completely fasting, but the reality is they were doing worse. During the five-week experiment, they would have lost more body fat sticking to their calorie-restricted diet than completely stopping eating in the middle of the trial.

Is Fasting Safe?

Eventually, after the third week of fasting, fat loss starts to overtake the loss of lean body mass in obese individuals, but is it safe to go that long without food? Proponents speak of fasting as a cleansing process, but some of what they are purging from their bodies are essential vitamins and minerals.[4086] Heavy-enough people can go up to 382 days without calories, but no one can go even a fraction that long without vitamins. Scurvy, for example, is diagnosable within as few as four weeks without any vitamin C.[4087] Beriberi is the disease caused by thiamine deficiency, the inadequate intake of vitamin B1. It may start even earlier than scurvy in fasting patients[4088] and, once manifest, can result in brain damage within days,[4089] which can eventually become irreversible.[4090] Even though fasting subjects report problems such as nausea and indigestion taking supplements,[4091] all the months-long fasting cases I've mentioned were given daily multivitamins and mineral supplementation as necessary. Without supplementation, hunger strikers and those undergoing prolonged fasts for therapeutic or religious purposes, like the Baptist pastor hoping to "enhance his spiritual powers for exorcism," have ended up paralyzed,[4092] comatose,[4093] or worse.[4094]

Nutrient deficiencies aren't the only risk of extended fasting. Reading about all the successful reports of massive weight loss from prolonged fasting in the medical literature, one doctor decided to give it a try. Of the first dozen patients he put on fasts, two died. His report, "Death During Therapeutic Starvation for Obesity," certainly put a damper on the enthusiasm for fasting.[4095] In retrospect, the two patients who died started out with heart failure and had been on diuretics. Fasting itself produces a pronounced diuresis, a loss of water and electrolytes through the urine, so it was the combination of fasting on top of the "water pills" that likely depleted their potassium and triggered their fatal heart rhythms.[4096] The doctor went out of his way to point out that "both the deaths in this series were admitted in severe heart-failure . . . but both had improved greatly whilst undergoing starvation therapy."[4097] Small consolation since they were both dead within a matter of weeks.

It would be one thing if all therapeutic fasting fatalities had come from complications of concurrent diuretic use, but that is not the case. "At first he did very well and experienced the usual euphoria," described one doctor about a fasting patient. His electrolytes remained fine, but, in the middle of the third week, he suddenly collapsed and died. "This line of treatment is certainly tempting because it does produce weight-loss and the patient feels so much better," the doctor concluded, "but the report of case-fatalities must make it a very suspect line of management."[4098]

Contrary to the popular notion that the heart muscle is specially spared during fasting, the heart appears to experience similar muscle wasting.[4099] This was noted in the victims of the Warsaw ghetto during World War II in a remarkable series of detailed studies carried out by the ghetto physicians before they themselves succumbed.[4100] In a case entitled "Gross Fragmentation of Cardiac Myofibrils After Therapeutic Starvation for Obesity," a twenty-year-old woman achieved her ideal body weight after losing 128 pounds fasting for thirty weeks. After a breakfast of one egg, she had a heart attack and died. On autopsy, the muscle fibers in her heart showed evidence of widespread disintegration. The pathologists suggested that "this regimen should no longer be recommended as a safe means of weight reduction."[4101]

Breaking the fast appears to be the most dangerous part.[4102] After World War II, as many as one out of five starved Japanese prisoners of war tragically died following liberation.[4103] Now known as *refeeding syndrome,* multi-organ system failure can result from resuming a regular diet too quickly.[4104] Some critical nutrients, such as thiamine and phosphorus, are used to metabolize food. In the critical refeeding window, if too much food is taken before these nutrients can be repleted, demand may exceed supply and whatever residual stores are still left can be driven down even further, with potentially fatal consequences.[4105] That's why rescue workers are taught to always give thiamine before food to victims who had been trapped or otherwise unable to eat.[4106] Thiamine is responsible for the yellow color of "banana bags," a term you might have heard used on medical dramas, used to describe an IV fluid concoction often given to malnourished alcoholics to prevent a similar reaction.[4107] Anyone with negligible food intake for more than five days may be at risk of developing refeeding problems.[4108]

Don't Try This at Home

Medically supervised fasting has gotten much safer now that there are proper refeeding protocols, we know what warning signs to look for, and we know who shouldn't be fasting in the first place[4109] (such as those with advanced liver or kidney failure, porphyria, or uncontrolled hyperthyroidism, and women who are pregnant or breastfeeding).[4110] The most comprehensive safety analysis of medically supervised, water-only fasting was recently published out of the TrueNorth Health Center in California. From the 768 visits to their facility for fasts up to forty-one days, were there any adverse events? Yes, 5,961 of them. Most were mild, known reactions to fasting, however, such as fatigue, nausea, insomnia, headache, dizziness, upset stomach, and back pain. Only two serious events were reported, with no fatalities.[4111]

Fasting longer than twenty-four hours and, particularly, for three or more days should only be done under the supervision of a physician and preferably in a live-in clinic.[4112] This is not just legalistic mumbo-jumbo. For example, your kidneys normally dive into sodium-conservation mode during fasting, but should that response break down, you could rapidly develop an electrolyte abnormality that may only manifest with nonspecific symptoms like fatigue or dizziness, which could easily be dismissed until it's too late.[4113]

The risks of any therapy must be premised on the severity of the disease. The consequences of obesity are considered so serious that effective therapies could have "considerable acceptable toxicity."[4114] For example, many consider major surgery for obesity to be a justifiable risk, but the key word is *effective*.

Therapeutic fasting for obesity has been largely abandoned by the medical community not only because of its uncertain safety profile but also because of its questionable short- and long-term efficacy.[4115] Remember, for a fast that only lasts a week or two, you might be able to lose as much body fat, or even more, on a low-calorie diet than a no-calorie diet. Abstinence may be easier to practice than temperance, though. Paradoxically, studies suggest people experience less hunger on a total fast compared to a low-calorie diet.[4116] This may be thanks to ketones.

We've discussed how blood sugar (glucose) is a universal go-to fuel for the cells throughout our bodies.[4117] Our bodies can break down proteins and make glucose from scratch, but most glucose comes from our diets in the form of sugars and starches. If we stop eating carbohydrates, most of our cells switch over to burning fat, but fat has difficulty getting through the blood-brain barrier.[4118] Our brains burn through about a half cup of sugar a day.[4119] That's up to a quarter of our resting metabolic rates (and up to 50 percent in children).[4120] To make that much sugar, we'd need to break down about a half pound of protein a day,[4121] which means we'd cannibalize ourselves to death within approximately two weeks. But people can fast for months. How is that possible?

The answer to the puzzle was discovered in 1967. Harvard researchers famously stuck catheters into the brains of obese subjects who had been fasting for more than a month and discovered that ketones had replaced glucose as the primary fuel for the brain.[4122] Your liver turns fat into ketones, which can then breach the blood-brain barrier and sustain your brain.

In this state of ketosis, when you have high levels of ketones in your bloodstream, your hunger is dampened. This may be why people's hunger can dissipate after a few days on a fast, as their brain switches over to ketones for fuel.[4123] When ketones are injected straight into people's veins, even those who are not fasting lose their appetites, sometimes even to the point of getting nauseated and vomiting.[4124] So ketones can explain why you might feel hungrier on a low-calorie diet than on a total fast. Can we then exploit the appetite-suppressing effects of ketosis by eating a ketogenic diet? If you ate too few carbs to sustain brain function, couldn't you trick your body into thinking you're fasting and start pumping out ketones? Yes. But is it safe? Is it effective?

Ketogenic Diets

Seizing Upon the Ketogenic Diet

The prescription of fasting for the treatment of epileptic seizures dates back to Hippocrates,[4125] and according to Mark 9:29, Jesus seems to have concurred.[4126] To this day, it's unclear why switching from blood sugar to ketones as a primary fuel source has such a dampening effect on brain over-activity.[4127] To prolong the therapy, in 1921, a distinguished physician and scientist at the Mayo Clinic suggested trying what he called a *ketogenic diet,* a high-fat diet designed to be so deficient in carbohydrates it could effectively mimic the fasting state.[4128] "Remarkable improvement" in seizures was noted the first time it was put to the test,[4129] efficacy that was later confirmed in randomized controlled trials.[4130] Ketogenic diets started to fall out of favor in 1938 with the discovery of the anti-seizure drug phenytoin (later sold as Dilantin),[4131] but they are still in use today as a third-line treatment for drug-refractory epilepsy in children.[4132]

Oddly, the success of ketogenic diets against pediatric epilepsy seems to get conflated by keto diet proponents into suggesting a ketogenic diet is beneficial for everyone.[4133] You know what else sometimes works for intractable epilepsy? Brain surgery, but I don't hear people clamoring to get their skulls sawed open. Since when do medical therapies translate into healthy lifestyle choices? Ketogenic diets are also being tested to see if they can slow the growth of certain brain tumors.[4134] Even if they are successful, you know what else can help slow cancer growth? Chemotherapy. Why go keto when you can just go chemo?

Promoters of ketogenic diets for cancer, paid by "ketone technology" firms[4135] or companies that market ketogenic meals,[4136] report "extraordinary" anecdotal responses in some cancer patients.[4137] I'm sure they do. But more concrete evidence is lacking.[4138] Even the theoretical underpinnings may be questionable. A common refrain is that "cancer feeds on sugar."[4139] True, but *all* cells feed on sugar. Advocating ketogenic diets for cancer is like saying Stalin breathed air, so we should boycott oxygen.

Cancer can also feed on ketones. Indeed, ketones have been found to fuel human breast cancer growth and drive metastases in an experimental model, more than doubling tumor growth.[4140] Some have even speculated that may be why breast cancer often metastasizes to the liver, the main site of ketone production.[4141] When ketones were dripped on breast cancer cells in a petri dish, the genes that got turned on and off made for a much more aggressive cancer and were associated with a significantly lower five-year survival in breast cancer patients.[4142] Researchers are even considering ketone-*blocking* drugs to prevent further cancer growth by halting ketone production.[4143]

High-fat diets in general are purported to increase breast cancer risk through "oxidative stress, hormonal dysregulation, or inflammatory signaling."[4144] A strong association has also been found between saturated fat intake and prostate cancer progression. Those in the top third of saturated fat consumption appeared to triple their risk of dying from prostate cancer.[4145] A meta-analysis of studies on diet and breast cancer mortality concluded that "saturated fat intake negatively impacts upon breast cancer survival," finding a 50 percent increase in the hazard of breast cancer–specific death for those with the most saturated fat intake compared to those women with the least.[4146] There's a reason the official American Cancer Society / American Society of Clinical Oncology Breast Cancer Survivorship Care Guidelines recommend a dietary pattern for breast cancer patients that's essentially the opposite of a ketogenic diet: "high in vegetables, fruits, whole grains, and legumes; low in saturated fats."[4147]

So far, not a single clinical study has shown a measurable benefit from a ketogenic diet for any human cancer.[4148] There are currently at least a dozen trials under way, however, and the hope is that at least some cancer types will respond.[4149] Still, that wouldn't serve as a basis for recommending ketogenic diets for the general population any more than would recommending everyone go out and get radiation, surgery, and chemo just for kicks.

Ketogenic Diet Put to the Test

By eschewing carbohydrates, you force your body to burn fat. And indeed, the amount of fat you burn shoots up when you eat a ketogenic diet.[4150] At the same time, however, the fat you *take in* shoots up when you eat a ketogenic diet. The question is *what happens to our overall body-fat balance?*[4151] You can't empty a tub by widening the drain if you're also cranking open the faucet. Low-carb advocates had a theory, though—the so-called carbohydrate-insulin model of obesity.

Proponents of low-carbohydrate diets, whether a ketogenic diet or some more relaxed form of carbohydrate restriction, suggested that the decreased insulin secretion would lead to less fat storage. So even if you were eating more fat, less of it would stick to your frame. You'd be burning more and storing less—the perfect combination for fat loss—or so the theory went.[4152] To their credit, instead of just speculating about it, they decided to put it to the test.

In 2012, Gary Taubes co-formed the Nutrition Science Initiative reportedly to sponsor research to validate the carbohydrate-insulin model.[4153] He's the journalist who wrote the controversial 2002 *New York Times Magazine* piece "What If It's All Been a Big Fat Lie?" which attempted to turn nutrition dogma on its head by arguing in favor of the Atkins diet and its bunless bacon cheeseburgers based on the carbohydrate-insulin model.[4154] (Much of Nina Teicholz's more recent *The Big Fat Surprise* is simply recycled from Taubes's earlier work.[4155]) Some of the very researchers Taubes cited to support his thesis accused him of twisting their words.[4156] "The article was incredibly misleading," one said. "I was horrified." "He took this weird little idea and blew it up, and people believed him," said another. "What a disaster."[4157] It doesn't matter what people say, though. All that matters is the science.

Taubes attracted $40 million in committed funding for his Nutrition Science Initiative in part to prove to the world that more body fat could be lost on a ketogenic diet and contracted noted NIH researcher Kevin Hall to perform the study. Seventeen overweight men were effectively locked in what's called a *metabolic ward* for two months to allow researchers total control over their diets. For the first month, they were placed on a typical carbohydrate-rich diet (50 percent carbohydrate, 35 percent fat, and 15 percent protein) and then switched to a low-carb ketogenic diet (5 percent carbohydrate, 80 percent fat, and 15 percent protein) for the second month. Both diets had the same number of daily calories. If a calorie is a calorie when it comes to weight loss, then there should be no difference in body fat loss on the regular diet versus the ketogenic diet. But, if Taubes were right, if fat calories were somehow less fattening, then body fat loss would become accelerated on the keto diet. What happened instead, in the very study funded by his Nutrition Science Initiative, was that body fat loss *slowed* upon switching to the ketogenic diet.[4158]

Just looking at the readings on their scales, the ketogenic diet would seem like a smashing success. The subjects went from losing less than a pound a week on the regular diet to losing three and a half pounds within seven days after switching to the ketogenic diet. What was happening *inside* their bodies, however, told a totally different story. On the keto diet, their rates of body fat loss were slowed by more than half, so most of what they were losing was water. The reason they started burning less fat on a ketogenic diet is presumably the same reason people who start fasting may start burning less fat: Without carbohydrates, the preferred fuel, their bodies started burning more of their own protein. Switching to a ketogenic diet made them lose less fat mass and more fat-free mass.[4159] That may help explain why the leg muscles of CrossFit trainees placed on a ketogenic diet may shrink as much as 8 percent.[4160]

The study subjects did start burning more fat on the ketogenic diet, but they were also eating so much more fat on that diet that they ended up retaining more fat, despite the lower insulin levels. This is "diametrically opposite"[4161] to what the keto crowd had predicted. In science-speak, the carbohydrate-insulin model "failed experimental interrogation."[4162]

In a separate experiment, Dr. Hall showed that if you cut about eight hundred calories of carbohydrates a day from your diet for six days, you lose fifty-three daily grams of body fat, but, if you cut eight hundred calories of *fat,* you lose eighty-nine daily grams of body fat. That's nine pats of butter worth of extra fat melting off their bodies every day. Same number of calories, but 68 percent more daily fat loss when they cut down on fat instead of carbs. The title of the study speaks for itself: "Calorie for Calorie, Dietary Fat Restriction Results in More Body Fat Loss Than Carbohydrate Restriction in People with Obesity."[4163]

Once again, the scale would mislead us into thinking otherwise. After six days on the low-carb diet, study subjects lost four pounds, but they lost less than three pounds on the low-fat diet. Less loss of body fat, but, stepping on the scale, it *looks* like the low-carb diet wins hands down, so it's easy to see why low-carb diets are so popular. But yet again, what was happening inside their bodies told the real story. The low-carb group was losing mostly lean mass—water and protein. This loss of water weight helps explain why low-carb diets have been such "cash cows"[4164] for publishers over the last 156 years.[4165] As one weight-loss expert noted, "Rapid water loss is the $33-billion diet gimmick."[4166]

What we care about is body fat, not water weight. Over those six days, the low-fat diet extracted a total of 89 percent more fat from the body than the low-carb diet.[4167] A meta-analysis of thirty-two controlled feeding studies swapping fat and carbs found the same thing: Less fat in the mouth means less fat on the hips, even when taking in the same number of calories.[4168]

In light of the "experimental falsification"[4169] of the low-carb theory, the Nutrition Science Initiative effectively collapsed in 2016,[4170] but not before Taubes personally pocketed in excess of a half million dollars.[4171]

Losing Your Appetite

The new data are said to debunk "some, if not all, of the popular claims made for extreme carbohydrate restriction."[4172] But what about the suppression of hunger? In that metabolic ward study where the ketogenic diet flopped, everyone was made to eat the same number of calories. So, yes—you may lose less body fat on a ketogenic diet than on a nonketogenic diet eating the same number of calories, but out in the real world, maybe all those ketones would spoil your appetite enough that you'd end up eating significantly less overall. On the low-carb diet, people ended up storing 340 more calories of fat every day,[4173] but outside the laboratory, being in a state of ketosis could allow you to offset that if you were able to sustainably eat sufficiently that much less.

The secret to long-term weight loss on any diet, of course, is compliance.[4174] Diet adherence is difficult, though, because, as you know, anytime you try to cut calories, your body ramps up your appetite to compensate. This is why traditional weight-loss approaches like portion control tend to fail. For long-term success, measured not in weeks or months but in years and decades, this day-to-day hunger problem must be overcome. On a wholesome plant-based diet, this can be accomplished, thanks in part to calorie density—you're just eating so much more food. On a ketogenic diet, it may be accomplished with ketosis. The answer to a systematic review and meta-analysis entitled "Do Ketogenic Diets Really Suppress Appetite?" was *yes*.[4175] What's more, ketogenic diets offer the additional advantage of being able to track dietary compliance in real time with ketone test strips you can pee on to see if you're still in ketosis.[4176] There's no pee stick that will tell you if you're eating enough fruits and veggies. All you have is the scale.

Keto compliance may be more in theory than practice, however. Even in studies where ketogenic diets are being used to control seizures, after a few months, dietary compliance may drop to less than 50 percent.[4177] This can be tragic for those with intractable epilepsy, but for everyone else, the difficulty in sticking to ketogenic diets long term may actually be a lifesaver.

Gut Reaction

Given the decades of use of ketogenic diets to treat certain cases of pediatric epilepsy, a body of safety data has accumulated. Nutrient deficiencies would seem the obvious issue.[4178] Inadequate intake of seventeen micronutrients has also been documented in those on ketogenic diets. Children have gotten scurvy,[4179] and some have even died from deficiency of the mineral selenium, which can cause sudden cardiac death.[4180] The vitamin and mineral deficiencies can be solved with supplements, but what about the paucity of prebiotics, the eight types of fiber and resistant starches found concentrated in whole grains and beans?[4181]

Not surprisingly, constipation is one of the most frequently cited side effects,[4182] but more seriously, starving our microbial selves can have myriad negative consequences, as I reviewed in the Microbiome-Friendly section. Ketogenic diets have been shown to reduce the richness and diversity of our gut flora.[4183] Microbiome changes can be detected within twenty-four hours of switching to a high-fat, low-fiber diet.[4184] It's not just the lack of fiber, though. We used to think dietary fat was nearly all absorbed in the small intestine, but we now know that about 7 percent of the fat in a fat-rich meal can make it down to the colon (based on studies using radioactive tracers).[4185] Saturated fat in particular appears to cause obesogenic and pro-inflammatory changes in gut flora, but most of the data are derived from animal models.[4186] Human studies have shown a drop in beneficial *Bifidobacteria* and a decrease in overall short-chain fatty-acid production, both of which would be expected to increase the risk of gastrointestinal disease.[4187]

Striking at the Heart

What might all that saturated fat be doing to the heart? A meta-analysis of four cohort studies following the diets, diseases, and deaths of more than a quarter million people found that those who eat lower-carb diets suffer a significantly higher risk of all-cause mortality, meaning they live, on average, significantly shorter lives.[4188] The risk of cardiovascular disease specifically appears to depend on the source of fat. In a Harvard study of heart attack survivors, those who adhered more to a lower-carb diet based on animal sources of fat and protein had a 50 percent higher risk of dying from a heart attack or stroke, but no such association was found for lower-carb diets based on plant sources.[4189] These studies were based on low-carb scoring systems, though, so they speak more to the risks of lower-carb eating rather than a truly low-carb ketogenic diet.

Cholesterol production in the body is directly correlated to body weight.[4190] Every pound of weight loss by any means is associated with about a one-point drop in cholesterol levels in the blood.[4191] But when people are put on ketogenic diets, the beneficial effect on bad LDL cholesterol is blunted or even completely neutralized.[4192] Counterbalancing changes in LDL size or HDL cholesterol are not considered sufficient to offset this risk.[4193] You don't have to wait until cholesterol builds up in your arteries to have an effect, though. Within three hours of eating a meal high in saturated fat (even from plant sources such as coconut oil), you can see a significant impairment of artery function.[4194] Even with about a dozen pounds of weight loss, artery function worsens on a ketogenic diet instead of getting better,[4195] which appears to be the case with low-carb diets in general.[4196]

How Not to *Die*-abetes

Ketogenic diets can certainly lower blood sugars,[4197] so much so that there is a keto product company that claims ketogenic diets can "reverse" diabetes,[4198] but that is confusing the symptom—high blood sugars—with the disease, which is carbohydrate intolerance. People with diabetes can't properly handle carbohydrates, and this manifests as high blood sugars. Sure, if you stick to eating mostly fat, your blood sugars will stay low, but you may actually be making the underlying disease worse.

We've known for nearly a century that if you put people on a ketogenic diet, their carbohydrate intolerance can skyrocket within just two days.[4199] One week on an 80 percent fat diet, and you can quintuple your blood sugar spikes in reaction to the same carb load compared to a week on a low-fat diet.[4200] Even one high-fat day can do it.[4201] If you're going in for a diabetes test, having a fatty dinner the night before can adversely affect your results.[4202] Just a single meal high in saturated fat can make the cause of diabetes, carbohydrate intolerance, worse within four hours.[4203] With enough weight loss by any means—whether cholera or a good meth habit—type 2 diabetes can be reversed, but a ketogenic diet for diabetes may not just be papering over the cracks but actively throwing fuel on the fire. One of the cofounders of MasteringDiabetes.org suggested it's like a CEO who tries to make the bad bottom line look better by borrowing tons of cash. The outward numbers look better, but on the inside, the company's just digging itself into a deeper hole.

The reason keto proponents claim they can "reverse" diabetes is that they can successfully wean type 2 diabetics off their insulin.[4204] The way they do it, however, is akin to faith healing someone out of the need for their wheelchair by putting them on permanent bed rest for the rest of their life. You won't have any more need for that wheelchair when you can't ever get out of bed! The diabetics' carbohydrate intolerance isn't gone—they're just not eating many carbs. Their diabetes isn't gone—it could be as bad or even worse. Type 2 diabetes is reversed when you have *normal* blood sugars on a *normal* diet off all medications. In other words, it is reversed when you're no longer intolerant to carbohydrates. Any diabetic can maintain normal blood sugars eating a stick of butter; only a *cured* diabetic can maintain the same feat eating a banana. As I detailed in *How Not to Die,* diabetes truly can be reversed this way with a healthy enough diet, sometimes in a matter of weeks and even *without* weight loss.[4205]

Spoiler alert: The true diabetes reversal diet, with more than three hundred grams of carbs a day, is practically the opposite of a ketogenic diet.[4206]

The irony doesn't stop there. One of the reasons diabetics suffer such nerve and artery damage is an inflammatory metabolic toxin known as *methylglyoxal,* which forms at high blood sugar levels. Methylglyoxal is the most potent creator of advanced glycation end products (AGEs),[4207] which are implicated in degenerative diseases from Alzheimer's disease and cataracts to kidney disease and strokes.[4208] One would expect high exposure to preformed AGEs on a ketogenic diet, since they are found concentrated in animal-derived foods that are high in fat and protein, but less internal, new AGE formation due to presumably low levels of methylglyoxal given the low blood sugars.[4209] Dartmouth researchers, however, were surprised to find *more* methylglyoxal. Two to three weeks on the Atkins diet led to a significant increase in methylglyoxal levels, and those in active ketosis did even worse, experiencing a doubling of the glycotoxin levels in the bloodstream.[4210] It turns out high sugars may not be the only way to create methylglyoxal.

One of the ketones you make on a ketogenic diet is acetone (known for its starring role in nail polish remover). Acetone does more than just make keto dieters fail Breathalyzer tests[4211] and develop what's described as "rotten apple breath."[4212] Acetone can oxidize in the blood to acetol, which may be a precursor for methylglyoxal.[4213] That may be why nondiabetic keto dieters can end up with methylglyoxal levels as high as those with out-of-control diabetes[4214] or end up with a heart attack.[4215] So the irony of "treating diabetes" with a ketogenic diet extends beyond just the potential of making the underlying disease worse, but by mirroring some of diabetes' dire consequences.

Bad to the Bone

An official International Society of Sports Nutrition position paper covering ketogenic diets notes "ergolytic" effects—that is, performance-impairing, the opposite of ergogenic—for both high- and low-intensity workouts.[4216] For nonathletes, ketosis can increase the feelings of perceived effort and fatigue during physical activity, which could potentially undermine exercise efforts.[4217] I already mentioned the shrinkage of measured muscle size among keto-dieting CrossFit trainees.[4218] A ketogenic diet may not only blunt the performance of endurance athletes[4219] but strength trainers, as well.[4220] This is why bodybuilding on a ketogenic diet has been referred to as an "oxymoron" in *Exercise and Sports Science Reviews,* a journal of the American College of Sports Medicine.[4221]

What about bone loss? Sadly, bone fractures are one of the side effects that disproportionately plague children placed on ketogenic diets, along with growth stunting and kidney stones.[4222] Ketogenic diets may cause a steady rate of bone loss (measured in the spine),[4223] presumably because ketosis can put people in a "chronic acidotic state."[4224] Ketones themselves are acidic[4225] and can result in a mild metabolic acidosis.[4226]

As with anything in medicine, it's all about risks versus benefits. Up to 30 percent of patients with epilepsy don't respond to anti-seizure drugs, and the alternatives aren't pretty, including procedures like brain surgery,[4227] which can involve implanting electrodes deep through the skull or even removing a lobe of the brain. This can obviously lead to serious side effects,[4228] but so can having seizures every day. So if a ketogenic diet helps, the pros can far outweigh the cons. For those just choosing a diet to lose weight, though, the cost-benefit analysis would clearly seem to go the other way.

Intermittent Fasting

In and Out of the Fast Lane

Rather than cutting calories day in and day out, what if, instead, you just ate as much as you wanted every other day? Or for only a few hours a day? Or what if you fasted two days a week or five days a month? These are all examples of intermittent fasting regimens, and they may even be the way we were built to eat. Three meals every day may be a relatively novel behavior for our species. For millennia, our ancestors often may have consumed only one large meal a day or went several days at a time without food.[4229]

Intermittent fasting is often presented as a means of stressing our bodies—in a good way. There is a concept in biology called *hormesis,* which can be thought of as the "that which doesn't kill you makes you stronger" principle. Exercise is the classic example: You put stress on your heart and muscles, and as long as there's sufficient recovery time, you are all the healthier for it.[4230] Is that the case with intermittent fasting? Mark Twain thought so: "A little starvation can really do more for the average sick man than can the best medicines and the best doctors. I do not mean a restricted diet; I mean *total abstention from food for one or two days.*"[4231]

Twain also said, "Many a small thing has been made large by the right kind of advertising."[4232] Is the craze over intermittent fasting just hype? Many diet fads have their roots in legitimate science, but over time, facts can get distorted, benefits overstated, and risks downplayed. As one medical journal news editor put it: "Science takes a back seat to marketing."[4233] At the same time, you don't want to lose out on any potential benefit by dismissing something out of hand based on the absurdist claims of overzealous promoters. You don't want to throw the baby out with the baby fat.

Alternate-Day Fasting: Efficacy

The most studied form of intermittent fasting is religious fasting,[4234] specifically Ramadan, a monthlong period during which devout Muslims abstain from food and drink from sunrise until sunset.[4235] The effects are complicated by a change in sleeping patterns, as well as thirst.[4236] The same dehydration issue arises with Yom Kippur, when observant Jews stop eating and

drinking for about twenty-five hours.[4237] The most studied form of intermittent fasting that deals only with food restriction is alternate-day fasting,
which involves eating every other day, alternating with days consuming little
or no calories.[4238]

At rest, we burn about a 50:50 mix of carbs and fat,[4239] but we usually
run out of our glycogen stores within twelve to thirty-six hours of when we
stop eating. At that point, our bodies have to shift to rely more on our fat
stores.[4240] This "metabolic switch" may help explain why the greatest rate
of breakdown and burning of fat over a three-day fast happens between the
hours of eighteen and twenty-four of the seventy-two-hour period.[4241] So
the hope is to reap some of the benefits of taking a break from eating without
the risks of prolonged fasting.[4242]

One of the potential benefits of alternate-day fasting over chronic caloric
restriction is that you get regular breaks from feeling constant hunger. Might
people become so famished on their fasting day, though, that they turn the
next into a *feasting* day and overeat? If you ate more than twice as much as
you normally would, then that presumably would defeat the whole point of
alternate-day fasting. Mice fed every other day don't lose weight. They just
eat roughly twice as much in one day than nonfasted mice would regularly
eat in two.[4243] That is not, however, what people do.[4244]

When study subjects were randomized to fast for thirty-six hours, from
8:00 p.m. on day one to 8:00 a.m. on day three, the thirty-six-hour fast only
led to people eating an average of 20 percent more the day after they broke
the fast, compared to a control group who didn't fast at all. That would leave
the thirty-six-hour fasters with a large calorie deficit, equivalent to a caloric
restriction of nearly a thousand calories a day.[4245] That particular study involved lean men and women, but similar results have been found among
overweight or obese subjects, typically only a 10–25 percent compensatory
increase in caloric intake over baseline.[4246] This seems to be the case whether
the fasting day was a true zero-calorie fast or a few-hundred-calorie "modified" fast.[4247]

Some studies found subjects appeared to eat no more[4248] or even eat *less*
on days after a daylong mini-fast.[4249,4250] Even within studies, however, great
variability is reported. In a twenty-four-hour fasting study where folks ate
dinner and then, the next day, skipped breakfast and lunch, the degree of
compensation at the dinner on day two ranged from 7 to 110 percent. This
means some got so hungry by the time the dinner rolled around the next

day that they ate more than twenty-four-hours' worth of calories in a single meal. The researchers suggested that perhaps people first try "test fasts" to see how much their hunger and subsequent intakes ramp up before considering an intermittent fasting regimen.[4251] Hunger levels can change over time, though, dissipating as our bodies habituate to the new normal.

In an eight-week study in which obese subjects were restricted to about five hundred calories every other day, they reported beginning to feel very little hunger on their slashed calorie days after approximately two weeks. This no doubt helped them lose about a dozen pounds on average over the duration of the study, but there was no control group with whom to compare.[4252] A similar study that did have a control group found a similar amount of weight loss—about eleven pounds—over twelve weeks in a group of "normal-weight" (that is, overweight on average) individuals.[4253] For these modified regimens where people were prescribed five hundred calories on their "fasting" days, researchers found that, from a weight-loss perspective, it did not appear to matter whether those calories were divided up throughout the day or eaten in a single meal, either at lunch or dinner.[4254]

Instead of prescribing a set number of calories on "fasting" days, which many people find difficult to calculate outside of a study setting, a pair of Iranian researchers came upon the idea of unlimited above-ground vegetables. Starchy root vegetables are relatively calorie-dense compared to veggies that grow above the ground, including stem vegetables like celery and rhubarb, flowering vegetables like cauliflower, leafy vegetables like, well, leafy vegetables, and all the fruits we tend to think of as vegetables, such as tomatoes, peppers, okra, eggplants, string beans, summer squash, and zucchini. So instead of just prescribing a certain number of calories for the "fasting" days, subjects alternated between their regular diets and helping themselves every other day to all-you-can-eat above-ground vegetables (along with naturally noncaloric beverages like green tea or black coffee). After six weeks, subjects lost an average of thirteen pounds and two inches off their waists.[4255]

The same variability discovered for calorie compensation was also found for weight loss. In a twelve-month trial in which subjects were instructed to eat only one quarter of their caloric needs every other day, weight changes varied from a gain of about eight pounds to a loss of around thirty-seven pounds. The biggest factor appeared to be not how much they feasted on their regular diet days but how much they were able to comply with the caloric restriction on their fast days.[4256]

Overall, ten out of ten alternate-day fasting studies showed significant reductions in body fat.[4257] Small, short-term studies show a 4–8 percent drop in body weight after three to twelve weeks.[4258] How does that compare with continuous caloric restriction? Zero-calorie, alternate-day fasting was compared head-to-head to a daily restriction of four hundred calories a day for eight weeks. Both groups lost the same amount of weight, about seventeen pounds, and, in the follow-up check-in six months after the trial had ended, both groups had maintained a similar degree of weight loss, still down about a dozen pounds.[4259]

The hope that intermittent fasting would somehow improve compliance or avoid the metabolic adaptations that slow weight loss doesn't seem to have materialized. The same compensatory reactions in terms of increased appetite and a slower metabolism plague both methods,[4260] and the largest, longest trial of alternate-day fasting found that it may be even less sustainable than more traditional approaches.[4261] By the end of a year, the dropout rate of the alternate-day fasting group was 38 percent compared to 29 percent in the continuous calorie-restriction group.[4262]

Though alternate-day fasting regimens haven't been shown to produce superior weight loss, for the individuals who may prefer this pattern of caloric restriction, are there any downsides?

Alternate-Day Fasting: Safety

Might going all day without eating impair our ability to think clearly? Surprisingly, the results appear to be equivocal. Some studies show no measurable effects, and the ones that do fail to agree on which cognitive domains are affected.[4263]

Might the fasting-feasting cycles cause eating disorder–type behavior like bingeing? So far, no harmful psychological effects have been found,[4264] though the studies that have put it to the test specifically excluded people with a documented history of eating disorders, for whom the effects may differ.[4265]

No change in bone mineral density was noted after six months of alternate-day fasting despite about sixteen pounds of weight loss, which would typically result in a dip in bone mass. However, there also were no skeletal changes noted in the control group who had lost a similar amount of weight using continuous caloric restriction. The researchers suggest this is because both groups tended to be more physically active than the average obese individual by one or two thousand steps a day.[4266]

Proponents of intermittent fasting suggest it can better protect lean body mass,[4267] but most of the intermittent trials have employed a less accurate method of body composition analysis (bioelectrical impedance), whereas the majority of continuous caloric-restriction trials used vastly more accurate technologies (dual-energy x-ray absorptiometry and magnetic resonance imaging).[4268] To date, it's not clear if there's a difference in lean mass preservation.[4269]

Improvements in blood pressure and triglycerides have been noted on intermittent-fasting regimens, though this is presumed to be due to the reduction in body fat, since the effect appears to be dependent on weight loss.[4270] Alternate-day fasting can also improve artery function, though that depends on what is eaten on the nonfasting day.[4271] Randomized to an alternate-day diet high in saturated fat, artery function worsened despite a twelve-pound loss in body fat, whereas it improved as expected in the lower-fat group. The decline in artery function was presumed to be because of the pro-inflammatory nature of saturated fat.[4272]

A concern has been raised about the effects of alternate-day fasting on cholesterol. After twenty-four hours without food, LDL cholesterol may temporarily bump up, but this is presumably just because so much fat is being released into the system by the fast.[4273] An immediate negative effect on carbohydrate tolerance may stem from the same phenomenon.[4274] After a few weeks, LDL levels start to drop as the weight comes off,[4275] but results from the largest and longest trial of alternate-day fasting have given me pause.

One hundred obese men and women were randomized into one of three groups: alternate-day modified fasting (25 percent of baseline calories on fasting days and 125 percent calories on eating days), continuous daily caloric restriction (75 percent of baseline), or a control group instructed to maintain their regular diets. So if you went into the trial eating 2,000 calories a day, you would continue to eat your 2,000 a day in the control group, you'd be prescribed 1,500 calories each day in the calorie-restriction group, and you would alternate between 500 calories one day and 2,500 calories the next in the intermittent-restriction group.

With the same overall average calorie-cutting prescribed in both weight-loss groups, each lost about the same amount of weight, but surprisingly, the cholesterol effects were different. In the continuous calorie-restriction group, as the pounds came off, the bad LDL dropped as expected compared to the control group. But in the alternate-day modified fasting group, they didn't. At the end of the year, the LDL cholesterol in the intermittent-restriction group ended up 10 percent *higher* than that of the constant calorie-restriction group, despite the exact same loss in body fat.[4276] Given that LDL cholesterol is a prime risk factor[4277]—or even *the* prime risk factor[4278]—for our number one killer, heart disease, this strikes a significant blow against alternate-day fasting. If you do want to try it anyway, I would advise you have your cholesterol monitored to make sure it comes down with your weight.

If you're diabetic, it's critical to talk with your physician about medication adjustment for any changes in diet, including fasting of any duration. Even with proactive medication reduction, advice to immediately break the fast should sugars drop too low, and weekly medical supervision, type 2 diabetics fasting even just two days a week were twice as likely to suffer from hypoglycemic episodes compared to an unfasted control group. We still don't know the best way to adjust blood sugar medications to prevent blood sugars from dropping too low on fasting days.[4279]

Consultation with one's medical professional is a good idea before fasting for anyone on medication. Even just fasting for a day can significantly slow the clearance of some drugs like the blood-thinning drug coumadin or increase the clearance of others like caffeine. Indeed, fasting for thirty-six hours can cut your caffeine buzz by 20 percent.[4280]

La Dieta de Hambre

Doctors have anecdotally attributed improvements in a variety of disease states to alternate-day fasting, including asthma, seasonal allergies, autoimmune disease (rheumatoid arthritis), osteoarthritis, infectious diseases (toenail fungus), periodontal disease, viral upper-respiratory-tract infections, neurological conditions (Tourette's syndrome, Ménière's disease), atrial fibrillation, and menopause-related hot flashes.[4281] However, the *actual* effect on chronic disease remains unclear.[4282]

Alternate-day fasting has been put to the test for asthma in obese adults. Asthma-related symptoms and control significantly improved, as did their quality of life, including objective measurements of lung function and inflammation. However, their weight also improved—about a nineteen-pound drop in eight weeks—so it's hard to tease out effects specific to the fasting beyond the benefits we might expect from weight loss by any means.[4283] Surprisingly, for the most remarkable study on alternate-day fasting, you have to go back more than a half century.

While that cholesterol finding was the most concerning data I could find on alternate-day fasting, the most enticing was published in Spain sixty-one years earlier in 1956. The title of the study translates as "The Hunger Diet on Alternate Days in the Nutrition of the Aged." Inspired by the data being published on life extension with caloric restriction on lab rats, researchers split 120 residents of a senior home in Madrid into two groups. Sixty residents continued to eat their regular diets, and the other sixty were put on an alternate-day modified fast. On the odd days of the month, they ate a 2,300-calorie, regular diet and, on the even days, were given only a pound of fresh fruits and a liter of milk,[4284] an estimated 900 calories.[4285] This continued for three years. What happened?

Over the duration of the study, thirteen died in the control group, compared to only six in the modified intermittent-fasting group, but those numbers were too small to be statistically significant. What was highly significant, though, was the number of days they spent hospitalized. Residents in the control group spent a total of 219 days in the infirmary, whereas those in the alternate-day fasting group were hospitalized for only 123 days.[4286] This is held up as solid evidence that caloric restriction in general, and alternate-day fasting in particular, may improve one's health span and potentially even one's life span. However, a few caveats must be considered. It's not clear how the residents were allocated to their respective groups. If instead of being randomized, healthier individuals were placed inadvertently in the intermittent-fasting group, the results could have been skewed in their favor. Also, it appears the director of the study was also in charge of medical decisions at the home. In that role, he could have unconsciously been biased toward hospitalizing more people in the control group.[4287] Given the progress that has been made regulating human experimentation, it's hard to imagine such a trial being run today, so we may never know if such impressive findings can be replicated.

The 5:2 Diet

Instead of eating every other day, what if you ate five days a week and fasted the other two? The available data are actually similar to those of alternate-day fasting. About a dozen pounds of weight loss were reported in overweight men[4288] and women[4289] over a six-month period with no difference found between those on the 5:2 intermittent-fasting regimen and those on a continuous five-hundred-calories-a-day restriction. The largest trial to date found an eighteen-pound weight loss within six months in the 5:2 group, not significantly different from the twenty pounds lost in the continuous calorie-restriction group. Weight maintenance over a subsequent six months was also found to be no different.[4290]

Though feelings of hunger may be more pronounced on the 5:2 pattern than an equivalent level of daily calorie cutting,[4291] it does not seem to lead to overeating on the nonfasting days.[4292] One might expect going two days without food may negatively impact mood, but no adverse effect was noted for those fully fasting (zero calories)[4293] or sticking to just two packets of oatmeal on each of the "fasting" days (approximately five hundred calories).[4294] Like alternate-day fasting, the 5:2 fasting pattern appeared to have inconsistent effects on cognition,[4295] no clear advantage for lean mass preservation,[4296] and it failed to live up to the popular notion that intermittent fasting would prove to be easier to adhere to than daily caloric restriction.[4297]

Fewer subjects on the 5:2 pattern expressed interest in continuing the diet after the study was over, compared to a continuous-restriction control group.[4298] This was attributed to quality of life issues, citing headaches, lack of energy, and the difficulty of fitting the fasting days into their weekly routine.[4299] However, there has yet to be a single 5:2 diet study showing elevated LDL cholesterol compared to continuous caloric restriction at six months[4300,4301] or a year,[4302] which offers a potential advantage over alternate-day regimens.

Alternate-Week Fasting

Some intermittent-fasting patterns employ longer alternating periods. Hundreds of pounds of weight loss have been documented in those who had had previously intractable obesity but were then fasted in blocks of ten days on, ten days off.[4303] Ten days of total fasting is too long to do safely on your own without medical supervision, so alternating weeks of caloric restriction were put to the test in the hope that giving your body weeklong breaks may prevent it from going into energy-conservation mode to slow weight loss. However, no significant weight-loss advantage was found in an eight-week study compared to the same degree of continuous calorie-cutting,[4304] and a fifteen-week study found a negative effect on lean body mass preservation.[4305]

Overweight postmenopausal women were randomized either to fifteen weeks of constant caloric restriction or the same fifteen weeks interspersed with two five-week periods of their baseline diets. Same overall length of the study and same overall number of calories restricted, so similar decreases in weight of about twenty-two pounds, but those on the intermittent regimen lost twice as much lean body mass, about four pounds compared to two.[4306] The longest such study, however, involving sixteen weeks of caloric restriction in middle-aged obese men, either uninterrupted or alternating two weeks on, two weeks off, found no significant difference in lean mass loss. What they discovered instead was 50 percent greater loss of body fat: twenty-seven pounds of fat loss versus eighteen pounds in the continuous calorie-restriction group despite an equivalent overall "dose" of caloric restriction. This was due at least in part to less metabolic slowing on the back-and-forth pattern.[4307]

Putting all such studies together, it appears to be a wash between intermittent and continuous caloric restriction.[4308] Until further data allow us to iron out the inconsistencies found in these studies, it may be prudent at least for postmenopausal women to refrain from using intermittent caloric restriction as a weight-loss strategy.[4309]

Fasting-Mimicking Diet

Instead of 5:2, what about 25:5, spending five days a month on a "fasting-mimicking diet"? Longevity researcher Valter Longo designed a five-day meal plan to try to simulate the metabolic effects of fasting by being low in proteins, sugars, and calories with zero animal protein or animal fat. By making it plant-based, he was hoping to lower the level of the cancer-promoting growth hormone IGF-1 related to animal protein consumption, which he accomplished, along with a drop in markers of inflammation, after three cycles of his five-days-a-month program.[4310]

One hundred men and women were randomized to consume his fasting-mimicking diet (FMD) for five consecutive days per month or maintain their regular diets for the duration of the study. After three months, the FMD group was down about six pounds compared to control, with significant drops in body fat and waist circumference accompanied by a drop in blood pressures. Three months after completion of the study, some of the benefit appeared to persist, suggesting the effects may last for several months. However, it's unclear if those randomized to the FMD group used it as an opportunity to make positive lifestyle changes that helped maintain some of the weight loss.[4311]

Dr. Longo created a company to commercially market his meal plan but says, to his credit, that he donates 100 percent of the profits he receives from it to charity.[4312] The whole diet appears to be mostly a few dehydrated soup mixes of vegetable, mushroom, and tomato, herbal teas like hibiscus and chamomile, kale chips, nut-based energy bars, an algae-based DHA supplement, and a multivitamin dusted with vegetable powder.[4313] But why spend fifty dollars a day on a few processed snacks when you could instead eat a few hundred calories a day of real vegetables?

Time-Restricted Feeding

Taking a Break

The reason many blood tests are taken after an overnight fast is that meals can tip our systems out of balance, bumping up certain biomarkers for disease, such as blood sugars, insulin, cholesterol, and triglycerides, yet fewer than one in ten Americans may even make it twelve hours a day without eating. As evolutionarily unnatural as eating three meals a day may be, most of us are eating even more than that. One study using a smartphone app to record more than twenty-five thousand eating events found that people tended to eat about every three hours over an average span of around fifteen hours a day.[4314] Might it be beneficial to give our bodies a bigger break?

Time-restricted feeding is defined as fasting for periods of at least twelve hours but less than twenty-four hours.[4315] This involves trying to confine caloric intake to a set window of time, typically three to four hours, seven to nine hours, or ten to twelve hours a day, resulting in a daily fast lasting twelve to twenty-one hours. When mice were fed high-fat diets of mostly lard,[4316] they gained less weight when restricted to a daily feeding window, even when fed the exact same amount.[4317] Rodents have such high metabolisms, though, that a single day of fasting can starve away as much as 15 percent of their lean body mass,[4318] which makes it difficult to extrapolate from mouse models.[4319] You can't know what happens in humans until you put it to the test.

Different as Night and Day

The dropout rates in time-restricted feeding trials certainly appear lower than in more prolonged forms of intermittent fasting, suggesting they're more easily tolerable,[4320] but do they work? When people stopped eating between 7:00 p.m. and 6:00 a.m. for two weeks, they lost about a pound each week compared to no time restriction. Note that no additional instructions or recommendations were given on the amount or type of food consumed. There were no gadgets, calorie counting, or record keeping. They were just told to limit their food intakes to the hours of 6:00 a.m. through 7:00 p.m. and they lost weight. A simple intervention, easy to understand and implement.[4321]

The next logical step was to try putting it to the test for months instead of just a couple of weeks. Obese men and women were asked to restrict eating to the eight-hour window between 10:00 a.m. and 6:00 p.m. Twelve weeks later, they had lost five pounds.[4322] This deceptively simple intervention may be operating from a number of different angles. People tend to eat more food[4323] and higher-fat foods later in the day,[4324] and the late-evening hours may represent a high-risk time for overeating.[4325] By eliminating eating in the late-evening hours, one removes prime-time snacking on the couch.[4326] And indeed, during the time-restricted weeks, the subjects in both studies were inadvertently eating about three hundred fewer calories a day.[4327]

There are also the chronobiological benefits of avoiding late-night eating. Remember how calories in the morning cause less weight gain than the same calories eaten in the evening?[4328] A diet with a bigger breakfast causes more weight loss than the same exact diet with a bigger dinner.[4329] Nighttime snacks are more fattening than the same snacks eaten in the daytime.[4330] Thanks to our circadian rhythms, metabolic slowing,[4331] hunger, carbohydrate intolerance, triglycerides, and our propensity for weight gain are all things that go bump in the night.[4332]

What about the fasting component? There's already the double benefit of consuming fewer calories and avoiding nighttime eating. Does the fact that the subjects in those two studies were fasting for eleven or sixteen hours a day play any role, considering that the average person may only make it about nine hours a day without eating?[4333] How would you design an experiment to test that? What if you randomized people into one of two groups and forced both to eat the same number of calories a day and also to eat late into the evening, but one group was designated to fast even longer, for twenty hours? That's exactly what researchers at the USDA and National Institute on Aging did.

Men and women were randomized to eat three meals a day or fit all those same calories into a single four-hour window between 5:00 p.m. and 9:00 p.m. and then fast the rest of the day.[4334] If the weight-loss benefits from the other two time-restricted feeding studies were due to the passive caloric restriction or avoidance of late-night eating, then presumably, both groups should end up the same in this study. That's not what happened. After eight weeks, the time-restricted feeding group ended up with nearly five pounds less body fat. About the same number of calories, but they lost more weight. A similar study with an eight-hour eating window resulted in three pounds of additional fat loss.[4335] So there does seem to be something to giving our bodies daily breaks from eating around the clock. Because the four-hour eating window was at night, though, the subjects suffered the chronobiological consequences—significant elevations in blood pressure and cholesterol levels—despite the weight loss.[4336]

The best of both worlds was demonstrated in 2018 with time-restricted feeding in a narrower window earlier in the day.[4337] Individuals randomized to stick to a six-hour eating window ending before 3:00 p.m. experienced a drop in blood pressure, oxidative stress, and insulin resistance even when all the study subjects were maintained at the same weight. The average drop in blood pressure was extraordinary, from 123/82 down to 112/72 in just five weeks, comparable to the effectiveness of potent blood pressure drugs.

The longest study to date on time-restricted feeding only lasted sixteen weeks, a pilot study with no control group that involved only eight people. Nonetheless, the results are worth noting. Overweight individuals who, like most of us, were eating more than fourteen hours a day, were instructed to stick to a consistent ten- to twelve-hour feeding window of their own choosing. On average, they were able to successfully reduce their daily eating duration by about four and a half hours, and within sixteen weeks, they had lost seven pounds. They also reported sleeping better and feeling more energetic. This may help explain why all the participants voluntarily expressed their interest in continuing the time-restricted feeding on their own after the study ended. You don't often see that after weight-loss studies. Even more remarkably, eight months later, they had retained their weight loss and improved energy and sleep—all from one of the simplest of interventions.[4338]

How did it work? As with the other time-restricted feeding trials, even though they weren't told to change calorie quality or quantity, they appeared to unintentionally eat hundreds of fewer calories a day. With self-selected time frames, you wouldn't necessarily think to expect circadian benefits, but because they were asked to keep the eating window consistent throughout the week, there may have been. Remember social jet lag, the discrepancy between eating and sleeping patterns on weekdays and weekends? Breakfast may get pushed back an hour or two on free days, as if you had just jumped time zones, so some of the metabolic benefits may have been due to maintaining a regular eating schedule.[4339]

Surviving the Test of Time

Early or midday time-restricted feeding may have other benefits as well. Prolonged nightly fasting with reduced evening food intake has been associated with lower levels of inflammation[4340] and better blood sugar control, both of which might be expected to lower the risk of diseases such as breast cancer.[4341] Data were collected on thousands of breast cancer survivors to see if nightly fasting duration made a difference. Those who didn't go more than thirteen hours every night without eating had a 36 percent higher hazard of cancer recurrence.[4342] These findings have led to the suggestion that efforts to "avoid eating after 8 pm and fast for 13 h[ours] or more overnight may be a beneficial consideration for those patients looking to decrease cancer risk and recurrence,"[4343] though we'd need a randomized controlled trial to know for sure.

Early time-restricted feeding may even play a role in the health of perhaps the longest living population in the world, the Seventh-day Adventist Blue Zone in California. Slim, vegetarian, nut-eating, exercising, nonsmoking Adventists live about a decade longer than the general population.[4344] Their greater life expectancy has been ascribed to these healthy lifestyle behaviors, but there's one lesser-known component that may be playing a role. Historically, eating two large meals a day, breakfast and lunch, with a prolonged overnight fast was a part of Adventist teachings. Today, only about one in ten Adventists surveyed was eating just two daily meals, but most (63 percent) reported breakfast or lunch was their largest meal of the day. Though this has yet to be studied with respect to longevity, frontloading one's calories earlier in the day with a prolonged nightly fast has been associated with significant weight loss over time, leading the researchers to conclude: "Eating breakfast and lunch 5–6 h[ours] apart and making the overnight fast last 18–19 h[ours] may be a useful practical [weight control] strategy."[4345]

Food for Thought

Because of the metabolic slowing and increased appetite that accompany weight loss, *sustained* weight loss requires a persistent calorie deficit of three hundred to five hundred calories a day,[4346] which can be accomplished without reducing portion sizes just by lowering the calorie density of meals. Doing so can result in the rare combination of weight loss with an increase in both quality—and even quantity— of food consumed.

Those who are pregnant or breastfeeding, have an active infection, or are already underweight should not consider a dramatic cut in calories by any means, and anyone on medications or with a chronic medical condition, including diabetes, heart, liver, or kidney disease, or a history of fainting, should do so only under guidance from their health-care providers.

Prolonged water-only fasting is no longer recommended as a clinical treatment option for obesity due to the associated risks of complications.[4347] Fasting more than a day or two should be done only under strict medical supervision.

Ketogenic diets are also not recommended. When you think of the ideal attributes of a diet for weight control—safe, effective, protective, healthful, wholesome, sustainable, nutritionally complete, and life-extending—typical keto diets guarantee none of them.

Some forms of intermittent fasting, on the other hand, may be safe and effective (and it's safe to say cost-effective when it comes to your grocery bills), but apparently no more so for weight loss than continuous caloric restriction.[4348] However, combining intermittent-fasting regimens, such as early or midday time-restricted feeding with a healthier diet during the feeding windows, may prove to be particularly powerful. The weight may be worth the wait.

MEAL FREQUENCY

Nibbling vs. Gorging

Since the 1970s, the size of our meals has increased about 10 percent, from 1.2 pounds of food to 1.3 pounds, but the number of our meals has gone up closer to 20 percent, from eating around four times a day to five.[4349] The typical time between meals has shrunk by an hour. On average, American adults are now eating every three waking hours.[4350] Given this, increased eating frequency may have played double the role of increased portion size in the current obesity epidemic.[4351] But don't the popular press[4352] and even weight management professionals advise people to eat frequent smaller meals throughout the day?[4353] Frequent eating is purported to reduce hunger, increase metabolic rate, and mobilize body fat, but might all that extra snacking just pile on the pounds?[4354] Let's see what the science says.

Population studies since the 1960s have often shown that those who report eating less frequently tend to be more overweight, leading to the suggestion that a "nibbling" pattern of grazing throughout the day may be better than a "gorging" pattern of trying to fit all our calories into a few large meals.[4355] Alternatively, as with all such epidemiological findings, the results could have been due to confounding factors or reverse causation. Indeed, those who report eating fewer meals also report eating unhealthier meals[4356] and engaging in less physical activity,[4357] so perhaps those habits, rather than the eating frequency, contributed to being overweight. And, as with the breakfast-skipping data, perhaps instead of fewer meals leading to obesity, obesity led to fewer meals, as folks tried to omit meals to lose weight.[4358] The most likely explanation, though, is massive underreporting bias.[4359]

Self-Deception

Obese individuals not only report eating fewer meals but also eating fewer calories. Most studies of reported caloric intake and body weight suggest that the *more* calories you eat, the *slimmer* you are. Let that sink in for a moment. Based on interviews and questionnaires asking people how much they eat, as well as monitored eating in restaurants or laboratory settings, there is said to be "overwhelming evidence" that those who are obese eat fewer calories, misleading people to proclaim that the presumption that obesity is caused by overeating is simply a myth.[4360] But if you objectively measure how much people are actually eating, the whole charade collapses.[4361]

For centuries, there have been claims of people thriving on little or no food.[4362] A Catholic "mystic," for example, reportedly not only survived for thirty-five years but even gained weight consuming nothing but a daily communion wafer.[4363] This reminds me of the founder of the Breatharian Institute of America. You could attend one of his workshops on how to live on air alone for the low, low price of $100,000—"no refunds"[4364]—that is, until he evidently got busted sneaking out of a 7-Eleven with a hot dog, Slurpee, and box of Twinkies.[4365]

When actual caloric intakes are measured, it turns out those who claim they can't lose weight no matter how little they eat are fooling themselves into thinking they're eating less than they actually are.[4366] A group of "diet resistant" obese individuals were found to be underreporting their actual food intakes by a whopping 47 percent and overreporting their physical activity by about the same amount.[4367] So, in reality, the failure to lose weight on a calorie-restricted diet is due to not actually being on a calorie-restricted diet. Were the subjects straight-up lying about their overeating? They didn't appear to be intentionally deceiving the researchers as much as they apparently were deceiving themselves. When they were informed of the results of the study, they were reportedly surprised and distressed by the findings. Interventional studies have shown for nearly a century that if you lock people in a room, everyone loses weight as predicted.[4368]

Dietary underreporting by overweight individuals has been called "one of the most robust biopsychological phenomena ever described."[4369] Since snacks appear to be "preferentially forgotten" when obese individuals underreport intake on diet surveys,[4370] it isn't difficult to see how obesity would be correlated with eating less frequently.[4371] When you control for the underreporting, the relationship gets flipped on its head, going from heavier individuals *appearing* to eat *less* frequently to *actually* eating *more* frequently.[4372] This would make sense if our bodies aren't able to fully compensate for snacks by eating that much less at subsequent meals, but you don't know until you put it to the test.[4373]

Three Squares or Seventeen?

The purported benefits of eating more frequent meals on appetite,[4374] metabolic rate,[4375] fat mobilization,[4376] and weight loss have failed to materialize. Randomizing people to eat the same number of calories in either a single daily meal or spread out all the way up to nine meals per day has failed consistently to yield differences in weight loss in studies ranging in duration from a week to a year.[4377] That doesn't mean there aren't other health impacts, though. Eating all our calories in a single evening meal is worse for cholesterol[4378] and blood sugar control,[4379] but that is presumably due to less of a meal frequency effect than an adverse chronobiology effect of pushing calorie intake to later in the day.

The most extreme meal frequency study switched people from three meals a day to seventeen. Each day, people were given a snack when they woke up and then another snack every hour for the next sixteen hours. This resulted in significantly lower average insulin levels, thought responsible for an 18 percent drop in bad LDL cholesterol. Insulin stimulates the same cholesterol-synthesizing enzyme that statin drugs block,[4380] so by lowering insulin levels, the same food resulted in a twenty-point drop in bad cholesterol within two weeks.[4381] The researchers went out of their way to say they "do not advocate"[4382] what has been called a "clearly . . . impractical"[4383] "extreme model."[4384] It was just a proof-of-principle study to show how leveling insulin spikes with a low-glycemic-index diet might end up lowering cholesterol levels,[4385] as has indeed been shown to be the case (though that may be primarily because lower-glycemic diets tend to have more fiber).[4386]

In an experimental setting, you can increase eating frequency without causing weight gain by doling out carefully measured portions. In the real world, though, the more times people eat, the more they tend to increase their daily caloric intakes.[4387] When that happens, meal frequency can have significant metabolic consequences. If you're going to add something to your diet that's going to spike your insulin, it's better to add it *to* meals rather than *between* meals. Men, for example, were randomized to add three liters of sugary soda to their daily diets either with meals or between meals as snacks. Looking at the scale, it didn't seem to make any difference: Both groups gained the same amount of weight. However, what was happening within their bodies told a different story. Increasing meal frequency by adding soda "snacks" between meals, instead of increasing meal size by adding the same amount of soda to meals, led to a 65 percent greater relative increase in liver fat,[4388] which, over time, could increase the risk of fatty liver disease and diabetes.[4389]

It need not be liters of soda. Drinking about two cups of 100 percent orange juice three times a day between meals is worse than drinking the same amount of juice with meals. Drinking juice between meals led to the accumulation of nearly three more pounds of body fat within two weeks compared to the same amount of juice taken with meals.[4390]

Food for Thought

Decreasing the number of times you consume calories a day, whether from dining, snacking, or drinking soda, juice, or the like, may help with weight control, especially if you're eating junk. If you're going to eat processed foods, tack them onto meals rather than having them as between-meal snacks.

The healthiest snacks are fresh fruits and vegetables, of course, but I also enjoy snacking on nori sheets, lentil sprouts, "air-fried" purple sweet potato fries, edamame, and seasoned air-popped popcorn.

The worst snacks, according to national snacking guidelines from around the world, are snacks that are sugary, fatty, or salty.[4391] One study found body fat benefits to nut-based snack bars. Compared to what, though? You could tell the study was funded by the nut bar company when researchers felt the need to use as a comparator the likes of Oreo Double Stuf cookies.[4392]

Tempted by unhealthy foods? There are "choice architecture" methods to help cut down on impulsive snacking. For example, placing healthier foods at eye level in the store or at the beginning of a buffet line may nudge people toward better choices. Similarly, when chocolate candies are left on the desks of office workers, more are eaten than if they are placed just out of reach or in an opaque container.[4393] In a large field study at Google headquarters, for instance, the separation of the snack station from the beverage station by less than a dozen feet appeared to cut down snacking rates by about 40 percent. The researchers concluded that employers or even families may be able to reduce snack consumption "easily, cheaply, and without backlash" just by adding mild inconvenience. In the Greger household, I am able to instill maximum inconvenience by just not keeping any junk in the house.

Unable to purge your surroundings? The next time cravings hit, try Tetris. A study entitled "Playing 'Tetris' Reduces the Strength, Frequency and Vividness of Naturally Occurring Cravings" found that three minutes of distracting oneself with a video game may help tackle cravings[4394]—though I imagine playing Candy Crush might be counterproductive.

METABOLIC BOOSTERS

Fighting a Losing Battle

Thermogenic drugs like DNP can increase resting metabolic rates by 300 percent or more but, as you may remember from the Fat Burners section, also caused people to overheat to death.[4395] A more normal range would vary about ten times less, from a 30 percent slower metabolism in people with an underactive thyroid to a 30 percent higher metabolism when the part of our nervous systems that controls our fight-or-flight response is activated.[4396] In response to a fright or other acute stressor, special nerves release a chemical called *noradrenaline* to ready us for confrontation. You experience that as your skin getting paler, cool, and clammy as blood is diverted to your more vital organs. Your mouth can get dry as your digestive system is put on hold, and your heart starts to beat faster. What you don't feel is the extra fat being burned to liberate energy for the fight. This is why people started taking ephedra for weight loss.

Ephedra is an evergreen shrub that has been used for thousands of years in China to treat asthma.[4397] It causes that same release of noradrenaline that offers relief to asthmatics by dilating their airways.[4398] In the United States, it was appropriated for use as a metabolic stimulant, shown to result in about two pounds of weight loss a month in nineteen placebo-controlled trials.[4399]

By the late 1990s, millions of Americans were taking it.[4400] The problem is ephedra had all the other noradrenaline effects, too, like increasing heart rate and blood pressure, so chronic use resulted in strokes, heart attacks, and death.[4401] The FDA warned the public of the risks in 1994, but it wasn't banned until a decade later after a Major League pitcher dropped dead.[4402]

As we've discussed, in the current Wild West of lax dietary supplement regulation, a supplement can be marketed without any safety data at all and the manufacturer is under no obligation to disclose adverse effects that may arise.[4403] Online vendors assured absolute safety: "No negative side effects . . . 100% safe for long-term use."[4404] The president of Metabolife International, a leading seller of ephedra, assured the FDA that the company had "never received one notice from a consumer that any serious adverse health event has occurred." Liar. In reality, Metabolife had received thirteen thousand health complaints, including reports of serious injuries, hospitalizations, and deaths.[4405]

This is not to say prescription obesity drugs have fared much better. Dozens have been pulled from the market, on average eleven years after the first reports of serious adverse effects.[4406] If only there were a way to speed your metabolism without suffering cardiovascular side effects.

Music to Our Ears

Music can impact our metabolisms. You can imagine how it might get you pumped up, but the original study showed the opposite effect. Published in the journal of the American Academy of Pediatrics, a study on preterm infants found that their resting metabolic rates slowed within ten minutes of researchers piping in Mozart. This was good news for the preemies, since that meant they could potentially put on weight faster and go home earlier.[4407]

Gaining weight faster is great for premature babies, but not so much for overweight adults. Could listening to music slow our metabolisms and contribute to weight gain? One study out of Sweden found no effect on adults, but the researchers used Bach, not Mozart.[4408] Bach doesn't cause a drop in energy expenditure in babies either. The researchers concluded it may be "more a 'Mozart effect' than a universal 'music effect.'"[4409]

What happens to our metabolisms when we just listen to music of our choice? We didn't know until 2014, when Brigham Young University researchers reported that listening to self-selected music appears to give our metabolic rates a tiny bump, such that you would burn around thirty extra calories if you listened all day.[4410] That's only about eight M&M's candies' worth, so it's better to use music to get up and start dancing or exercising. Music may not only improve exercise enjoyment but also power output,[4411] touted as a "legal method" to improve athletic performance.[4412]

What about making music? In terms of calorie expenditure, playing piano or a brass or woodwind instrument isn't much better than taking a casual stroll, though trombone is the exception given all the associated arm movement, making it equal to light calisthenics.[4413] Rock drummers, however, can burn more than six hundred calories an hour.[4414] One study concluded, "The metabolic demands required during heavy metal drumming meet the American College of Sports Medicine guidelines for the development of health related fitness."[4415]

The Diving Reflex

Picture walking across a frozen lake and suddenly falling through the ice, plunging into the frigid depths. It's hard to think of a greater instantaneous fight-or-flight shock than that. Noradrenaline would be released, causing the blood vessels in our arms and legs to constrict to bring blood back to our cores. You can just imagine how fast your heart might start racing. That would be counterproductive, though, because you'd use up more oxygen. Remarkably, what happens instead is that your heart rate actually slows down. That's called the *diving reflex,* first described in the 1700s.[4416] Air-breathing animals are born with this automatic safety feature to help keep us from drowning.

In medicine, we can exploit this physiological quirk with what's called a *cold face test.* To test whether a comatose patient has intact neural pathways, you can apply cold compresses to their face and see if their heart immediately starts slowing down.[4417] Or, more dramatically, it can be used to treat people who flip into an abnormally rapid heartbeat.[4418] Remember that episode of *ER* where Carter dunked the patient's face into a tray of ice water? (*ER* was on the air when I was in medical school, and a group of us would gather around and count how many times the doctors and nurses violated "universal precautions.")

What does this have to do with weight loss? The problem with noradrenaline-releasing drugs like ephedra is the accompanying rise in heart rate and blood pressure. What the diving reflex shows is that it's possible to experience *selective* noradrenaline effects, raising the possibility there may be a way to get the metabolic boost without risking stroking out. Unbelievably, this intricate physiological feat may be accomplished by the most simple of acts—instead of nearly drowning in water, simply drink it.

How to Prevent Yourself from Fainting

We know how important it is to stay hydrated, enough so that this book has an entire Hydration section. But did you know that when you drink three or four cups of water, within three minutes, the level of noradrenaline in your bloodstream can shoot up 60 percent?[4419] Have people drink two cups of water with needle electrodes stuck in their legs, and within twenty minutes, you can document about a 40 percent increase in bursts of fight-or-flight nerve activity.[4420] Chug two or three cups of water, and blood flow clamps down in your calves[4421] and arms[4422] as arteries to your limbs and skin[4423] constrict to divert blood to your core. That's why drinking water can be a safe, simple, effective way to prevent fainting.[4424]

Fainting (known medically as *syncope*) is the sudden, brief loss of consciousness caused by diminished blood flow to the brain. About one in five people experience this at least once, and about one in ten may have repeated episodes, causing millions of emergency room visits and hospitalizations every year.[4425] Though fainting can be caused by heart problems, it is most often triggered by prolonged standing, as blood pools in our legs, or by strong emotions, which can cause our blood pressures to bottom out.

About one in twenty-five people has what's called *blood, injury, or injection phobia,* where getting stuck with a needle, for example, can cause you to faint. More than 150,000 people experience fainting or near-fainting spells each year when donating blood.[4426] All you have to do to help prevent yourself from getting woozy, though, is simply chug two cups of water five minutes before you get stuck with the needle.[4427] The secret isn't in bolstering overall blood volume; drinking two cups of water or even a whole quart doesn't change our blood volume more than 1 or 2 percent.[4428] Rather, a fainting spell can be dispelled due to the shift in the distribution of blood toward our centers, caused by the noradrenaline-induced peripheral artery constriction. Might all that noradrenaline help with weight loss in the same way ephedra did, but without the side effects?

Be Still Your Beating Heart

Drinking water stimulates as much of a noradrenaline release as drinking a couple of cups of coffee or smoking a couple of unfiltered cigarettes.[4429] If the simple act of drinking water causes such a profound fight-or-flight reaction, why doesn't it cause your heart to pound and your blood pressure to shoot through the roof? It's like the diving reflex—when you drink water, your body shoots out noradrenaline while simultaneously sending signals to your heart to slow it down. Try this at home: Measure your heart rate before and after drinking two cups of water. Within ten minutes of drinking the water, your heart rate should slow by about four beats per minute, and by fifteen minutes, you should be down six or seven beats.[4430]

One of the ways scientists figured this out is by studying heart transplant patients. When a heart is moved from one person to another, all the attached nerves first have to be severed. Amazingly, some of the nerves can grow back, but even so, give healed heart transplant patients two glasses of water and their blood pressures go up as much as twenty-nine points.[4431] The body is unable to sufficiently quell the effect of that burst of noradrenaline. Some people have a condition known as *autonomic failure,* in which blood pressure regulation nerves don't work properly, and their pressures can skyrocket dangerously more than one hundred points after drinking two cups of water.[4432] That's how powerful an effect the simple act of drinking a glass of water can be, and the only reason that doesn't happen to all of us is that we have an even more powerful counterresponse to keep our hearts in check. It reminds me of the poor woman who had a stroke after taking the ice bucket challenge due to an insufficient diving reflex to tamp down all that extra noradrenaline.[4433]

The remarkable water effect can be useful for people suffering from milder forms of autonomic failure, such as orthostatic hypotension, which causes dizziness when people stand up suddenly. Drinking some water before getting out of bed in the morning can be a big help.[4434] But what about that metabolic boost? With so much noradrenaline being released, might drinking a few glasses of water cause you to burn more body fat? Could tap water be a safe alternative to ephedra, with all the weight loss but a nice slowing of your heart rate instead? Researchers decided to put it to the test.

A Tall Drink of Water

Published in *The Journal of Clinical Endocrinology & Metabolism*,[4435] the study's results were described as "uniquely spectacular."[4436] Drinking two cups of water increased the metabolic rate of men and women by 30 percent. The increase started within ten minutes of water drinking and reached a maximum within an hour. In the ninety minutes after drinking a single tall glass of water, the subjects burned an extra twenty-four calories.[4437] Simply drinking a tall glass of water four times throughout the day would wipe out nearly one hundred extra calories, more than the calories burned by taking weight-loss doses of the now-banned ephedrine three times a day.[4438] Plain, cheap, safe, and legal tap water!

Using the Ten-Calorie Rule I explained in the Intermittent Fasting section, unless we somehow compensated by eating more or moving less, drinking that much water would cause us to lose ten pounds over time. "In essence," concluded one research team, "water drinking provides negative calories."[4439]

A similar effect was found in overweight and obese children. Drinking about two cups of water led to a 25 percent increase in metabolic rate within an hour.[4440] So just getting the recommended, daily "adequate intake" of water—about five cups a day for children aged four through eight and seven cups a day for girls and eight daily cups for boys aged nine through thirteen[4441]—may offer more than just hydration benefits.

Not all research teams were able to replicate these findings, though. Others found only about a 10–20 percent increase,[4442] a 5 percent increase in metabolic rate,[4443] or effectively none at all, pouring cold water on the whole concept.[4444] What we care about, though, is weight loss, and the proof is in the pudding.

Testing the Waters

According to some researchers, "The increase in metabolic rate with water drinking could be systematically applied in the prevention of weight gain."[4445] Talk about a safe, simple, side effect–free solution—in fact, free in every sense. Pharmaceutical companies may spend billions getting a new drug to market.[4446] Surely a little could be spared to test something that, at the very least, couldn't hurt, right? That's the problem, though. Water is a "cost-free intervention."[4447]

As I discussed in the Hydration section, there are observational studies suggesting those who drink four or more cups of water a day, for example, appear to lose more weight independent of confounding factors, such as less soda or more exercise.[4448] As always, you can't really know until you put it to the test.

In 2013, a study entitled "Effect of 'Water Induced Thermogenesis' on Body Weight, Body Mass Index and Body Composition of Overweight Subjects" was published.[4449] Fifty overweight women aged eighteen through twenty-three were asked to drink, over and above their regular water intakes, two cups of water three times a day a half hour before meals without otherwise changing their diets or physical activity. They lost an average of three pounds in eight weeks. What happened to those in the control group? There was no control group, which is a fatal flaw for any weight-loss study, due to the Hawthorne effect, where just knowing you're going to be watched and weighed may subtly affect behavior.[4450] Of course, we're just talking about water, so, with no downsides, you might as well give it a try. Nevertheless, I'd feel more confident if there were some randomized controlled trials to *really* put it to the test. Thankfully, there are.

Overweight and obese men and women randomized to two cups of water before each meal lost nearly five pounds more body fat in twelve weeks than those in the control group.[4451] Both groups were put on a calorie-restricted diet, but the group with the added water lost weight 44 percent faster. A similar randomized controlled trial found that about one in four in the water group lost more than 5 percent of their body weight compared to only one in twenty in the control group.[4452] This is comparable to some commercial weight-loss programs, and all they did was drink a couple of extra cups of water.[4453] The average weight-loss difference was only about three pounds, but those who adhered to the three-times-a-day instructions lost about eight more pounds compared to those who only drank the extra water once a day or less.[4454]

Optimum Dose, Type, and Temperature

A single cup of water may be sufficient to rev up the noradrenaline nerves, but additional benefit is seen at two or more cups.[4455] To get the metabolic boost, do you have to drink straight, plain water? Water is water, whether flavored or sweetened in a diet drink, right? No. When trying to prevent fainting before blood donation, juice doesn't work as well as plain water,[4456] and when trying to keep people from getting dizzy when they stand up, water works, but the same amount of water with salt added doesn't.[4457] What's going on?

We used to think the trigger was stomach distension. When we eat, our bodies shift blood flow to our digestive tracts, in part by releasing noradrenaline to pull in blood from the limbs. This has been called the *gastrovascular reflex*.[4458] So drinking water was thought to be a zero-calorie way of stretching our stomachs. But if you instead drink two cups of saline (essentially salt water), the metabolic boost vanishes, so stomach expansion can't explain the water effect.[4459]

We now realize our bodies appear able to detect osmolarity, the concentration of liquid. You can demonstrate this by monitoring sweat production (used as a proxy for noradrenaline release) after covertly slipping liquids of varying concentrations into people's stomachs via a feeding tube.[4460] This uncanny ability may be a spinal reflex, as it's preserved in quadriplegics,[4461] or picked up by the liver, as we see less noradrenaline release in liver transplant patients who've had their liver nerves severed.[4462] Whichever the pathway, our bodies can tell. Thought we only had five senses? The current count is upward of thirty-three.[4463] (Maybe the Bruce Willis movie should have been called *The Thirty-Fourth Sense!*)

In my Daily Dozen recommendation, I rank certain herbal teas as among the most healthful beverages. After all, they would seem to have all the benefits of water with an antioxidant bonus. But from a weight-loss perspective, plain water may have an edge. One research team even suggested this may help explain the results of a series of diet soda studies I document in the Wall Off Your Calories section.[4464] Basically, overweight and obese individuals randomized to replace diet beverages with water lost significantly more weight.[4465,4466] This was chalked up to getting rid of all those artificial sweeteners, but could it be that the diet drinks were too concentrated to offer the same water-induced metabolic boost? Diet soda, like herbal tea, has about ten times the concentration of dissolved substances compared to tap water.[4467] So plain water on an empty stomach may be best.

Does the temperature of the water matter? In a journal published by the American Society of Mechanical Engineers, an engineering professor proposed that the "secret" of a raw food diet for weight loss was the temperature at which the food was served. To bring two cups of room-temperature water up to body temperature, he calculated the body would have to dip into its fat stores and use up about six thousand calories. But his math was faulty.[4468] In nutrition, a "calorie" is actually a kilocalorie, a thousand times bigger than the same word used in the rest of the sciences. Confusing, right? Still, I'm shocked the submission was published.

Drinking two cups of water at room temperature actually only takes six calories to warm up to body temperature, not six thousand. If you were a hummingbird drinking four times your body weight in chilly nectar, you could burn up to 2 percent of your energy reserves warming up the nectar,[4469] but it doesn't make as much of a difference for us. What about really cold water, though? A letter called "The Ice Diet" published in the *Annals of Internal Medicine* estimated that eating a quart of ice—like a really, really big snow cone without syrup—could rob our bodies of more than 150 calories, the "same amount of energy as the calorie expenditure in running 1 mile."[4470] You don't directly burn fat to warm up the water, though. What our bodies do is just corral more of the waste heat we normally give off by constricting blood flow to our skin.[4471] How do they do that? Noradrenaline!

If you compare drinking body-temperature water to room-temperature water to cold water, a significant constriction in blood flow to the skin occurs only after drinking room-temperature water and cold water, and neither the warm nor tepid water could boost metabolic rate as much as cold (fridge temperature) water.[4472] So it turns out our bodies do end up—at least indirectly—burning off more calories when we drink our water cold.

Food for Thought

Drink two cups of cold water on an empty stomach a few times a day. Does it matter when? I'll cover that question in the Negative Calorie Preloading section.

Caution: Never drink more than three cups in an hour, since that starts to exceed the amount of fluid our kidneys can handle.[4473] If you have kidney or heart failure, your physician may not want you drinking extra water at all, but even with healthy kidneys, any more than three cups an hour can critically dilute the electrolytes in your brain with potentially critical consequences. (The first patient I ever lost in the hospital was a man who tragically drank himself to death—with water. He suffered from a neurological condition that causes pathological thirst. I knew enough to order his liquids be restricted and shut off his sink, but didn't think to turn off his toilet.)

Note if you're on a beta-blocker drug, the entire strategy may fail. If you give people the drug metoprolol (sold as Lopressor) before they chug their two cups of water, the metabolic boost is almost completely prevented.[4474] This makes sense since the "beta" being blocked are the beta receptors triggered by noradrenaline. Beta blockers are often prescribed for heart conditions or high blood pressure, and typically end with the letters *lol,* such as *atenolol, nadolol,* or *propranolol,* sold as Tenormin, Corgard, or Inderal, respectively.

MILD TRENDELENBURG

The Way to a Person's Stomach Is Through the Heart

In the Hydration section, I detailed what happens when our kidneys detect a drop in blood volume. What happens when our blood capacity expands? Upswings in blood volume are detected by our hearts, which, in response, release a hormone called *atrial natriuretic factor,* or *ANF.* We used to think the heart was just a pump, but we now know it's a gland too. There are stretch receptors in the first chamber of the heart that can detect when excess blood pours in, triggering the release of ANF directly into the bloodstream. What does the hormone do? As the title of a review in an obesity journal puts it: "Heart Hormones Fueling a Fire in Fat."[4475]

If you drip ANF on human fat and muscle tissue, fat is released rapidly[4476] and muscle cells ramp up their capacity to burn it.[4477] Infuse ANF into people, and the rate at which fat is mobilized and burned can bump up by 15 percent.[4478] You can take muscle biopsies from people and show how much better their muscles burn fat in the presence of elevated ANF levels.[4479] No surprise, then, that obese and overweight individuals tend to have considerably lower levels in their bloodstreams.[4480]

Why would this stretch-sensitive heart hormone tap into our fat stores? Well, when does the heart get stretched? During intense physical activity. We used to think adrenaline-type hormones were released when we exercise to mobilize fat from our tissues, but we now know ANF from our hearts also plays a key role.[4481] If you inject people with the amount of ANF they'd normally get in their systems by exercising, their whole-body-fat burning goes up even if they're just lounging on the couch.[4482]

How else can we stretch our hearts that extra little bit to release ANF? By expanding our blood volume through drinking extra water.[4483] If you don't drink any water for twelve hours straight, the ANF levels in your blood may fall by about 25 percent,[4484] but if you chug about four glasses of water, your levels can jump 50 percent within ninety minutes.[4485] That's too much to drink at one time,[4486] but it can offer a sense of how much potential control we have over this fat-burning hormone.

A New Slant on Weight Loss

How else might we trick our bodies into producing this "exercise hormone" without lacing up our gym shoes? If it's all about pooling extra blood into our hearts, what about lying down at an angle with your head lower than your feet? It sounds a little funny, but researchers took the possibility seriously enough to run the experiment. They laid people on a slanted surface with their heads down at a six-degree angle, which is enough of a tilt for gravity to pull extra blood up into their torsos. Within an hour, their ANF levels doubled and stayed elevated for the four hours the experiment lasted. Did they suddenly start burning more fat? Yes, the proportion of fat they were burning as fuel shot up by 40 percent—and they were just lying down the whole time.[4487]

Certainly, if you have a heart condition, such as congestive heart failure, you won't want to lie tilted back. As many as eight to twelve cups of blood may be displaced into the torso from the extremities,[4488] so you have to have the cardiovascular fitness to handle that. Acid reflux could also be a problem. In fact, we typically tell heartburn patients to do the reverse and put a few bricks under the posts at the *head* of their beds to have gravity work in their favor to keep stomach acid down where it belongs. But for those without medical problems, is there a harm in lying tilted back for a few hours? Well, it could give you a "space headache."

It *Is* Rocket Science

In movies, astronauts are shown training underwater, but the gold standard for simulating the physiological effects of the weightlessness of outer space is HDTBR, head-down-tilt bed rest.[4489] On Earth, our blood tends to collect in our legs, so our bodies are designed to force blood headward. In outer space, our bodies still try to push our blood "up," but without Earth's gravity, blood pushes upward in our heads and chests, just as it does when we lie tilted back. This realization came from cosmonauts returning from the space station feeling as though they were slipping toward the foot of the bed and only feeling "normal" when they were tilted back six degrees.

All the extra blood pooling in the head is thought to contribute to the headaches reported by up to 70 percent of astronauts during spaceflights, and a similar percentage of individuals suffer headaches from prolonged head-down-tilt bed rest. This was after days, though. In preparation for a Mars mission,[4490] space agencies put people through head-down-tilt bed rest for prolonged periods, having subjects eating, bathing, and toileting all while lying in bed tilted back for literally months at a time.[4491]

Extended stretches for weeks may impair brain,[4492] lung,[4493] and immune function[4494] and cause a loss of muscle mass.[4495] On the last Apollo mission, the astronauts lost about five pounds of fat over the twelve-day trip, but they also lost about two pounds of lean body mass.[4496] Prolonged weightlessness or bed rest, regardless of tilt, can result in muscle and bone loss,[4497] but simply sleeping on a slant for a few hours could theoretically offer the boost in fat metabolism without the long-term adverse effects.

The Pressure to Succeed

Do *not* try this at home if you have any heart or lung issues or problems with your brain (like head trauma) or eyes[4498] (even a family history of glaucoma disqualifies you). And first ask your physician if they think it's safe for you to sleep in "mild Trendelenburg." Friedrich Trendelenburg was a pioneering surgeon who popularized the use of what was formerly referred to as *head-down position* for certain abdominal and pelvic procedures. Angling the operating table back fifteen to thirty degrees pulls some abdominal organs out of the way to help declutter the surgical field, resulting in what is now widely known as the *Trendelenburg position.*[4499]

Steep Trendelenburg (twenty-five or thirty degrees) has been associated with transient visual problems, thought due to the increase in pressure within the eyeball.[4500] Cautions have been issued for those at risk for glaucoma, a disease of increased eye pressure, to avoid "inversion" therapy, where people hang upside down,[4501] as well as yoga positions like headstands that can have a similar effect.[4502]

Lying back in mild Trendelenburg (less than fifteen degrees) can cause a fleeting bump in eye pressure[4503] that normalizes within a few hours,[4504] but the pooling of blood in the head may reduce blood flow to the retina[4505] sufficient to impair nerve impulses.[4506] Similar effects have been noted within the brain. Intracranial pressure normalizes after a few hours at a six-degree head-down tilt,[4507] but the uphill outflow of blood through the jugular veins slows.[4508] This is why you should skip this booster if you have eye or brain pathology.

Good to the Bone

Sleeping in mild Trendelenburg was actually put to the test to prevent bone loss in sedentary individuals. Restrict people's activity to under an average of two miles of walking a day, and, within a year, they can lose as much as 15 percent of their bone mineral density. What happened to those randomized to the same exercise restriction but combined with sleeping first at a two-degree head-down tilt, which was increased by two degrees about every two months so they ended up at the end of the year sleeping at a fourteen-degree slant (or at whatever angle they found comfortable)? Not only did it completely block the bone loss, they built *more* bone. Despite the movement restriction, they ended up with about 12 percent greater bone mineral density than when they had started. Note this bone-building effect was only apparent in sedentary individuals. Another group randomized to the same mild Trendelenburg but also assigned to run an average of five or six miles a day just maintained their same skeletal integrity.[4509]

The study was repeated, and the same remarkable effects were found. There is something about the "periodic fluid redistribution" that comes with sleeping tilted back at night that actively builds both bone density and volume after the daylong stagnant pooling of blood in the legs in sedentary individuals.

The research team claims this is just the beginning to the benefits, citing "unpublished studies" asserting a near panacea of perks to sleeping in Trendelenburg.[4510] I can't be too critical of this apparent dodge when I can't point to a single study supporting my supposition that it will help with weight loss. As far as I can tell, tilting the scales with a head-down tilt has never been tried or even proposed. What I can promise is that any researchers who take up the gauntlet of putting it to the test will definitely have their study featured in a video on NutritionFacts.org!

FOOD FOR THOUGHT

If you want to try losing weight like an astronaut, you can try putting three or four bricks under the posts at the foot of your bed to achieve those six degrees of separation from the floor. Expect to experience symptoms such as stuffiness in the nose or ears and puffiness in the face[4511] (a common occurrence among astronauts[4512]).

My biggest concern, however, is the orthostatic intolerance I talked about in the Metabolic Boosters section. You know how sometimes when you stand suddenly after sitting or lying down for a while you can get a head rush and feel dizzy, faint, or light-headed? This is thought to be because the blood drains from your brain down into your legs before your body has a chance to compensate for the change in position. This can be exacerbated by lying with your head tilted back, so you need to be careful and get up gradually. After four hours of a six-degree head-down tilt, most people experience these symptoms if they get up too fast.[4513] Though it may be impractical, drinking two cups of cold water thirty minutes before rising may also help.[4514]

At a six-degree tilt, the 50 percent rise in fat-burning ANF occurs within the first four hours and then starts to drop back down to baseline once your heart gets used to the new normal, so you may be able to get the full benefits sleeping just half the night at that angle.[4515] If this really works for weight loss, maybe someone will design a bed that slowly dips you down for a couple of hours and then brings you back up. Again, just be really careful and take it slowly when stand-ing back up, and don't try this at all if you have any issues with your heart, lungs, brain (such as head trauma), or eyes (or even a family history of glaucoma). And make sure to ask your physician if they think it's safe for you to sleep in mild Trendelenburg.

NEGATIVE CALORIE PRELOADING

Timing of Water Before Meals

When timed properly, drinking water may be able to affect both sides of the calorie-balance equation. In the Metabolic Boosters section, I explored how drinking two cups of water could increase the calories-out side of the equa-tion. If we time it right before a meal, might we fill ourselves up enough to cut down on the calories-in side too?

Older obese men and women were randomized to drink about two cups of water thirty minutes before a buffet-style meal.[4516] Compared to no pre-load, the water group ate 13 percent less, resulting in seventy-four fewer calories consumed, but this may only work for older individuals. A study of young adults found they ate a similar amount whether or not they preloaded with water thirty minutes before the meal.[4517] This discrepancy was pre-sumed to be because stomach emptying slows when we get older. It takes about a third longer for liquids to empty from our stomachs as we age, keep-ing us fuller for longer.[4518] Give some young whippersnappers a few cups of water, and in just ten minutes, half is nearly gone. After thirty minutes, nearly 90 percent of it has already drained out of the stomach.[4519] Okay, so what if you don't wait a half hour?

What if you give young adults two cups of water immediately before a meal? Do they then eat less? Indeed, they eat about 20 percent less, taking in more than one hundred fewer calories.[4520] Is this why overweight men and women randomized to two cups of water before each meal lost weight 44 percent faster?[4521] Not entirely. They may have been taking in slightly fewer calories, but not enough to explain the five extra pounds of body fat the water group lost.[4522] So the metabolic boost from water intake may be the main effect, but if you're going to drink two cups of water a few times every day, you might as well do it before meals to take the added advantage of its stomach-filling effect.

Sparkling or Still?

If it's all about filling up your stomach, wouldn't sparkling water work even better than still? One cup of highly carbonated water can release nearly four cups of gas, so it's no surprise sparkling water makes you feel fuller than drinking the same volume of still water.[4523] But does that translate into eating less?

The first study to put it to the test found that drinking a high-fizz beverage (carbonated close to the level one might find in tonic water) ten minutes before a meal resulted in 15 percent lower caloric intake than preloading with a low-fizz beverage (carbonated to the level one might find in lightly carbonated fruit drinks). The effects of a medium-fizz beverage (carbonated to the level one might find in colas) was less consistent.[4524] A subsequent study, however, found no difference between a higher-fizz drink and one that was completely flat.[4525] That study only used a 300 ml preload (about 1¼ cups), though, whereas the first study used 400 ml (more like 1⅔ cups), which would mean about 1½ cups more gas in the stomach, but it's unclear if this plays a role in explaining the contradictory findings.

Another potential factor favoring fizz is the oral sensory stimulation. Remember in the Eating Rate section how that helped explain the satiating effects of prolonged chewing? What could be more stimulating than the effervescent tingle of all those bubbles? When people "sham drink" club soda, spitting it out rather than swallowing it, they experience a temporary feeling of fullness in their stomachs even though they didn't drink anything.[4526] The craziest such study involved measuring the temperatures of people's toes.

If you have people drink a glass of regular water, the temperature of their toes drops about 5°F within thirty minutes. Why? Because of that release of noradrenaline constricting peripheral blood flow. Even just swishing carbonated water in our mouths, though, can have nearly the same effect.[4527] This suggests sparkling water may have a metabolic edge, but it has never been tested directly. What matters in the end is weight loss, and as of yet, there haven't been any studies comparing sparkling water to still.

Aperitif?

Carbonated or not, drinking a beverage that has calories as a preload could defeat the purpose. Even high-protein beverages, such as liquid yogurt or chocolate skim milk, which were presumed to be satiating, didn't reduce subsequent meal intake any more than did, respectively, a chocolate bar[4528] and Coca-Cola.[4529] Given that, they would be expected to increase total caloric intake in the end.[4530] Alcoholic beverages, however, may be even worse.

Not only does alcohol carry its own calories, it may end up increasing intake. I mean, the whole purported point of an aperitif is to stimulate appetite. When people drink a glass of wine or beer before lunch, they may eat more food than if they had drunk the same volume and calories of grape juice and other nonalcoholic beverages.[4531] Those drinking a beer with quadruple the regular alcohol content ate two hundred calories more at a subsequent meal compared to those drinking a regular beer—and that was above and beyond the beer's own calories.[4532] So it's like a reverse-preload effect that just makes things worse.

At that level of alcohol intake, judgment may be affected as well. Women given about one shot of vodka were covertly observed eating nearly 50 percent more chocolate chip cookies in one study, which was chalked up more to a loss of control than an increase in appetite.[4533] Even if alcohol had a neutral effect on consumption, it would still pile on its own calories.[4534] That's one of the benefits of a zero-calorie preload like water.

What About Fiber Supplements?

Higher-fiber foods are more satiating for all the reasons I laid out in the High in Fiber-Rich Foods section. Preload people with a chicken appetizer, for example, and they eat significantly more at the subsequent meal than after eating the same appetizer made with more fiber-rich options, either tofu or a meat-free chicken (Quorn).[4535] What if you just gave people straight fiber isolated into pills or powders?

The data on fiber supplements for weight loss have been inconsistent[4536] and largely disappointing.[4537] Randomizing people to mix sachets of wheat bran with water before meals didn't seem to help,[4538] and neither did water mixed with alginate, the main type of fiber in brown seaweed.[4539] Even in studies showing an advantage, the benefits were relatively modest—for example, less than a pound a month in those randomized to eat a total of fifteen daily grams of yellow split pea fiber thirty minutes before meals.[4540]

Have you seen those shirataki noodles? They are translucent, gelatinous strands made from a fiber derived from the konjac plant (also known as *voodoo lily, snake palm,* and *devil's tongue*). Their claim to fame is that they can be up to 97 percent water and boast as few as ten calories per serving. With so few calories, they might seem like a good candidate for a negative-calorie preload, which I define as one that contributes fewer calories than it reduces. In actuality, though, they don't seem to result in a reduction of subsequent caloric intake.[4541] If you do eat them, please chew thoroughly, as they can gum together and cause a stomach outlet obstruction requiring surgical intervention.[4542] (And while we're on the subject, never let kids slurp down those little fruit-flavored konjac gel cups often sold in Asian markets.[4543] Though they've been banned for sale in Australia, Europe, and the United States for choking children to death, they can still be found on store shelves.[4544])

What about PGX, a favorite of diet doctors who also, not so coincidentally, sell it? PGX is short for *PolyGlycopleX,* a brand name for α-D-glucurono-α-D-manno-β-D-manno-β-D-glucan, α-Lgulurono-β-D-mannuronan, β-D-gluco-β-D-mannan, α-D-glucurono-α-D-manno-β-D-manno-β-D-gluco, α-L-gulurono-β-D-mannurono, β-D-gluco-β-D-mannan.[4545] PGX is a designer fiber created through a patented process purported to produce some special properties, but even most of the manufacturer-sponsored trials failed to show weight-loss benefits.[4546] One study that did—six pounds lost in twelve months—failed to beat out psyllium,[4547] a fiber supplement that's more than ten times cheaper.

Sold generically and under the brand name Metamucil, psyllium has been shown to decrease body weight up to four pounds in twelve weeks when taken with a cup of water before each meal. Study subjects just advised to eat more healthfully lost as much weight, though, and there was no additional benefit found for psyllium on top of healthier eating advice.[4548] By six months, however, a different study found that twice-a-day psyllium preloading could edge out healthier eating advice by about five pounds.[4549] One of the reasons all that extra fiber may not have worked better is that psyllium isn't fermented in the human gut like the fiber found in whole foods, so we may miss out on all the auxiliary microbiome benefits of high-fiber diets.[4550]

"Negative Calorie" Salads

A bona fide "negative caloric effect"[4551] is easy for water because it doesn't provide any calories of its own. If drinking water gets us to eat just one fewer calorie or burn just one more calorie, then we're left with fewer calories to store as fat. And remember: It wasn't just one fewer calorie, but up to one hundred fewer calories consumed after drinking two cups of water. If preloads can have such a dramatic effect on intake, then what about filling up at the beginning of a meal with low-calorie-density foods?

Celery is the classic example of a food with lots of bulk with few calories, due to its high fiber and water content. There's even a myth that celery contains fewer calories than the energy required for our bodies to digest it. A cup of celery, about two stalks, has sixteen calories. Digesting that much celery takes about fourteen calories.[4552] So, no: The consumption of celery does not induce a negative-energy balance, but you are only left with two calories. If eating a cup of celery before a meal led you to eat even three fewer calories, then celery could end up providing "negative calories" after all.

In a famous series of experiments, researchers at Penn State decided to put water-rich vegetables to the test. Study subjects were served a pasta meal for lunch and told to eat as much or as little as they'd like. On average, they consumed about nine hundred calories. What do you think would happen if as a first course you gave them one hundred calories of salad composed largely of lettuce, carrots, cherry tomatoes, celery, and cucumber? Would they go on to eat the same amount of pasta and end up with a thousand-calorie lunch? Or would they eat one hundred fewer calories of pasta, effectively canceling out the added salad calories? It was even better than that. They ate more than two hundred fewer calories of pasta.[4553] One hundred calories in; two hundred calories out. So, in essence, the salad had *negative one hundred* calories.

Preloading with vegetables can effectively subtract one hundred calories out of our diets. That's how you can lose weight by eating more food.

Of course, the kind of salad matters. The researchers repeated the experiment, adding a fatty dressing and extra shredded cheese, which quadrupled the salad's calorie density. Eating this version of the salad as a first course didn't turn the nine-hundred-calorie meal into one with fewer than eight hundred calories. Instead, it turned it into a meal with calories in the quadruple digits.[4554] It's like preloading pizza with garlic bread. You could end up with more calories overall, whereas a pre-pizza salad may cut calories even more than preloading with water,[4555] presumably in part because of the combination of water and fiber in vegetables.

We've learned from studies on preloading that eating about a cup of food before a meal decreases subsequent intake by about one hundred calories, so to get a "negative calorie" effect, the preload has to contain fewer than one hundred calories per cup.[4556,4557] As you can see in the Calories per Cup chart in the Low in Calorie Density section, that would include most fresh fruits and vegetables. So is that it? Are we simply diluting the calories of a meal by adding low-calorie-density foods, or does the timing matter? To figure that out, you'd have to randomize people to either preload with a salad before a meal or eat that same salad during a meal, and that's exactly what researchers did.

Those on a diet randomized to eat a preload of a salad comprised mostly of vegetables fifteen minutes before lunch and dinner for three months lost four more pounds than the group given the same extra foods, but with instructions they be eaten alongside their meals and not before.[4558] This showed that the "negative-calorie"-preload strategy can indeed lead to weight loss, and the effect appears to extend beyond merely adding more low-calorie-density foods. That actually may be one of the secrets of preloading, though. It's thought that preloading works by allowing time for our satiety hormones to start ramping up before we dive into the main meal. By frontloading the most healthful foods first, when you're hungriest, you may also eat more of them.[4559] Those given a salad before a meal ate more salad than when it was competing for their attention during the meal.[4560] So part of the magic of preloading may indeed lie in eating more low-calorie-density foods after all.

Celery Sun Rash

A warning for those who eat a lot of celery, celery juice, or celeriac (celery root): There are compounds called *psoralens* in the celery/parsnip/parsley family that can make you sensitive to sunlight.[4561] Without skin protection, farmworkers can suffer from a condition known as *celery blisters* when handling the plants in the sun,[4562] and even grocery store workers who go from the produce aisle to the tanning salon can get into trouble.[4563] These compounds can make their way into our skin from the inside out as well, and they are not destroyed by cooking. So too much time in the sun after commencing a "celery soup diet"[4564] or spending time in a tanning bed an hour after eating just one large celery root may be enough to result in a serious blistering burn.[4565]

Apple-tizer

What about a fruit salad? We've explored preloading with water and vegetables, but what about fruits? Give people a large apple to eat before that same pasta meal instead of the salad, and rather than consuming about two hundred fewer calories, they consumed more than *three hundred* fewer calories.[4566] So how many calories does an apple have? *It depends on when you eat it.* Before a meal, it may effectively have negative two hundred calories!

Baked and puréed, the same amount of apples preloaded in the form of applesauce only knocked out about two hundred calories from the meal, but that still left people with about a one-hundred-calorie deficit.[4567] Preload experiments with other fruits weren't as successful. Kiwifruit didn't beat out white rice,[4568] melon didn't do much better than cheese and crackers,[4569] and about a cup of fruit smoothie or mixed fruit salad did no better than about the same volume of water in decreasing subsequent intake.[4570] The proof is in the pudding, though. What about weight loss over time?

There was that premeal tomato study showing weight loss that I discussed in the Inflammation Quenchers section, but tomatoes are more often viewed as vegetables. There was also the study that showed that adding three apples or three pears to people's daily diets decreased body weights compared to adding the same number of calories and amount of fiber in oat cookie form, but participants were just told to consume the fruits as snacks between meals, so the timing is unclear.[4571] Those told to eat half a grapefruit three times a day before meals lost as much weight as those in the apple and pear study—a few pounds in a few months—but no more than preloading instead with half cups of water.[4572] This would seem to confirm that it is but a "long-held myth"[4573] that grapefruits have any sort of special fat-burning property, but one could argue that the grapefruit might have had a bit of an edge since it produced roughly the same weight loss, even while adding about 125 calories a day.[4574]

Soup's On! Weight's Off?

The United States is not a nation of soup eaters. Even during the winter months, most Americans don't eat soup more than a few times a month, whereas in France, for example, about half eat soup at least a few times a week[4575] and in Japan, the average is soup every day.[4576] In the United States, soup eaters tend to be slimmer on average[4577] and significantly less likely to be overweight,[4578] but as I discussed in the Low in Calorie Density section, soup eaters also tend to consume healthier diets (with the exception of excess sodium).[4579]

When put to the test, those randomized to eat more soup lost up to 50 percent more weight,[4580] but those weren't preload studies. It's like the water and apples—soup anytime is good, but it may work even better right before a meal. If you feed someone a radioactive omelet—that is, one with the egg labeled with an isotope to track it with a gamma-ray camera through the body—those randomized to precede it with about a cup and a half of soup slowed stomach emptying by about 25 percent.[4581] This may be why those who have soup as a first course eat so much less throughout the rest of the meal.

Let's go back to the preeminent preloaded pasta experiments. With no first course, about 900 calories were eaten. When people were given about two cups of vegetable soup totaling around 150 calories before the meal, they ate about 250 fewer calories of pasta.[4582] So a healthy soup, like the healthy salad, can end up offering negative 100 calories. A similar study that tracked people's intake throughout the day found that overweight subjects randomized to prelunch vegetable soup deducted an additional 100 calories at dinner, too, a whole seven hours later.[4583] So the next time you sit down to some soup, you can imagine calories being veritably sucked out of your system with every spoonful. Vegetable soup would seem to be the perfect weight-loss food.

Similar results were found for young children. Without any soup, the kids ate about 400 calories of mac 'n cheese. When they first started their meals with about a half cup of tomato soup, though, they ate about 100 fewer calories of mac 'n cheese.[4584] Since the soup only contained about 50 calories, it effectively subtracted, rather than added, calories to their diets when used as a first course.

There's just something special about soup. If you give people about 250 calories of a casserole and a glass of water before eating a buffet meal, they eat about 250 fewer calories at the buffet, effectively just swapping the different foods, calorie for calorie. But take that same casserole and glass of water and blend them into a soup, and once again serve it before the same buffet meal, people went on to eat 350 fewer calories at the buffet. Same calories, same ingredients, same food, but they were just as satiated eating 100 fewer calories when eaten as a soup.[4585] Is it simply because soup takes longer to eat? No, the researchers made people eat the actual casserole and the soupified casserole at the same rate. So it's not that soup is just salty or served hotter or eaten slower. It could be cognitive factors: Soup seems to be perceived as being particularly filling.[4586] It may be the sieving effect I talked about in the High in Water-Rich Foods section.[4587] We aren't quite sure, but we do know there's just something special about soup.

FOOD FOR THOUGHT

Starting a meal with foods containing fewer than one hundred calories per cup can result in fewer overall calories consumed. This includes many fruits, vegetables, soups, salads, or simply a tall glass of water.

SLEEP ENHANCEMENT

Epidemic Proportions or Distortions?

Conventional wisdom has it that over the last fifty years or so, sleep duration has declined in parallel with the increasing prevalence of obesity, suggesting that an epidemic of sleep loss is associated with the epidemic of weight gain.[4588] Today, our triple-digit TV channels, personal computers, smartphones, and tablets keep us entertained well into the night. "The hurry and excitement of modern life is quite correctly held to be responsible for much of the insomnia," concluded one medical journal editorial.[4589] But that was an editorial published in 1894. Are we really sleeping that much less?

Over the last century, sleep duration in children and adolescents has declined by an average of nearly two hours.[4590] Child labor wasn't outlawed until 1938, though, so much of that may be due to the exhaustion of sweating it out in mines, farms, and factories in the early part of the last century.[4591] Indeed, sleep duration in youth has declined only about fifteen minutes per night, and it's not clear it's changed much at all in adults. Based on 168 studies of objective measurements of sleep duration (instead of just self-report), sleep duration in adults has remained relatively steady since 1960.[4592] If anything, since 2003, average sleep duration in the United States even seems to have gone up.[4593]

Just because we don't have evidence there has been a growing epidemic of sleep deprivation doesn't necessarily mean we're getting enough sleep.[4594] Maybe we weren't getting enough sleep fifty years ago either, or since the advent of Edison's light bulbs, or since candles were invented about five thousand years ago. How might we determine the optimal sleep duration? One way would be to study millions of people and see how many hours a night is associated with the longest life span.

Sleeping in the Sweet Spot

Sleep is a great mystery. A trait shared across animal species, sleep must be of vital importance to survive natural selection pressures to eliminate such a vulnerable state.[4595] Indeed, cringeworthy experiments have shown that keeping animals awake long enough can be fatal within eleven to thirty-two days.[4596] One function of sleep that has been elucidated in recent years is the clearance of toxic waste substances[4597] through a newly discovered drainage system in the brain.[4598] This could help explain why those who routinely get fewer than seven hours of sleep a night are at increased risk of developing cognitive disorders such as dementia.[4599] Even a single all-nighter can cause a significant increase in accumulation of beta amyloid, a gummy substance implicated in the development of Alzheimer's disease, in critical brain areas.[4600]

The lowest risk for developing cognitive impairment was found for those getting seven to eight hours of sleep a night, based on nine studies following twenty-two thousand people for up to twenty-two years.[4601] The same range was found for diabetes, based on thirty-six studies following more than a million people, with increasing risk found for those sleeping either six hours a night or less, or nine hours a night or more. Remarkably, the increased risk associated with getting six hours of sleep a night versus seven hours is comparable to the increase in diabetes risk linked to physical inactivity.[4602]

For death from all causes combined, there have been more than fifty studies following more than three million people for up to thirty-four years. Sleeping too little and for too long are both associated with cutting one's life short, with the apparent sweet spot at seven hours a night.[4603] Seven hours may seem short, but that may actually be what's natural for our species. Scientists studied three isolated preindustrial societies across two continents and found a surprising uniformity. Despite no electric lighting or electronic gadgets, they stayed up until approximately three hours after sunset and then typically rose before dawn, accumulating about a solid six and a half hours of sleep out of about seven and a half hours in "bed."[4604]

A mechanism by which excess sleep might be harmful remains elusive, so the association between increased risk of death and disease with sleeping nine or more hours a night has largely been dismissed as implausible.[4605] Could it be reverse causation, like sickness leading to more time in bed instead of vice versa, or confounding factors such as employment status?[4606] After all, who tends to sleep in? Those without a job. There is, however, experimental evidence showing negative health effects from insufficient sleep, including weight gain.

Midnight Munchies

Population studies have found short sleep duration has been associated with obesity in both children[4607] and adults.[4608] Observational studies can never prove cause and effect, though. Maybe the obesity is leading to sleep loss instead of the other way around. Obesity can cause arthritis, acid reflux, and apnea, all of which can interfere with sleep.[4609] The relationship between obesity and sleep apnea, where breathing repeatedly stops and starts throughout the night, may be explained by increased tongue fat—fat deposited inside the base of the tongue. This may contribute to obstructing your airway when sleeping on your back.[4610] The reverse causation explanation of the link between obesity and inadequate sleep is bolstered by the findings that weight-loss interventions can improve daytime sleepiness.[4611]

Potential confounding factors also abound. For example, people with lower socioeconomic status often work less desirable hours, such as rotating or overnight shifts,[4612] or may live in noisier neighborhoods with lesser air quality.[4613] The link between inadequate sleep and obesity persists after controlling for these factors,[4614] but you can't control for everything. You can't know for certain if sleep deprivation leads to weight gain until you put it to the test.

If you have people pull an all-nighter, they get hungrier[4615] and choose larger portions.[4616] If you randomize people to shave off a couple of hours of sleep every night, they can start eating an average of 677 more calories a day compared to the normal-sleep control group.[4617] Although individual responses vary widely—anywhere from eating 813 fewer calories per day to as many as 1,437 more calories—on average,[4618] sleep deprivation tends to lead people to overeat by about 180–560 calories a day.[4619]

Restrict people's sleep, and they also start craving unhealthier choices: more snacks[4620] and more sugary and fatty foods.[4621] And if you stick people in a brain scanner after staying awake all night[4622] or after a few nights of four hours of sleep,[4623] their reward pathways light up brighter in response to high-calorie foods. Sleep deprivation bumps up the levels of the chief endocannabinoid in the body, the natural chemical we synthesize that binds to the same receptors as an active ingredient in marijuana.[4624] This may help explain the nighttime nibbling.

On the calories-out side of the equation, some short sleepers may take the extra time to exercise, while others will be so sleepy they exercise less.[4625] The extra wakefulness may raise calorie expenditures up to about one hundred calories a day,[4626] but if sleep-deprived individuals are overeating hundreds of calories, over time, sleep deprivation may end up putting the "wide" in wide awake.[4627]

Sleep Less, Gain More

With insufficient sleep inadvertently leading to such higher caloric intake, it's no surprise that four out of five studies involving as few as two to five nights of sleep restriction found an increase in body weight.[4628] Even if you control caloric intake, though, you still lose more fat when you get more sleep.

In an NIH-funded study performed at the University of Chicago Sleep Research Laboratory, overweight subjects who normally got between six and a half to eight and a half hours of sleep a night were randomized to either eight and a half hours of sleep a night or five and a half hours on the same calorie-controlled diet. After two weeks, the groups switched and spent another two weeks on the opposite regimen. They spent a month living in the lab so their diets and sleep could be totally controlled and monitored. By just looking at the scale, sleep duration didn't seem to matter. During both two-week periods, the subjects ate the same number of calories and lost the same amount of weight, but most of the weight lost when getting eight and a half hours of sleep a night was fat, whereas most of the weight lost when only getting five and a half hours was lean body mass. With the same diet but more sleep, they ended up losing more than twice as much body fat.[4629]

To get better insight into what was going on, researchers took fat and muscle biopsies from people after a night of sleep loss. In terms of the genes that were being turned on and off by the sleep deprivation, molecular signatures were discovered suggesting muscle breakdown and fat buildup.[4630] That was after an all-nighter, though, and in the weight-loss study, the sleep-restricted groups ended up getting little more than five hours a night.[4631] What about a more realistic scenario?

Overweight adults were randomized to eight weeks of either a calorie-restricted diet or the same diet combined with five days a week of one less hour of sleep a night. The sleep-restricted group slept one less hour each night on weekdays and ended up sleeping one more on weekend days. So, overall, they just cut about three hours of sleep out of their week. Was that enough to result in any weight-loss difference? On the scale, no, but in the normal sleep group, 80 percent of the weight loss was fat, whereas in the group missing a few hours of sleep a week, it was the opposite with 80 percent of the loss being lean body mass.[4632] This shows that a few hours of "catch-up sleep" on the weekends is insufficient. Indeed, it may in fact be contributing to the problem based on the social jet lag effect I described in the Chronobiology section.

A comparable study was designed for kids, but the sleeping periods only lasted a week. Eight- to eleven-year-olds were randomized to either increase or decrease their time in bed by ninety minutes per night for a week and then switch the following week. On the days they slept less, they ate an average of 134 more calories and gained about a half pound compared to the sleep-more week.[4633] The exciting question then becomes: Would sleeping more facilitate weight loss?

Sleep It Off

A benefit of interventional studies is that they can demonstrate cause and effect, but observational studies can more easily allow for the tracking of people and their behaviors over a longer time span. In one such study, researchers followed a group of mostly overweight individuals for six years. At the start of the study, the subjects averaged fewer than six hours of sleep a night. During the five years of the study, however, about half maintained that schedule, but the other half increased their sleep duration up to seven or eight hours a night and ended up gaining five fewer pounds of fat.[4634] A study entitled "Sleeping Habits Predict the Magnitude of Fat Loss in Adults Exposed to Moderate Caloric Restriction" found that every extra hour of sleep at night was associated with an extra one and a half pounds of weight loss over a period of about three to six months.[4635] That's not the same as randomizing people to extra sleep, though. Maybe the subjects were sleeping more because they were exercising more, and that was the real reason they lost more weight. That's why we need randomized controlled trials.

Getting people to bump up their sleep from about five and a half hours to seven can lead to an overall decrease in appetite within two weeks, particularly for sugary and salty foods.[4636] A four-week study randomizing habitually short sleepers to sleep about an extra hour a night led them to consume about two fewer spoonfuls' worth of sugar a day compared to the control group, but this didn't translate into any changes in body composition.[4637] A twelve-week study that randomized overweight and obese individuals to a weight-loss intervention with or without a sleep component, on the other hand, found that the sleep group lost weight significantly faster.[4638]

A six-month randomized trial to improve household routines for obesity prevention among young children resulted in a lower BMI.[4639] A national cross-sectional survey had suggested lower obesity rates among kids in households where they regularly ate dinner together as a family, got adequate sleep, and limited screen times,[4640] so Harvard researchers decided to put those behaviors to the test. Normally, it's hard to tease out the effects of multicomponent interventions, but in this case, exhortations to limit overall TV watching didn't work, and the families were already eating together six days a week. The only component the researchers were able to get the kids to alter significantly was their sleep, so the improved weight outcomes may be attributed at least in part to the three-quarters of an hour average increase in nightly slumber.[4641]

Overall, most sleep improvement interventions tend to show improved weight loss, giving a positive spin to the phrase *You snooze, you lose*.[4642] I was intrigued, though, to look up the one study in a published systematic review that failed to show a benefit. The nice thing about systematic reviews—unlike so-called narrative reviews—is that they exhaustively include mention of every study that meets some prespecified criteria. While this keeps reviewers from cherry-picking, it can also lead to the inclusion of some strange studies. Case in point: a randomized controlled trial of playing the didgeridoo, the indigenous Australian wind instrument. Those randomized to the didgeridoo to improve their sleep quality weren't reported as losing any weight, but they also failed to improve the quality of their sleep[4643] (or, likely, their neighbors').

How to Get a Good Night's Sleep

In the Harvard Nurses' Health Study, women who got five or fewer hours of sleep a night gained about six more pounds over the subsequent sixteen years than those getting seven hours of sleep a night.[4644] Even if that were due solely to the difference in sleep, that's still only six pounds for more than ten thousand additional hours of sleep. If even a tiny fraction of that time were spent on diet and exercise, such as biking to the nearest farm stand, more weight could have been lost in sixteen weeks than during those sixteen years. Every little bit helps, though, which is the theme of this entire Weight-Loss Boosters section, and getting at least seven hours of sleep is probably healthier anyway.[4645]

The biggest reason to lose sleep over losing sleep is motor vehicle accident risk.[4646] Driving while drowsy increases your risk of killing yourself and others.[4647] People might think twice about getting behind the wheel after staying awake for forty-eight hours straight, but even just two weeks of sleeping only six hours a night impairs our cognitive performance as much as pulling two all-nighters in a row.[4648] So what's the best way to sleep better?

Sleeping pills are a nonstarter. People prescribed fewer than eighteen pills a year of hypnotics, the class of sleeping pills that includes Ambien, appear to have triple the hazard of dying prematurely.[4649] Since up to 10 percent of the adult population is prescribed these drugs,[4650] if those pills really are killing people, that could mean a six-figure death toll every year.[4651] Ambien's manufacturer questioned the study,[4652] but it was just one of two dozen studies that found a significant association between sleeping pills and premature death.[4653] When the principal investigator at the Scripps Clinic Sleep Center was criticized for "reporting alarmingly high death risks from commonly used medications,"[4654] he replied: "We cannot hide risks, even if they might frighten patients out of taking hypnotics. Patients have a right to know."[4655]

What's more, nonpharmacological methods have been found to work as well or even better than the drugs.[4656] The recommended first-line treatment for insomnia is "cognitive behavioral therapy," which combines conditioning techniques to reassociate the bed with sleep and education surrounding optimal sleep hygiene.[4657]

Four Rules of Sleep Conditioning:[4658]
1. Go to bed only when you're sleepy.
2. Only use the bed for sleep (and sex). No reading, eating, or screen time.
3. If you can't fall asleep within fifteen to twenty minutes or so, get up, leave the bedroom, and don't go back until you're sleepy again. Repeat as necessary.
4. Get up at the same time every morning no matter how little sleep you have had.

Although avoiding napping is often added to the list, contrary to expectations, the majority of research does not show that daytime naps interfere with nighttime sleep.[4659]

Four Rules of Sleep Hygiene:[4660]
1. Exercise regularly.
2. Avoid caffeine, nicotine, and alcohol before bedtime.
3. Make the bedroom dark, cool, comfortable, and quiet.
4. Establish a relaxing bedtime routine.

The best time to exercise to improve sleep appears to be four to eight hours before bedtime,[4661] though it appears to be a myth that exercising right before bed is somehow disruptive to sleep.[4662]

Efforts to replicate the nearly quarter-century-old study I mentioned in the Fat Burners section on page 419 showing even morning coffee may impair sleep[4663] have yet to be attempted.[4664] However, it's clear that hefty caffeine doses up to six hours before bedtime interfere with sleep. Late-afternoon alcohol consumption (six hours before bedtime) may also impair sleep.[4665] Additionally, nicotine, whether from gum, pill, patch, vape, or cigarette, may have negative sleep effects[4666]—though active nicotine withdrawal may as well.[4667]

Nocturnal noise can adversely impact sleep even if you're not consciously aware of it. Within a few days, you can become habituated to noises such that they no longer wake you up, but EEG studies and subjective sleep surveys show the quality of our sleep can still be affected.[4668] Earplugs and sound masking, such as with a white noise machine, have been shown to help.[4669] I was kicking myself after I ordered a white noise machine to try out only to then realize there are around a gazillion free white noise apps available for my phone.

Relaxation techniques, such as massage,[4670] mindfulness meditation,[4671] and soothing music,[4672] may also help. So, too, may taking a relaxing hot bath or shower. One of the reasons late-night eating can delay sleep is that it may interfere with the drop in core body temperature that normally occurs around bedtime,[4673] which is thought to be one of the cues that it's time for bed. So wouldn't that make a hot shower counterproductive? No. As soon as you step out of the bath, your rapid decline in skin temperature can accentuate the natural nighttime drop and improve sleep.[4674] Even just a warm footbath may help you fall asleep about fifteen minutes faster.[4675]

Food-wise, low fiber intake and high saturated fat and sugar intakes are associated with lighter, less restorative sleep.[4676] Meat intake is associated with napping, suggested to be a proxy for inadequate sleep.[4677] This may help explain why insomnia has been reported as a side effect of ketogenic diets.[4678] I talked about melatonin-rich foods and supplements in the Chronobiology section. Megadoses of vitamin D were found to improve sleep duration and quality in men and women aged twenty through fifty with sleeping disorders, though no associated weight loss was reported.[4679]

FOOD FOR THOUGHT

Aim for at least seven hours of regular sleep a night. Have trouble sleeping? Try the Four Rules of Sleep Conditioning and the Four Rules of Sleep Hygiene. *Sweet dreams!*

STRESS HORMONE RELIEF

Stressed Out, Calories In

According to national surveys conducted by the American Psychological Association, the majority of Americans report moderate to high levels of stress.[4680] Though the prevalence of full-blown anxiety disorders hasn't changed much over the last few decades, the level of general psychological stress appears to be getting worse.[4681] After following thousands of people and their stress levels over time, there does seem to be a connection between stress and modest weight gain.[4682] In fact, the increased risk of diabetes in veterans with post-traumatic stress disorder (PTSD) may be explained by the link between PTSD and weight gain.[4683] Effects on both sides of the calorie-balance equation have been used to explain the stress-obesity relationship.

For many who are stressed, structured exercise may be viewed as a disruptive inconvenience, just one more demand on their time, and indeed, the majority of observational studies have found that stress is associated with less physical activity.[4684] Stress may also reduce the thermic effect of food and reduce how much fat is burned after a meal. In one study, those reporting a stressful event the day before testing burned about one hundred fewer calories in the six-hour period after eating compared to days not preceded by anything particularly stressful.[4685]

People who are stressed may eat more too. Though some people eat less when stressed, the majority not only eat more,[4686] they tend to gravitate toward foods high in sugar, fat, and calories.[4687] If you give people their own private snack buffet, those with high chronic stress levels eat less fruits and veggies and more chocolate cake.[4688] We suspect it's cause and effect because you can demonstrate the acute effects of stress in a lab. Randomize people between solvable and unsolvable word puzzles, for example, and food choice shifts from a healthy snack (grapes) to a less healthy snack (M&M's) in the more stressful condition.[4689] The stress of public-speaking challenges or being made to plunge and keep your hand in ice water has been found to dull your ability to sense sweetness, tempting you to eat more to achieve the same taste.[4690] Even just watching a video with distressing scenes, including traffic problems, financial hardship, and sexual harassment, can evoke the same shift in eating behavior toward chocolate.[4691]

They don't call it a comfort food for nothing. Overeating may be a sign that something is eating us.

Stress Belly

Under stress, we tend not only to eat more food but worse food, and we seem to deposit more fat in the worst place, in and around our abdominal organs. Cortisol, known as the *stress hormone,* may be the reason stress levels correlate with visceral obesity (deep belly fat).[4692] Cortisol has been alleged to be a potential "kingpin" in the obesity epidemic.[4693]

We are now at a time in human history where most of our stressors may be psychological rather than physical. These days, we're more likely to fight with our spouses than a saber-toothed tiger, but our bodies respond the same way—we produce cortisol.[4694] Within seconds of a stressor, we get that fight-or-flight burst of adrenaline release, followed within minutes or hours with a rise in cortisol, which is secreted by our adrenal glands above our kidneys.[4695] One effect of cortisol is to boost our appetites, which is adaptive if the stress is a physical threat, such as a predator or famine, but maladaptive if that stress is just trouble at work or financial insecurity—and particularly if the stressor is worrying about your weight!

If you covertly inject people with a drug that increases cortisol levels and then give them a basket of snacks, they eat about 140 more calories than if they had been injected with a placebo instead.[4696] That's why cortisol-like drugs are sometimes given to cancer patients who are wasting away: Corticosteroids may stimulate their appetites,[4697] explaining why weight gain is a common side effect of these drugs.[4698] Four days on the cortisol-like drug methylprednisolone (sold as Medrol, which is used in many autoimmune diseases) can boost daily intake nearly 60 percent, resulting in more than 1,000 extra calories consumed a day.[4699] Cortisol has been implicated as a factor in motivating food intake even when we're not really hungry.[4700]

The weight gain caused by cortisol isn't uniform across the body, however. Fat cells deep in our bellies have a greater density of cortisol receptors,[4701] which activate the enzyme that stuffs our fat cells with fat.[4702] There's a disease called *Cushing's syndrome* that is characterized by an extreme excess of cortisol (for example, due to an adrenal gland tumor). The distribution of cortisol receptors of different regions of fat explains why abdominal obesity is a hallmark symptom of Cushing's, which can be resolved once cortisol levels are brought under control.[4703] There's even been the suggestion that the accumulation of visceral fat is the body's way of sopping up excess cortisol to help buffer the effects of stress.[4704]

So are people with higher levels of cortisol in their bloodstreams more likely to gain weight and become obese? This has actually been a difficult research question to answer because there are such wide, day-to-day fluctuations in cortisol based on stress levels.[4705] Even just getting stuck in traffic on the day of the blood test could throw things off. But a new, noninvasive method has been developed to measure long-term average cortisol levels, involving a snip of hair rather than a vial of blood. As our hair grows, it traps a snapshot of cortisol in our bloodstreams at the time. Each inch of hair on our heads represents about three months of cortisol levels, growing out like rings in a tree trunk.[4706] With this new research tool, scientists have been able to show that high cortisol levels over time are indeed associated with measures of abdominal fat.[4707] One study of thousands of children found that higher hair cortisol levels were linked to a whopping nine times the odds of obesity by age six.[4708]

Might the stress of dieting increase cortisol levels? Although total fasting can dramatically increase cortisol levels—as much as doubling them within five days[4709]—less severe caloric restriction does not.[4710] There is a way stress and obesity could turn into a vicious cycle, though: weight stigma.[4711]

It Can Weigh on You

Even after controlling for body size, those who report weight discrimination may end up with 33 percent higher chronic cortisol levels, meaning even at the same weight, those who experience stigma appear significantly more stressed.[4712] That may account for some of the correlation between stress and obesity.[4713] The researchers suggest, "Chronic exposure to elevated levels of cortisol may play a role in generating a vicious circle of weight gain and discrimination."[4714]

The weight of the stigma can be demonstrated experimentally. Researchers from Rutgers and UCLA set up an ethically questionable test. Women were invited to participate in a study allegedly designed to examine the "hormonal responses to shopping." The study subject entered a staging area along with a "thin female confederate" who posed as just another study participant but was actually in on the experiment. The slim conspirator was then congratulated on the great news that she qualified to participate in a group shopping activity for designer clothing and was escorted into a celebration. After returning to the staging area, the researcher told the real study subject one of two manipulations. In the control condition, she was told, "Unfortunately, the group shopping activity is full now, and since you were the last to sign up, we can't include you in the activity." However, those randomized to the stigma condition were instead told, "Unfortunately, your size and shape just aren't ideal for this style of clothing and we really do want everyone to have fun and feel good. Plus, we want to return the clothing to the designer in good condition." Ouch. Irrespective of their actual weight, study subjects who perceived themselves to be heavy experienced a rise in cortisol within thirty minutes in the stigma compared to control condition.[4715]

Even just observing weight stigma can be stressful. Compared to cortisol levels measured after watching an emotionally neutral video (like a clip about the invention of the radio), women watching a stigmatizing scene, such as an actress in a fat suit dancing seductively for a group of repulsed construction workers, experienced greater cortisol secretion.[4716] Does this then translate into increased calorie consumption? Yale researchers found that when normal-weight women are provided with bowls of M&M's, jelly beans, and chips to snack on after watching clips of stigmatizing material like clumsy, loud, lazy stereotypes getting teased about their weight, they eat about the same amount compared to watching neutral material such as insurance commercials. But when overweight women watch the same two sets of videos, they *triple* their caloric intakes after watching the stigmatizing scenes.[4717] A similar finding was reported for overweight youth, who were more likely to respond to being socially ostracized with overeating compared to normal-weight kids.[4718]

You can dress up skinny people in fat suits and get the same result. The UCLA research team who had helped design the shopping study published a paper entitled "Putting on Weight Stigma" in which slim men and women were randomized to appear obese by wearing a fat suit. Just walking around in public for a few minutes while wearing a fat suit led to hurt feelings of rejection, anger, anxiety, and sadness.[4719] Immediately afterward, those in fat suits went on to consume nearly two hundred more calories of chips, chocolate, and soda—and that all occurred even without the internalized stigma, self-blame, and shame that too often plague the truly obese.[4720] Ironically, this experience of "walking a mile in their shoes" appeared to have zero effect on the skinny study subjects' own anti-fat attitudes.

No one should ever be discriminated against unfairly, but given the current reality, the most effective way to lose the weight stigma may be to lose the weight. That's what this entire book is about, but what are some of the best ways to deal with stress, whether from stigma or otherwise?

Sweat It Out?

Exercise can have a powerful stress-buffering effect. People who regularly exercise report significantly lower stress levels, and when put to the test, randomized controlled trials have shown that acute bouts of exercise are effective in reducing self-reported stress levels and improving quality of life. Physically active individuals have lower cortisol levels and a healthier cortisol response to stressors.[4721]

One of the most popular experimental methods to induce psychological stress is the Montreal Imaging Stress Task protocol. It involves timed arithmetic challenges with failure built in by manipulating the difficulty and time limits to be just beyond the individual's mental capacity.[4722] When you put a group of sedentary individuals through the test, their cortisol spikes higher than aerobically fit subjects, but have them walk on a treadmill for thirty minutes before the test, and their cortisol responses drop right down.[4723]

Is the drop in cortisol from even just a single exercise session enough to blunt stress-induced eating? To find out, researchers put people though a mental challenge stressful enough to increase post-test pizza consumption by an additional hundred calories. If you first have them do fifteen minutes of high-intensity interval training, though, they end up eating less than they would have without doing the mental challenge. Combined with the calories burned by the exercise, they ended up with about one hundred fewer calories than they would have had they just sat down to the pizza alone.[4724] So exercising to relieve stress can help control weight from both sides of the calorie equation.

Laugh It Off?

Exercising your funny bone doesn't appear to do much on paper. Genuine voiced laughter only causes about a 10–20 percent increase in calorie expenditure above resting metabolic rate, which is not much more than such activities as light clerical work, writing, or playing cards. Ten to fifteen minutes of laughter a day may only burn about an extra ten to forty calories, depending on body weight and laughter intensity,[4725] but laughter can have an oversized effect on lowering stress.

The very evolution of laughter is thought to have been as an antidote to stress, the release of nervous energy.[4726] Within sixty minutes of people watching a comedy video (complete with "Gallagher's classical Sledge-O-Matic finale"), cortisol levels in their bloodstreams were cut by more than half.[4727] This has been offered as an explanation as to why mirthful laughter has been shown to improve immune function.[4728] Cortisol acts as an immunosuppressant, which is why cortisol-like steroids such as prednisone are used for inflammatory autoimmune diseases. This may explain why those laughing heartily at a humorous video had improvements in natural killer cell function—critical for anticancer and antiviral immunity—compared to those randomized to a control group watching tourism videos.[4729] (Replicating the results these days may be difficult given the original researchers' choice of comedic stimulus: Bill Cosby.)

Under the assumption that our bodies can't tell the difference between real and fake laughter, "laughter yoga" was developed[4730] in which participants force themselves to laugh as a form of exercise "akin to internal jogging."[4731] Drops in cortisol levels have been noted when it has been put to the test, but would spontaneous laughter be better?[4732] Researchers in Japan decided to find out. They compared the cortisol changes in people randomized either to simulated laughter in a laughter yoga session, genuine laughter watching a funny video, or no laughter in a control group given some dry reading instead. Both laughter groups actively reduced cortisol levels within half an hour compared to the reading group, but the comedy group beat out the laughter yoga.[4733] Maybe our bodies can tell if we're faking it after all.

Strike a Pose?

What about regular yoga? Practiced by as many as twenty million Americans every year,[4734] yoga in the United States is comprised mainly of body postures, breathing exercises, and meditation.[4735] A meta-analysis of randomized controlled trials found that yoga interventions can lower cortisol levels, but does this translate into weight loss?[4736] A cross-sectional study found that practicing yoga for four or more years was associated with less weight gain over time, but yoga practitioners also tended to exercise twice as much in general and eat more healthful diets (for example, 45 percent higher consumption of fruits and vegetables).[4737] This may all be related, though. Yoga practitioners often claim they feel "more connected" to their bodies, which may translate into healthier choices.[4738] However, you can't tell what role yoga itself plays until it's put to the test.

There are randomized controlled yoga trials showing weight loss, but they're often in comparison to control groups who did nothing. Indeed, compared to no changes in physical activity, doing about thirty hours of yoga has been shown to lead to about five pounds of weight loss and an inch off the waist.[4739,4740] But are there some supplemental benefits to yoga beyond just the three or so calories burned per minute[4741] due to the physical exertion alone? Researchers decided to find out.

Yoga was compared head-to-head to resistance exercise and walking for weight loss. Doing thirty-six hours of resistance training with rubber exercise bands, weights, and balance balls led to a 1 percent drop in body fat compared to the sedentary control group. Doing the same amount of yoga led to the same 1 percent drop.[4742] In the walking study, fulfilling my Daily Dozen recommendation to walk at least a total of ninety minutes a day on a plant-based diet also led to similar amounts of weight loss compared to swapping in the same amount of yoga—about five pounds and an inch off the waist in fifteen days.[4743] The walking group were told to walk at their own pace, which ended up being more of a leisurely stroll, but that matched the metabolic cost of most yoga, which is classified by American College of Sports Medicine criteria as a light-intensity physical activity.[4744]

What about Bikram—or hot—yoga, practiced at a humid 100°F and purported to burn a thousand calories a session? That's a bit of a stretch. (*Ahem.*) When put to the test, calorie expenditure during hot yoga was no more fat-burning than room-temperature yoga.[4745] Overall, yoga doesn't appear to have any special weight-reducing benefits,[4746] but the best form of exercise is the one you'll actually do, so if you enjoy it, go for it. *Namaste.*

Rub It In?

Yoga can be thought of as self-massaging our internal organs, but what about getting a regular massage as a stress-management technique for weight loss? In both term and preterm infants, massage leads to weight *gain,*[4747] which is great for babies, but not necessarily for adults. Repeated massage-like stroking "on the ventral side" of rats (that is, giving them belly rubs) also increases weight gain,[4748] but what about human adults? No effect. Getting weeks[4749] or months[4750] of massages appears to have no effect on body weight or waist circumference.

Turn It Up?

What about music to soothe the savage beast of stress? We've been playing music since at least the Paleolithic era forty thousand years ago,[4751] and music as therapy has been documented at least since biblical times (1 Samuel 16:23). The first music therapy experiment I could find was published in *The Journal of the American Medical Association* in 1914. Explaining why a phonograph was placed in the operating room as his patients lay fully conscious and awake during surgery, the surgeon said it was "a means of calming and distracting my patients from the horror of the situation."[4752]

Now that we have good general anesthesia, music is used to calm nerves *before* surgery. Normally, we use Valium-type drugs like midazolam (sold as Versed), but they can have a variety of side effects, including, ironically, sometimes making people even more agitated.[4753] A study from Sweden sought to determine if relaxing music has a greater anxiety-reducing effect than a standard dose of midazolam. Researchers whipped out some Kenny G, and the music indeed worked significantly better than the drug. Those listening to soft jazz, relaxing pop, classical, new age, and nature sounds all had lower anxiety scores, heart rates, and blood pressures. This was heralded as the first time any antianxiety therapy worked not only as well as but even better than Valium-type drugs, and it didn't leave patients with the typical "post-operative hangover." The researchers noted that the "difference in side effects of relaxing music and midazolam is obvious."[4754]

Listening to music while eating does not seem to affect intake,[4755] and though I couldn't find any studies putting music to the test for weight loss, more than a dozen studies have found that listening to recorded music can reduce cortisol levels.[4756] Not all music, though. Subjectively, Mozart has been found to lead to a greater self-reported reduction in tension than grunge rock (Pearl Jam).[4757] When cortisol lowering was measured, Beethoven beat out techno (Techno Magnetiko's *Cyber Trip Techno Shock*), but that may just be a function of the tempo.[4758] People get the same bump in breathing and blood pressure listening to fast classical music, such as Vivaldi's "Summer Presto," which was as stimulating or even more so, researchers found, than the Red Hot Chili Peppers (the band, not the plants).[4759]

What about heavy metal? Kenneled dogs were provided with various Spotify options for audio enrichment.[4760] Soft rock and reggae appeared to reduce stress, but the "loud and sudden nature of heavy metal may be unsuitable for dogs" as well as the "general experience of shelter employees and potential adopters."[4761] (Maybe they should have played Ozzy's "Bark at the Moon.") When people were randomly assigned to self-selected music, classical, heavy metal, or silence, the self-selected and classical music produced increased feelings of relaxation, as did sitting in silence, but heavy metal had the opposite effect.[4762]

Compared to relaxing and pleasant Renaissance music, exposure to "arousing and unpleasant" heavy metal caused a heightened amylase response in men.[4763] Amylase is an enzyme in our saliva that digests starch into simple sugars. When we go into fight-or-flight mode, we immediately start churning out the enzyme to provide blood sugar for quick energy, so you get a spike when you go skydiving,[4764] if someone dunks you in near-freezing water,[4765] or, apparently, if you just listen to heavy metal for ten minutes.[4766] With all that extra enzyme, if you're eating bread while banging your head, you may end up digesting it faster.

Change Your Mind?

Mindfulness-based stress reduction involves cultivating a nonjudgmental, accepting, moment-by-moment awareness.[4767] In the context of food, mindful eating is the practice of being fully present for a meal. This may involve slowing down the pace, savoring every bite, and getting in tune with your body's fullness cues.[4768] When we're distracted, we tend to eat faster and for longer. For example, men and women randomized to eat while watching TV averaged an extra slice of pizza or 71 percent more mac 'n cheese, totaling nearly three hundred additional calories.[4769] This may help explain why one survey found overweight individuals reported they ate almost half their meals while watching television.[4770] Researchers at the Stanford Prevention Research Center found that on the weekends, about a quarter of a child's calories may be consumed in front of the TV.[4771]

Even just being distracted listening to something can have an impact. Study subjects told to eat while giving their full attention to a radio conversation[4772] or a detective story recorded on cassette tapes (old-school podcast!) ended up eating significantly more, for instance up to 77 percent more ice cream compared to undistracted eating.[4773] Even just engaging in conversation while eating with friends can inadvertently boost intake.[4774]

Distracted eating may also affect subsequent consumption. Have people play computer solitaire while eating a fixed-calorie meal, and they eat nearly twice as many cookies a half hour later, as if they hadn't fully consciously registered how much they ate while they were distracted by the game.[4775] Conversely, if you have people listen to an audio clip encouraging them to eat mindfully and focus on the look, smell, taste, and texture of the food, they eat fewer cookies hours later than those who had either eaten in silence[4776] or while listening to neutral audiobook content.[4777] Another way mindful eating may help prevent overeating is by sharpening the memory of each meal. Those who could more reliably recall an experimental lunch have been shown to average lower afternoon snack intake.[4778] Most but not all such studies found focused attention during a meal decreased later food intake, at least in a research lab setting.[4779]

How to Deal with Cravings

Attending to the sensory qualities of food and our bodies' reactions is just one aspect of mindful eating. Mindfulness has been described as a "moment-to-moment awareness, cultivated by paying attention in a specific way, in the present moment, as non-reactively, nonjudgmentally, and openheartedly as possible."[4780] Just being aware may not be enough, though. Practicing mindfulness is said to involve three steps: awareness, acceptance, and then something called *cognitive defusion*.

When we are struck with a craving, a typical reaction is *cognitive restructuring,* a psychological term for challenging our thoughts and replacing them with alternative ones.[4781] For example, if we're hit with a pang for chocolate, instead of reaching for a candy bar, a restructuring response might be: *No, I don't need chocolate. I can have something healthier instead.* Unfortunately, this rarely works. More than one hundred self-identified chocolate cravers were randomized to an hour of cognitive restructuring instruction and then given a bag of chocolates to carry around with them for a week to see how well they could resist the temptation. Despite the hour-long instruction at the start of the week, they didn't do much better than the control group who tried the same exercise but without any instruction at all.

The mindful eating approach, on the other hand, involved cognitive defusion. People are taught to defuse their thoughts as "merely thoughts" and place mental distance between themselves and their thoughts. A defusion response to the thought of needing chocolate would involve simply observing the thought (*I notice I'm having the thought that I need to eat some chocolate*) and thanking one's mind for the thought (*Thanks, mind*).[4782] A "mindbus" metaphor is used, in which people are taught to imagine themselves as the driver of a bus and their thoughts as mere passengers.[4783] You visualize yourself taking control as you stop the bus and let off the negative passengers. *Thanks for the feedback, folks, but this is my bus.*

Cognitive defusion was tested head-to-head against cognitive restructuring in the same chocolate experiment, and those who had gotten an hour of defusion instruction had three times greater odds of remaining "chocolate abstinent" in the face of a week of constant temptation.[4784] Defusion was then pitted against acceptance: Instructing people to observe a thought or feeling, accept its presence, and build up a degree of tolerance for uncomfortable feelings. Study subjects were randomized to less than a half hour of coaching on either defusion or acceptance, or to a control group who spent the time learning a muscle-relaxation technique. They were then asked to carry a bag of chocolate candy with them for five days— untouched. The acceptance group failed to beat out the control group, but the defusion group did.[4785] Of all the mindfulness skills, cognitive defusion, also known as *disidentification,* appears to be the most effective.

Putting Your Mind at Rest

Mindfulness is a major part of the billion-dollar meditation industry,[4786] with as many as one in five Fortune 500 companies implementing some kind of workplace mindfulness program.[4787] It has been rebranded from "hippy dippy nonsense" to portrayals such as "brain training" said to "sell it better."[4788] These reductionist, commodified forms have been derided as "McMindfulness,"[4789] but who cares what they call it if it works? But does it?

Research into mindfulness has been complicated by the fact that the term can mean anything from informal practices, such as conscious awareness while eating, to structured meditation programs involving designating set times to sit in a specific posture attending to your breathing, for instance.[4790] This has made an understanding of the efficacy hard to capture. It can't hurt, though, right? Well . . .

There have been more than twenty observational studies or case reports documenting instances of adverse effects, such as meditation-induced psychosis, mania, anxiety, and panic.[4791] One study at an intensive meditation retreat assessed participants' negative experiences since they had begun meditation. They found that seventeen of twenty-seven participants—more than 60 percent—reported at least one adverse effect, including an individual who was hospitalized for a psychotic break.[4792] Even outside of an immersive retreat environment, as many as 12 percent of meditators recall negative side effects within ten days of initiating the practice.[4793]

It's considered plausible that adverse effects occur at rates approximating that of psychotherapy,[4794] with about one in twenty patients reporting lasting negative effects of psychological treatment.[4795] With about twenty-five million Americans practicing meditation[4796] and as many as a million new meditators a year,[4797] even a 5 percent adverse-event rate could mean hundreds of thousands of negative side effects a year. As with any medical intervention, though, it's all about risks versus benefits. Unfortunately, many of the benefits have been overstated.[4798]

A commentary in a psychiatry journal entitled "Has the Science of Mindfulness Lost Its Mind?" notes that even the books on mindfulness written by scientists are "bursting with magical promises of peace, happiness and well-being."[4799] Contrary to the popular perception, however, the evidence for even the most well-founded benefits is not entirely conclusive.[4800] This is not an issue unique to meditation. There is a "replication crisis" across the entire field of experimental psychology,[4801] where many of the landmark findings in the social sciences published in even the most prestigious journals don't appear to be reproducible.[4802]

Drug companies aren't the only ones to suppress the publication of studies that don't come out the way they wanted. The majority of mindfulness-based trials apparently never see the light of day, raising the specter of a similar publication bias.[4803] Presumably, if the studies showed promising results, they would have been released rather than shelved. What's more, many of the ones that do make it into the scientific record are underwhelming. The federal Agency for Healthcare Research and Quality published a systematic review of the available data and concluded that mindfulness meditation worked best for improving anxiety, depression, and pain, but even then, the quality of evidence was only "moderate."[4804] What about weight loss?

Mindfulness-based modalities can help with stress management[4805] and self-control,[4806] and can decrease impulsive,[4807] binge, and emotional eating, all of which might facilitate weight management.[4808] However, the first review of the available evidence published five years ago failed to find evidence of significant or consistent weight loss.[4809] Part of the problem is compliance.

Like any other diet or lifestyle intervention, mindfulness only works if you do it.

For instance, women were randomized to attend four two-hour workshops that taught mindfulness techniques such as cognitive defusion. After six months, they lost no more weight on average than the control group. However, if those who reported "never" applying the workshop principles at all were excluded and only those who used the techniques at least some of the time were considered, their weight loss *did* beat out the control group by about five pounds.[4810]

Other studies showed a lack of weight gain rather than loss. For example, one study found that obese subjects in the control group continued to gain weight at about a pound a month, whereas the weight of those in the mindfulness intervention group remained stable.[4811]

Putting all the studies together, the latest and largest review published in 2018 did find that mindfulness-based interventions can lead to weight loss compared to doing nothing, an average of about seven pounds over four months or so.[4812] Pitted head-to-head, however, they didn't beat out other lifestyle-change interventions, but the nice thing about stress management and mindfulness is they can be practiced on top of whatever else you're doing.

Get Planted

A single high-fat meal can exacerbate the effects of stress. People randomized to eat a sausage-and-egg McMuffin with hash browns experienced a heightened cardiovascular reactivity to both psychological stress (public speaking) and bodily stress (submerging their hand in ice water for minutes) two hours later. How do we know it wasn't just the carbs in the english muffin and hash browns? Because the control meal was a sugary mess of Frosted Flakes and Froot Loops, and those randomized to the breakfast candy reacted significantly better to the stressors than those in the high-fat group. The McMuffin meal also had more than ten times the cholesterol, thanks to the egg, and the researchers suggest this may also have contributed to the effect.[4813] Population studies show that higher dietary cholesterol is associated significantly with increased risk of impaired cognitive function and memory, effectively mimicking accelerated brain aging. The effect of eating an additional 80 mg of cholesterol a day—which is less than half an egg[4814]—was similar to the effect of being approximately three years older, appearing to effectively accelerate brain aging.[4815]

Though effectively all dietary cholesterol comes from animal foods, saturated fat is not exclusive to the animal kingdom. Remember the packs-a-punch study from the Anti-Inflammatory section showing just a few days of a breakfast high in saturated fat can cause learning and memory problems? The researchers used palm oil, so it's not just animal fats. Tropical oils, including palm and coconut oils, are highly saturated, too, though the vast majority of saturated fat in the American diet continues to come from meat and dairy. Every single one of the top fifteen sources of saturated fat is meat, dairy, or junk.[4816] What would happen if we instead centered our diets around whole, healthy, plant foods?

In a study published in *Nutritional Neuroscience* entitled "Vegans Report Less Stress and Anxiety Than Omnivores," those eating completely plant-based do seem to be significantly less stressed, but it may not necessarily be their diets. The researchers suggest it's because they're eating less pro-inflammatory animal fats, but those eating more plant-based also tended to exercise more, spend more time outdoors, and practice more yoga. The om-nivores also reported dieting more often, which alone can be stressful.[4817]

Even if it is the diet, it could be the anti-inflammatory compounds in fruits and vegetables rather than the "cascade of neuroinflammation" (brain inflammation) potentially caused by the arachidonic acid[4818] (an inflamma-tory omega-6 fat) concentrated in chicken and eggs[4819] or the saturated fat in red meat and dairy.[4820] It could also be because of all the beneficial prebiotics in whole grains and beans. Researchers performed a fecal transplant between stress-prone mice and normal mice by feeding them each other's stool, and the normal mice started exhibiting anxiety and the stressed mice relaxed.[4821] You don't know for sure until you put it to the test—in people. No studies as of yet trading poop with the Dalai Lama, but there have been interventional trials using plant-based diets.

Five hundred men and women suffering from anxiety and depression were placed on a whole food, plant-based diet and lifestyle program. Most dropped out within the first two weeks because they felt the program was "too rigor-ous" for them. However, the majority of those who stuck with the program experienced substantial improvements in mood and a "large improvement or full remission" of anxiety symptoms. Most who had been suffering from fatigue and pain got better and, over the twelve-week study period, lost an average of six pounds. What was most remarkable is that three months after the study ended, they were down a total of fifteen pounds, suggesting they stuck with it on their own. Exercise and twenty minutes of relaxation a day were also prescribed with the whole food, plant-based diet, though, so it's impossible to isolate out the effects of what they ate.[4822]

There are randomized controlled trials of plant-based diets that have resulted in significant improvements in anxiety, fatigue, depression, and emotional well-being utilizing dietary changes alone,[4823] but is that directly because of the diet or indirectly due to the augmented weight loss? Even placed on similar caloric intakes, plant-based diets can result in superior weight loss, with significant reductions in all compartments of body fat.[4824] Maybe that's why the subjects reported a greater improvement in quality of life compared to the control group.[4825] The reason we suspect the causal link may be direct is that if you randomize people to remove all meat and eggs from their diets, you can get a significant drop in stress levels within just two weeks, compared to those who kept eating fish or a third group who continued to include all animal foods. So even before significant weight loss could occur, the researchers suggest "individuals who eliminate meat, fish, and poultry may cope better with mental stress."[4826]

The Meat of the Matter

A single meal high in animal protein can nearly double the level of the stress hormone cortisol in the blood within a half hour of consumption, more than twice that of a meal closer to the recommended level of protein.[4827] Give someone a meal of crabmeat, tuna, and cottage cheese, and the level of cortisol in their saliva shoots up within the hour. Instead, give someone some barley soup and a vegetable stir-fry, and cortisol levels drop *down* after the meal.[4828] Imagine eating meat or dairy meal after meal, day after day. The concern is you might "chronically stimulate" your adrenal glands.[4829] We don't always have control over the stress in our lives, but at least we can make some dietary tweaks to help keep cortisol under control.

Chronic high cortisol levels don't just increase obesity risk. Blood cortisol strongly predicts cardiovascular death in men and women—even among those without any known preexisting cardiovascular disease.[4830] This may help explain "death from a broken heart," the heightened heart attack and stroke risk in the weeks immediately following the loss of a spouse.[4831] The higher cortisol levels days, months, or even years after losing someone you love may increase cardiac risk and reduce immune function. Remarkably, the rise in stress hormone levels after losing a spouse[4832] is less than the bump you may get eating a high-meat diet.[4833]

If you feed men a high-protein diet packed with fish, poultry, other meat, and egg whites, and then switch them to a lower-protein diet centered around bread, fruits, and vegetables, their cortisol levels drop about a quarter within ten days.[4834] Interestingly, at the same time, their testosterone levels shoot up by about the same amount. Contrary to the "flagrant misuse of scientific information" in *Men's Health* magazine,[4835] high-protein diets suppress testosterone.[4836] That's why if men eating plant-based diets begin eating meat every day, their testosterone levels go down,[4837] which, over time, might itself contribute to the accumulation of belly fat.[4838]

Controlling Cortisol from Birth

The spikes in cortisol levels that occur each time we eat a meaty meal[4839] may not just affect our health but that of our children. Substantial evidence now suggests that high-protein diets during pregnancy have adverse effects on the fetus.[4840] Take, for example, the infamous Harlem Trial of 1976. Poor black pregnant women were randomized into one of three groups, either getting forty grams of added animal protein a day, an additional six grams, or none. The added-protein groups suffered an excess of very early premature births, with infant death rates doubling in the six-gram group and quadrupling in the forty-gram group. The babies who survived suffered "significant growth retardation."[4841]

In a similar experiment in Scotland, pregnant women were told to eat a high-meat diet in hopes of preventing a disease of pregnancy known as *preeclampsia*.[4842] It didn't work. In fact, the lowest preeclampsia rates I've ever come across were among women eating completely plant-based diets: only 1 case out of 775 pregnancies.[4843] Preeclampsia normally strikes about 1 in 20,[4844] so a plant-based diet might "alleviate most, if not all, of the signs and symptoms of this potentially serious condition."[4845]

What happened when the Scottish women went from eating about one daily portion of meat to around two a day? The mothers who ate more meat during pregnancy gave birth to children who grew up to have higher blood pressures.[4846] One explanation for the adverse effects of high meat consumption, including fish, is that this may have increased maternal cortisol concentrations, which in turn affected the developing fetus, resetting their stress hormone "thermostat" to a higher level. Indeed, researchers found higher blood cortisol levels in both the sons and daughters of women who had reported higher consumption of meat, including fish—about a 5 percent increase for every daily serving.[4847] This may help explain why animal protein intake during pregnancy has been associated with children becoming overweight later in life.[4848]

You Are What Your Mother Ate

Whereas babies of meat-free mothers have lower cortisol levels,[4849] higher-meat diets are considered to present a "metabolic stress" to the mother, effectively reprograming the adrenal glands of their children, leading to lifelong elevations of stress hormones in their blood.[4850] Every daily portion of meat consumed during late pregnancy was linked to about a 1 percent greater fat mass in their children by the time they reached adolescence.[4851]

The adult children of mothers who ate more meat during pregnancy don't just walk around with higher baseline stress hormone levels but also appear to react more negatively to whatever life throws at them. Researchers tracked down the now grown-up kids whose mothers had been part of the double-the-meat experiment and measured their cortisol levels after a stressful public-speaking challenge. If their moms had eaten fewer than two daily servings of meat (fish included) while carrying them, they got relatively small surges of stress hormones from their adrenal glands. The cortisol levels in those whose moms had eaten fourteen to sixteen servings a week rose 30 percent higher, and those whose moms had eaten the most meat—seventeen or more servings a week—had their cortisol levels jump more than 50 percent higher in response to the same imposed stress.[4852]

It's no surprise then that animal-protein intake during pregnancy may lead to greater weight gain for her children later in life,[4853] but remarkably, it may even impact her grandchildren. Recent evidence suggests that the long-term adverse consequences may not be limited to one generation, potentially affecting the ovaries and future eggs of her unborn daughter. "Ultimately," one review concluded, "these findings will shed light on the transmission of diabetes, obesity, and cardiovascular disease that are rapidly expanding in Western countries."[4854]

FOOD FOR THOUGHT

The best way to relieve the effects of stress is to relieve the stress itself. To the extent possible, we should try to reorient our lives to avoid major stressors and use exercise to work off what's unavoidable. This can include yoga, walking, or resistance band stretches. Mindfulness techniques can be used to reduce stress and deal with cravings. To buffer the release of the stress hormone cortisol, we can reduce our intake of saturated fats and animal protein, and pile on the plants.

WALL OFF YOUR CALORIES

Liquid Candy Crush

In the Eating Rate booster section, I discussed the classic jelly bean-versus-soda study that showed our bodies may not register calories in liquid form as well as they do calories from solid foods. If you're given an extra one hundred calories, your body tries to take that into account, adjusting your appetite over the remainder of the day so you stay in relative calorie balance. This response isn't perfect, though; your body isn't able to completely compensate calorie for calorie. In studies where this has been measured, those given an extra one hundred calories of food end up eating an average of only sixty-four fewer calories later on, not the full hundred. But if you *drink* those hundred extra calories, your body hardly seems to notice, only downregulating your subsequent appetite by about nine calories.[4855] So by the end of the day, you may be left with a ninety-one-calorie surplus. Our brains just don't seem wired to recognize liquid calories. After all, for millions of years, the only thing on tap was water.

This may help explain why sugary drinks have been blamed as perhaps the single largest driver of the obesity epidemic,[4856] accounting for at least one-fifth of the weight gained between 1977 and 2007 in the United States.[4857] By the year 2000, Americans were drinking an estimated 190 calories a day of sweetened beverages.[4858]

It would be bad enough to eat 190 empty calories' worth of candy a day, but it may be even worse to drink it.

It's been estimated that just removing soda and other sugary drinks from the SNAP program (formerly known as *Food Stamps*) would prevent hundreds of thousands of cases of obesity.[4859] Through the program, the soda industry is snatching up billions of taxpayer dollars every year.[4860] The USDA has denied state requests for excluding soda from SNAP, arguing, "No clear standards exist for defining foods as good or bad, or healthy or not healthy."[4861] The fact that the federal government can't even agree that sugar water is unhealthy explains a lot about the sad state of the U.S. Dietary Guidelines.

Industries argue that removing soda subsidies would disproportionately hurt the poor, like tobacco taxes. Of course, the public health community sees ending the subsidies as disproportionally *helping* the poor, but it might be more consistent to restrict the use of federal dollars across the board, such as at cafeterias in federal buildings and military bases, for example.[4862] When those actually affected by the policy were asked (*what a concept!*), the majority of SNAP participants surveyed *supported* removing sugary drinks, especially if it led to additional benefits for healthful foods like fruits and vegetables.[4863]

Obesity, like lung cancer, is not an equal-opportunity killer. Those living in poverty are significantly more likely to become obese.[4864] Predatory industries such as fast food,[4865] alcohol,[4866] and tobacco have long targeted low-income neighborhoods and communities of color.[4867] The soda industry appears to be no exception.[4868] As one tobacco industry executive was recorded saying, "We don't smoke that s***. We just sell it. We just reserve the right to smoke for the young, the poor, the black and the stupid."[4869]

Wining and Dining

Speaking of liquid calories, what about wine? Alcohol and obesity may be a dangerous mix. Up to nine out of ten obese individuals already have nonalcoholic fatty liver disease,[4870] and by age fifty, two-thirds end up with advanced liver scarring from the resultant chronic inflammation.[4871] No wonder medical journal editorials have referred to obesity and alcohol consumption as "the double peril."[4872] Given the dual threat, those who drink alcohol are cautioned to "take care to not become overweight."[4873] Might drinking alcohol undermine that goal on its own?

Population studies suggest the term *beer belly* is apropos, with drinking about a pint or more of beer a day associated with abdominal obesity. In some populations, drinking beer is associated with more sedentary lifestyles and poorer dietary choices,[4874] though, so it's hard to tease out cause and effect until you put it to the test.

Six interventional studies comparing regular beer head-to-head with nonalcoholic beer found more average weight gain on the alcoholic beer. Since the body has no capacity to store alcohol, it may temporarily switch from burning fat to burning alcohol to help clear it out of the system, leaving a small excess fat balance.[4875] However, no such difference was found in a study comparing consumption of wine to grape juice.[4876]

(continued)

Thinking an aperitif might help patients with advanced cancer slow weight loss, researchers randomized subjects to a glass of wine a day, but it didn't appear to make a difference. One study on wine and appetite showed a significant bump in caloric intake, but not for the reason the researchers were expecting.[4877] When study participants were randomized to drink wine, beer, or soda with a meal, they ended up consuming more calories with the wine—but not because they ate more food. It was because they drank more wine. A quarter of the subjects drank the entire bottle, the "maximum allowed for ethical reasons."[4878]

What about weight gain over time? When people who don't normally imbibe were randomized to drink a glass of red wine, white wine, or sparkling water with dinner for two years, they ended up with no significant differences in body fat among the three groups.[4879] What about all the other long-term randomized studies on wine and weight? There aren't any, so the best available balance of evidence suggests a single daily glass of wine, 150 ml or about two-thirds of a cup, does not appear to affect body weight. Although from a health standpoint "the safest level of drinking is none,"[4880] inordinate weight gain may not be one of wine's adverse effects.

Particle Physics

Liquefied meats, fruits, and vegetables appear to be less satiating than the same foods in solid form. Part of this is due to eating speed. You can eat applesauce four times faster than you can eat the same amount in whole-apple form.[4881] However, even at approximately the same rate of ingestion, a chicken smoothie,[4882] blended carrots,[4883] and apple purée[4884] were found to be less satisfying than their solid equivalents.

Part of it may be psychological. When researchers have tricked study subjects into falsely believing they had just consumed a liquid that would instantly gel in their stomachs, the subjects felt so much fuller that they ended up eating hundreds of fewer calories over the course of a day compared to those who had been given the same liquid without the lie.[4885] However, there are also physiological reasons why the form food takes may be important for weight control.

Nuts are the classic example. Comparing the absorption of fat from peanuts to the exact same number of peanuts ground into peanut butter, you flush more than twice the amount of fat down the toilet when you eat the peanuts themselves.[4886] No matter how well you chew, small bits of nuts trapping some of that oil make their way all the way through our systems and are lost out the other end.[4887] Same number of calories going into our mouths, but because of the food structure—whole versus blended—fewer calories stay in our bodies. This introduces the concept of *metabolizable energy*. Remember, it's not what you eat but what you absorb. For some foods, the calorie count on the label may not accurately reflect the calories that make it into your bloodstream.

Based on macronutrient content—4 calories per gram of protein or carbohydrate, and 9 calories per gram of fat—a can of almonds may list 180 calories per ounce. However, if you rummage through people's stools after they had eaten an ounce of almonds, you may find that 55 almond calories had escaped. So the metabolizable energy of almonds is really only 125 calories per ounce, not the listed 180. Given that, whole nuts may have 30 percent fewer calories than you'd expect. In contrast, the calculated calories and metabolizable calories in almond butter are nearly identical.[4888] You absorb the full complement of calories from nut and seed butters because none of the oil is trapped inside unchewed fragments.

Which has more calories? Raw almonds or dry, roasted almonds? They may have the same number listed on their respective labels, but raw almonds are harder nuts to crack. Roasting makes nuts more brittle, so they fracture into tinier pieces in our mouths. If you have people chew almonds and then spit them out without swallowing, the size of the particles of chewed raw almonds is twice the size of chewed roasted almonds. And indeed, you end up getting about 10 percent more metabolizable calories when eating roasted almonds than raw, since the roasted nuts get broken down so much smaller when you eat them.[4889]

Does this mean you absorb more calories from nuts if you chew them more? Researchers in Indiana decided to put it to the test. People ate about two ounces of nuts every day for four days while their stools were collected. Those instructed to chew ten times per mouthful lost about 25 percent more fecal fat compared to those told to chew twenty-five times.[4890] Same food, same amount of food, yet nearly two hundred fewer calories absorbed based on how they ate them. One would expect the extended orosensory exposure from the extra chewing to suppress appetite, but the meal amounts were fixed so the study can't show how much this might have compensated for the calorie deficit.

In Bad Form

The physical form of food can alter not only fat absorption but carbohydrate absorption as well. It comes as no surprise that Rice Krispies and Corn Flakes cause a much greater spike in blood sugars than rice or corn on the cob,[4891] but it's not just the added sugar in the cereals. Even with identical ingredients, food structure can make a big difference. For example, rolled oats have a significantly lower glycemic index than unsweetened instant oatmeal, which is also just straight oats but in thinner flakes,[4892] and oat *flakes* cause lower blood sugar and insulin spikes than *powdered* oats.[4893] The same single ingredient, oats, in different forms can have different effects.

Why do we care? As I noted in the Low Glycemic Load section, the overly rapid absorption of carbohydrates after eating a high-glycemic-index meal can trigger a sequence of hormonal and metabolic changes that promote excessive eating. In a study out of Harvard's Children's Hospital, a dozen obese teen boys were fed instant oatmeal versus steel-cut oatmeal. After the instant oatmeal, the teens went on to eat 53 percent more than after eating the exact same number of calories of steel-cut oatmeal. The instant oatmeal group was snacking within an hour after the meal and went on to accumulate significantly more calories throughout the rest of the day.[4894] Same type of food, but different form, yielding different effects.

Steel-cut oatmeal is considered a low-glycemic-index food, averaging under 55. The glycemic index of instant oatmeal is 79, making it a high-glycemic-index food, but not as bad as some breakfast cereals, which can get into the 80s or 90s. This is even true of zero-sugar cereals like shredded wheat.[4895] The new industrial methods used to create breakfast cereals, such as extrusion cooking and explosion puffing, accelerate starch digestion and absorption, causing an exaggerated blood sugar response.[4896] Shredded wheat has the same ingredients as spaghetti—straight wheat—but twice the glycemic index.[4897]

When you eat spaghetti, you get a gentle rise in blood sugars.[4898] If you eat the same amount of wheat baked into bread form, however, you get a big spike in blood sugars. All the little bubbles in bread allow our bodies to break it down so fast that it can cause our bodies to overreact with an insulin spike so large it can drive down our blood sugars below fasting levels. This hypoglycemic dip two hours after breaking bread can then trigger hunger sensations. Experimentally, if you infuse someone with insulin so their blood sugars fall, you can cause their hunger to rise[4899] and, in particular, spike cravings for high-calorie foods.[4900] In short, lower-glycemic-index foods may help us feel fuller longer than equivalent higher-glycemic-index foods.[4901]

A dramatic illustration of this effect was demonstrated by researchers at Columbia University. Individuals were randomized into one of three breakfast conditions—oatmeal made from quick oats, the same number of calories of Frosted Flakes, or just plain water—and then the researchers measured how much the subjects ate for lunch three hours later. Unsurprisingly, those who had eaten the oatmeal felt significantly fuller and less hungry after a few hours and indeed went on to eat significantly less lunch. Overweight participants in the oatmeal group ate less than half as many calories at lunch, hundreds of fewer calories compared to the other groups. How did the cereal group fare? The breakfast cereal was so unsatiating that the Frosted Flakes group ate as much lunch as the breakfast-skipping water-only group.[4902] It's as if the cereal group hadn't eaten any breakfast at all.

Saving Scraps for Our Friendly Flora

White rice has a lower glycemic index than white potatoes, but only, evidently, because you end up swallowing larger particles. If you blend rice into a slurry, its glycemic index rises to match that of the potato.[4903] The same is not true, however, of beans. Blended lentils have the same low glycemic index as whole lentils.[4904] Even when cooked into a creamy dal, lentils have the same flattened blood sugar curve.[4905] Whole beans, puréed beans, and powdered beans (like you'd find in bean pastas) all have the same low-glycemic response.[4906] Legumes have thicker, fibrous cell walls that protect the inner starch from disruption during processing,[4907] such that the early metabolic response to blended beans is the same, but it may be a different story hours later.

Researchers in Australia randomized people to eat the same whole foods, but during one week, the seeds, grains, beans, and chickpeas they were given were in more or less intact form, and during a different week, the foods were ground up. So, for example, for breakfast, the intact-grain group got muesli, while the ground-grain group got the same muesli but blended into a porridge. In the intact group, beans were added to salads, whereas in the ground group, they were blended into hummus. Note that during both weeks, the subjects were eating the same, whole, unrefined foods but, in one of the weeks, the whole grains, beans, chickpeas, and seeds were just made into flour or blended up.[4908] So what happened?

The intact-grain diet doubled their stool size. They ate the same food and the same amount of food, yet ended up with twice the fecal bulk compared to the ground-grain diet.[4909] Remember, most of our stool is pure bacteria. No matter how well we chew, when we eat the way nature intended, the little bits and pieces left behind when we swallow transport a smorgasbord of starch and other prebiotic nutrients straight down to our good bacteria, who get fruitful and multiply. Short-chain fatty-acid production shoots up, and we can bask in all the benefits I detailed in the Microbiome-Friendly section.

Just as our bodies weren't designed to handle liquid calories, powdered grains also represent a novel challenge to our systems. In *How Not to Die*, I encouraged everyone to eat whole grains, but from an optimal weight-loss standpoint, that may be insufficient. Intact whole grains are superior to milled whole grains in the same way that whole grains are superior to refined grains. Whole-wheat bread is better than white bread because it has more fiber to feed our good bacteria. If we just ate refined grains, we would starve our microbial selves. But fiber is pretty much all whole-wheat flour has to offer our colonic colleagues. When whole grains are finely milled into flour, the rest of the nutrients are absorbed rapidly high up in the small intestine, leaving few leftovers. It still has the fiber, at least, so 100 percent whole-grain flour won't leave our good gut bacteria completely starving, but they'll certainly be left malnourished compared to if you had eaten an intact whole grain like brown rice, where you eat the entire kernels of grains instead of powder.

Structural Integrity

There's a big difference between how small we can get food particles when we chew and how small they can be ground in a mill. The chomping of our teeth and the churning of our stomachs reduce the size of anything we eat down to under about two millimeters, about one-sixteenth of an inch, before entering our intestines.[4910] That may sound small, but a two-millimeter particle of wheat would contain about 10,000 plant cells filled with starch, of which only approximately 3,800 would be ruptured open on their surface.[4911] That would still leave 62 percent of the starch in that grain particle locked inside indigestible plant walls. Our starch-eating enzymes can diffuse through those walls and get at some of the starch inside, but a bounty will still be left over for our microbiomes.[4912] In contrast, flour particles can be one hundred times smaller, even smaller than the size of the cells themselves, so nearly all may be ruptured open to spill their contents early, leaving our gut flora relatively high and dry.[4913]

The same goes for nuts and nut butters. Even a tiny two-millimeter nut particle has more than three hundred thousand oil-rich cells, less than 10 percent of which are exposed on the surface for early digestion.[4914] This leaves a residual horn of plenty, shown experimentally to boost the growth of our gut flora.[4915] In contrast, the specks found in ground nut butters average a thousand times smaller than the chewed particles of whole or chopped nuts, obliterating the cell walls and opening them for easy access.[4916] This explains why feeding people almonds can alter their microbiomes for the better, boosting the growth of bugs that produce short-chain fatty acids, but feeding people the same amount of almond butter appears to have no prebiotic influence.[4917]

Remember the amazing second-meal effect where people fed beans at dinner aren't as hungry at breakfast the next morning?[4918] When you eat nuts whole, not only do you feel fuller at the time compared to nut butter[4919] (presumably because of all that extra chewing and orosensory stimulation), but you may also feel fuller hours later throughout the day.[4920] If you feed people at dinner boiled rye berries, which are the intact rye kernels before they're milled into rye bread, they eat less at *lunch* the next day, more than twelve hours later.[4921] You do not, however, see that same second-meal effect on long-term satiety—or, in this case, a *third*-meal effect—with the same amount of milled rye porridge made from rye flour. The researchers suspect the appetite-suppressing benefits of eating structurally intact foods derive from the afterparty effects in our colons from the bountiful abundance.[4922]

The Matrix

To claim "whole grain" on a label, the food just has to contain more than 51 percent whole-grain ingredients.[4923] So a "whole grain" product could be nearly half white flour and straight sugar. This is why you see "whole grain" plastered across the likes of Froot Loops, Trix, Lucky Charms, and Cocoa Puffs. Even most "100 percent" whole-wheat flour these days starts out as white flour and then has some bran and germ added to approximate the proportions of the original grain.[4924] Stone-ground flour, which really is just crushed grains, can be 100 percent whole grain though the cellular structure is still obliterated.

Nearly a half century ago, the *dietary fiber hypothesis* was proposed, suggesting that fiber was the reason that diets centered around whole plant foods were so protective against chronic disease.[4925] Predictably, this gave rise to a multibillion-dollar fiber supplement market.[4926] (People could just eat real food, but where's the money in that?) The problem is it didn't work.[4927] Yes, fiber supplements can help with constipation, but all the other purported benefits didn't seem to materialize. Studies associating high fiber intake with lower risk of disease and death relate only to fiber from *food* intake rather than from fiber isolates or supplements.[4928] You can't just take your magic bullet of Metamucil with your Wonder Bread. That's not how fiber works.

Fiber is a smuggler.

Dietary fiber alone has certain benefits, but its primary role may be to encapsulate nutrients for special delivery to our gut microbiomes. If there's one recurring theme in this book, it's *wall off your calories*. Make sure as many of your calories as possible—your protein, your carbs, your fat—are encased in cell walls. Cell walls are made out of fiber, which acts as an indigestible physical barrier, so when you eat structurally intact plant foods, many of the calories remain trapped. Chew all you want—you're still going to end up with calories completely surrounded by fiber, which then blunts the glycemic response, activates the ileal brake, and delivers sustenance to your friendly flora. That's what nature intended to happen.

The primary *utility* of fiber may be more as a vehicle to transport cached calories and nutrients. Fiber is a ferry. Now you can see why apples, "contrary to expectations," were found to be more satiating than apple juice enriched with an identical amount of added fiber.[4929] You can't just sprinkle on the fiber. That's not how fiber works. Fiber is the carrier. Fiber is the matrix.

The word *matrix* comes from the Latin *matricis,* derived from *mater,* meaning *mother.*[4930] We should strive to preserve the matrix (the *blue* pill, Neo) by choosing not just whole grains but *intact* grains.

As one review title put it, "Food Structure Is Critical for Optimal Health."[4931] We can preserve this "botanical integrity" of grains by sticking to whole kernels.[4932] I was amused to see a paper in a journal published by the Royal Society of Chemistry entitled "The Anti-Obesity Effect of Starch in a Whole Grain-Like Structural Form."[4933] Researchers at the Institute of Biotechnology and a food science lab found they could reduce weight gain in obese mice by embedding starch microspheres "in a biopolymer-based artificial matrix to form a whole g[r]ain-like structure." If only Mother Nature had a ticker symbol on the stock exchange.

Broken Bread

Oil and sugar are examples of concentrated forms of "acellular" calories,[4934] which have been blamed as a contributor to the obesity crisis.[4935] Not only have the cells' walls that once held them been ruptured, they've been removed completely. White flour is not far behind, with most of its fiber stripped away. Though 100 percent whole-wheat flour may have all its original fiber, the cellular structure has been disintegrated such that while the fiber is there, it's not protectively wrapped around the starch. That's why the glycemic index of intact wheat kernels (wheatberries) or even cracked wheat (like bulgur found in tabbouleh) is down around 45, but whole-wheat bread is nearly as bad as white bread with both up about 70.[4936] There's fiber floating around in that whole wheat, but the starch is still out there flapping in the breeze. (The sciency way of saying that is milling disrupts the "physical encapsulation of intracellular nutrients by cell walls of plant foods."[4937])

Researchers funded with dough from Big Bread assert that white bread's weight-control concerns are "one of the most common mistakes and myths about nutrition."[4938] But what does the conflict-of-interest-free science say? In that famous satiety index study where dozens of foods were tested, three slices of bread were found to be less satisfying than the same number of calories of all foods except croissants, cake, donuts, and candy bars. Even jelly beans appeared a bit more satiating.[4939] Whole-wheat bread does appear to be more filling than white,[4940] but do these results translate into changes in weight?

Ecological studies, such as country-by-country comparisons of per capita bread supply and obesity rates, show no clear link.[4941] They are considered a rather weak form of evidence, though, since data are analyzed at a population level, rather than an individual level. So while it's true that average bread consumption has been declining in some countries while obesity rates have been rising, that doesn't necessarily exonerate bread since we don't know if the particular individuals who are eating more or less bread are the ones losing or gaining more weight. You could do a cross-sectional study to see if, in a snapshot in time, those who ate more bread are thinner or fatter, but you'd never know which came first, like in the candy and diet soda studies where one's weight status may determine consumption, rather than the other way around.

Enter cohort studies, following individuals and their diets over time. Researchers in Spain found that over a period of four years, those who increased their white-bread consumption appeared to gain weight and abdominal fat, but no such effect was found for whole-grain bread.[4942] The challenge with cohort studies is confounding. Maybe people who cut down on white bread also made other dietary changes. Indeed, those who stopped eating so much bread also tended to stop eating so much meat and started eating more fruits and vegetables. So maybe the bread itself had nothing to do with it. Maybe it was skipping the bologna in the bologna sandwich.

Whole-grain consumers exhibit a variety of other healthy dietary behaviors as well,[4943] but statistical tools used to adjust for some of these other factors suggest white-bread consumption does indeed have negative health consequences.[4944] Consistent results were also found in two other cohort studies that looked into bread. White-bread consumption appeared to be associated with greater belly fat and a significantly higher risk of becoming overweight or obese, whereas no such relationship was found for whole-grain bread.[4945,4946]

Aside from just whole-grain over white, which breads are better than others? From a glycemic-index standpoint, breads made from sprouted grains[4947] or with added cracked wheat[4948] are preferable. If you simply just must eat white bread, freezing and defrosting it lowers the blood sugar response, as does toasting[4949] and the use of sourdough fermentation.[4950] If you make your own bread at home, you can shorten the final rising time (proofing) to make a denser loaf, which has been found to lower the glycemic index and improve satiety.

Perhaps one way to test the healthfulness of a loaf is to see if it hurts if you drop it on your foot.

I was disappointed to learn that frozen bagels, even though the dough seems denser and they have the freeze-defrost cycle going for them, appear to cause the same exaggerated blood sugar spike as Wonder Bread.[4951,4952]

Some breads don't just incorporate cracked grains but entire kernels. Bread with added wheatberries results in a lower glycemic index[4953] and improved satiety compared to straight whole-wheat bread,[4954] and pumpernickel bread, which often includes whole rye kernels, has comparably blunted blood sugar and insulin responses.[4955] I thought the glycemic index of wheatberries was low at 45.[4956] Rye berries are even lower at 34, perhaps due to their higher fiber content,[4957] which is down around legume territory. This may explain why those randomized to eat whole-grain rye products for six weeks lost significantly more weight than those given refined wheat, but those given whole-wheat products instead did not.[4958]

The Pasta Exception

There's no need to completely deflour your diet. Unlike bread, whose structure collapses into a slurry of starch that is rapidly absorbed,[4959] the compact structure of pasta caused by the high-pressure compression during production slows down digestion.[4960] The glycemic index of pasta is in the moderate range, at 55, compared to the glycemic index of even whole-wheat bread, which may exceed 70. Feed diabetics bread, and over the next five hours, their blood sugar curve is about 60 percent greater than had they had the same amount of carbohydrate in pasta form.[4961]

We used to think it might be the type of wheat that's used. Pasta is typically made from harder varieties like durum wheat, which gets milled into coarser particles called *semolina*.[4962] But if a batch of bread is made from the exact same flour used to make a batch of pasta, there's still a dramatic difference in how our bodies react metabolically.[4963] Another way to demonstrate that the structure is key is by testing "spaghetti porridge," a rather unappetizing-sounding concoction—blenderized spaghetti—dreamed up by researchers. Though the porridge may have spared research subjects some fork twirling, significantly higher blood sugar spikes were noted.

When you eat bread, the particles you swallow can be a thousand times smaller than when eating spaghetti. Bread tends to break down into particles under a millimeter, many of which are too microscopic to be seen by the naked eye. On the other hand, when subjects were instructed to chew some spaghetti, then spit it out instead of swallowing it, researchers found segments up to an inch long.[4964] Our bodies' starch-munching enzymes can start superficially eroding the surface of these pieces, but it takes longer for spaghetti to get fully digested.

Is some pasta better than others? Macaroni is digested much quicker than spaghetti for some reason. Maybe we chew the elbows into smaller pieces? Thick linguini tested a bit better than thin.[4965] Surprisingly, though, there was no glycemic difference between undercooked spaghetti boiled for five minutes and overcooked spaghetti boiled for fifteen.[4966]

Greater glycemic impact doesn't necessarily translate into reduced satiety, however. Remember how white potatoes took home the gold for the most satiating food on a calorie-for-calorie basis? Tested head-to-head, boiled and mashed potatoes beat out pasta for satiety, despite their bread-like glycemic index. Children consumed about 35 percent fewer calories at meals served with mashed potatoes than those served with pasta or rice.[4967]

Greater satiety also doesn't necessarily translate into reduced calorie consumption. People feel fuller eating whole-grain pasta compared to refined-grain pasta, but apparently not enough to affect subsequent meal intake hours later.[4968] Similarly, people fed pasta for breakfast don't appear to eat any less at lunch than after a bready breakfast,[4969] so do the short-term metabolic effects make any long-term difference?

Eating higher-glycemic-index diets is associated with a small to medium increase in breast cancer and colorectal cancer.[4970] This is thought to be because regularly eating high-glycemic loads can cause a small increase in the blood of levels of IGF-1, the cancer-promoting growth hormone related to animal protein consumption I discussed in *How Not to Die*.[4971] Researchers zeroed in on bread versus pasta intake. Two case-control studies comparing the past diets of cancer cases to the diets of matched cancer-free controls found that bread consumption was more strongly associated with cancer of the breast and colon than was the consumption of pasta.[4972] Pasta consumption is associated with other healthy habits, though, like greater tomato consumption. The studies were performed in Italy, so presumably they weren't eating Day-Glo mac 'n cheese out of a box.

These confounding factors also make it difficult to tease out the effects of pasta on body fat. Pasta consumers do tend to be slimmer,[4973] but that could be due to related diet and lifestyle factors or possibly a chicken-or-the-egg phenomenon arising from overweight individuals disproportionately cutting down. You don't really know until you put it to the test.

Recently, two systematic reviews were published that compiled all the randomized controlled trials ever done on pasta and body weight.[4974,4975] Neither found a single such trial. There aren't any randomized trials assessing the effects of pasta intake on any health parameter. All they could find were trials that tested pasta in the context of broader dietary patterns. There are dozens of studies randomizing people to low-glycemic-index diets that often include switching people from breads to pastas as a component. That swap is an easy way to change the glycemic index without changing the nutrient composition as much, so researchers can better isolate the glycemic effects. Though the switch to more pasta was just part of a constellation of dietary changes, when all those studies were put together, they did show significantly more weight loss compared to those randomized to higher-glycemic diets.

FOOD FOR THOUGHT

If you could only make one dietary change, getting rid of sugary beverages would be a good choice and one that is consistent with my advice to wall off your calories. That means eliminating soda sweetened with sugar or corn syrup, as well as other sugary drinks, both carbonated and uncarbonated, such as sports and energy drinks.

As I mentioned in the Fat Blockers section, I defined my Green Light category in How Not to Die as foods of plant origin to which nothing bad has been added and from which nothing good has been taken away. How is this different from my recommendation to wall off your calories, to ensure your protein, carbs, and fat are trapped within cell walls? After all, only plants have cell walls. (Animals are made up of cells with fluid membranes, requiring bones to hold them up, whereas plants have rigid cell walls made out of fiber.) So isn't walling off calories the same as saying choose whole plant foods? The difference becomes apparent with examples of formless foods like powdered whole grains. Imagine a whole-grain cream of wheat cereal with one ingredient: 100 percent whole wheat. Or almond butter with one ingredient: almonds. Green Light, right? Plant foods to which nothing bad has been added and from which nothing good has been taken away. But now we know something good *has* been taken away: the structure.

The reason I have always considered whole-grain pasta to be a Green Light food, but whole-grain bread, even if it's 100 percent whole grain, as a Yellow Light food, had nothing to do with the structure. It was all due to Green Light's "nothing bad added" caveat. Bread-makers add salt, making bread a leading contributor of sodium intake, second only to chicken for most American adults.[4976] If we all just reduced our salt intake by about a half teaspoon a day, we could potentially prevent between 86,000 and 165,000 strokes and heart attacks and save 44,000 to 92,000 lives in the United States every year.[4977]

Eating whole grains is good, but eating whole-grain *kernels* is better. Former Harvard nutrition chair Walter Willett has argued that the term *whole grain* should probably be reserved for only whole intact grain kernels.[4978] So eat the wholiest of grains: intact grains, also known as *groats*.

Take oats, for example. They're found out in the fields as oat groats and then have their inedible outer husks removed during processing.[4979] Groats can then be sliced into two to four pieces to make steel-cut (also known as *pinhead* or *Irish*) oats, coarsely ground into Scottish oatmeal, or steamed and flattened into "old-fashioned" rolled oats.[4980] Quick-cooking oats are just old-fashioned oats rolled even thinner, and instant oats are steamed longer and rolled even more thinly.[4981] Then, at the bottom of the list, the most processed would be powdered oats, which you might find in oat-based breakfast cereals. Instead of buying boxed breakfast cereals, make oatmeal out of whole, intact oats. *They're gr-r-oat!*

I like to start my mornings with what I call my *BROL bowl. BROL* stands for *barley, rye, oats, and lentils.* Most people are only familiar with pearled barley, which is partially refined by having some of its bran polished off. You can buy barley groats, sold as hulled or hull-less barley. If your budget allows, go for purple barley, which naturally contains some of the antioxidant pigments found in berries as a bonus. Rye groats are typically sold as rye berries. Oat groats are just oat groats, though I've also seen the terms *hull-less* and *hulled oats*. And since I know I should probably check off a morning legume box on my Daily Dozen, I add black lentils, which are the most antioxidant-packed,[4982] sold as *beluga* lentils due to their resemblance to expensive caviar.

I have them all premixed in an unimaginative 1:1:1:1 ratio and then, in an electric pressure cooker, just cook one scoop of dry BROL to two scoops of water. There's probably a quicker way to do it, but I simply press a default one-touch button for thirty minutes, and it comes out fine. Of course, that's just the base. It has a great texture but very little flavor. Depending on my mood, I go savory with greens and mushrooms or sweet with frozen dark red cherries, cocoa powder, dates, and walnuts, giving me more of a chocolate-covered-cherry sensation. I'll make sure to include a bunch of these recipes in my forthcoming cookbook.

With all the new data on the importance of food form, I'm starting to sour on flour, so I advise not living by bread alone. The new structure created by the pasta-making process can mediate these effects, though, so you don't have to say *basta* to pasta.

V. Dr. Greger's
Twenty-One Tweaks

Too Much Food, Not Enough Calories

In *How Not to Die,* I compiled the healthiest of the Green Light foods into my Daily Dozen checklist of foods I encourage people to try to fit into their daily routines. I made it into a free app, Dr. Greger's Daily Dozen, available for iPhone and Android, so anyone and everyone can try to check off all the boxes every day and track their progress over time.

As the feedback poured in from people giving the app a try, two themes of complaints arose. The first was that it was just too much food. There was no way they could eat all that food in one day. In response, I explained that the Daily Dozen was aspirational, something to shoot for, just a tool to inspire people to include some of the healthiest of healthy foods into their daily diets. The vast volume of food I prescribed was on purpose. I was hoping that by telling people to eat so much healthy stuff, it would naturally crowd out some of the less-healthy stuff. After checking off all twenty-four servings in the Daily Dozen, there's only so much room left for a pepperoni pizza.

Ironically, the second major complaint we got is that it doesn't have enough calories. I had to explain that the Daily Dozen just represented the minimum I encourage people to eat, not the maximum, and that, certainly, training athletes requiring thousands more calories would have to eat much more. This all got me thinking, though. Too much food but too few calories? Sounds like the perfect weight-loss diet!

The Daily Dozen is by definition all Green Light foods, all whole plant foods, so that right there bakes in all seventeen of the ideal weight-loss diet ingredients listed on page 269. What about the calorie count? A systematic review of successful weight-loss strategies concluded that given the metabolic slowing and increased appetite that accompanies weight loss, to achieve *significant* weight loss, calorie counts may need to drop as low as 1,200 calories a day for women and 1,500 calories a day for men.[4983] I set up a spreadsheet and tried a bunch of common foods in each of the categories, and what do you know: The Daily Dozen averages about 1,200 calories, with the higher-calorie food choices nailing 1,500 calories.

The Daily Dozen Diet

There are a number of tweaks necessary to optimize the Daily Dozen for weight loss. A typical breakfast of Green Light foods that would check off a few of the Daily Dozen boxes would be a big bowl of oatmeal sweetened with raisins. Based on what we learned in the Low in Calorie Density, High in Water-Rich Foods, Eating Rate, and Wall Off Your Calories sections, we could optimize that meal for weight loss by making the oatmeal from steel-cut or whole groats rather than rolled or instant, cooking it thick, and switching the dried fruit for fresh, for example, swapping in strawberries for the raisins. If we did want to use dried, as we learned in the Amping AMPK and Inflammation Quenchers sections, barberries or gojis might be a better choice.

Similarly, when choosing vegetables, we can steer toward above-ground veggies highest on the water scale. Bell peppers have that nicotine edge I described in Amping AMPK, and uncooked vegetables in general offer more orosensory stimulation. If you want to go underground, based on what we learned about glycemic load, sweet potatoes would be preferable to white. We certainly want to mix it up, though, to take advantage of our built-in striving for variety, and since vegetables represent the healthiest class of foods with the fewest calories, we should aim to eat them earlier in the meal.

In the Appetite Suppression section, we learned yet another reason to include ground flaxseeds in our daily diets. Nuts are a great complement to greens to boost the absorption of fat-soluble nutrients, but they ideally should be eaten raw and whole or coarsely chopped rather than blended into butters. Miss the taste of peanut butter? A sprinkle of any one of the myriad powdered peanut butters on the market can help satisfy that craving. This is not to say something like almond butter or tahini is unhealthy by any stretch, but for weight-loss acceleration, structurally intact nuts and seeds would be better.

My free Dr. Greger's Daily Dozen app has become so popular that I decided to completely revamp it with new features for this book, so I've incorporated all these tweaks to the Daily Dozen to optimize it for weight control. You just have to switch over to the weight-loss setting. Now, you can not only track your progress, graphing your momentum day to day and month to month to see how well you're nailing each of the Daily Dozen, but since so many seemed to really appreciate having a list of reminders to check off throughout the day, I decided to add an entirely new checklist to capture the weight-loss boosters I documented here in part IV. With this new, expanded version of the app, you can toggle over to weight-loss mode and make a game out of how many of the new fat-busting boosters you can squeeze in every day, along with your Daily Dozen checkboxes.

Boxes of Tricks

Some of the weight-loss boosters are automatically taken care of with the Daily Dozen. For example, fat-blocking thylakoids and calcium are covered with my recommendation to eat lots of low-oxalate greens. But for the others, I've developed my Twenty-One Tweaks, practical takeaways from the boosters collected into one simple list on the next page.

You may have noticed that not all the strategies I covered in part IV are included in the list. Some only apply to certain individuals. For example, asking people to get into the NEAT habit of using steppers, fidget bars, or bouncing their knees during prolonged sitting may only apply to those with desk jobs. Other accelerants may be too risky for general consumption. For example, while the 25:5 modified fasting shows promise, you probably shouldn't drop below a thousand calories a day for more than twenty-four hours without medical supervision.[4984] Finally, there are options that show theoretical promise but haven't been sufficiently vetted in clinical trials, such as pistachios for circadian synchronization or mixing peppermint oil into hand lotion to facilitate BAT activation.

So here's the list of strategies that made the cut—broadly applicable, relatively safe, and evidence-based. See how many of these easily actionable tweaks you can incorporate into your daily routine.

Dr. Greger's Twenty-One Tweaks

At Each Meal

☑☑☑ preload with water

☑☑☑ preload with "negative calorie" foods

☑☑☑ incorporate vinegar (2 tsp with each meal)

☑☑☑ enjoy undistracted meals

☑☑☑ follow the twenty-minute rule

Every Day

take your daily doses

  ☑ black cumin (¼ tsp)

  ☑ garlic powder (¼ tsp)

  ☑ ground ginger (1 tsp) or cayenne pepper (½ tsp)

  ☑ nutritional yeast (2 tsp)

  ☑☑ cumin (½ tsp with lunch and dinner)

  ☑☑☑ green tea (3 cups)

☑ stay hydrated

☑ deflour your diet

☑ front-load your calories

☑ time-restrict your eating

☑ optimize exercise timing

☑☑ weigh yourself twice a day

☑☑☑ complete your implementation intentions

Every Night

☑ fast after 7:00 p.m.

☑ get sufficient sleep

☑ experiment with mild trendelenburg

At Each Meal

Preload with Water

Time your metabolism-boosting two cups of cool or cold unflavored water before each meal to also take advantage of its preload benefits.

Preload with "Negative Calorie" Foods

As the first course, start each meal with an apple or a Green Light soup or salad containing fewer than one hundred calories per cup.

Incorporate Vinegar (2 tsp with each meal)

Never drink vinegar straight. Instead, flavor meals or dress a side salad with any of the sweet and savory vinegars out there. If you want to drink it, make sure to mix it in a glass of water and, afterward, be sure to rinse your mouth out with water to protect your tooth enamel.

Enjoy Undistracted Meals

Don't eat while watching TV or playing on your phone. Give yourself a check for each meal you're able to eat without distraction.

Follow the Twenty-Minute Rule

Whether through increasing viscosity or the number of chews, or decreasing bite size and eating rate, dozens of studies have demonstrated that no matter how we boost the amount of time food is in our mouths, it can result in lower caloric intake. So extend meal duration to at least twenty minutes to allow your natural satiety signals to take full effect. How? By choosing foods that take longer to eat and eating them in a way that prolongs the time they stay in your mouth. Think bulkier, harder, chewier foods in smaller, well-chewed bites.

Every Day

Take Your Daily Doses

Black Cumin (Nigella sativa) (¼ tsp)

As noted in the Appetite Suppression section, a systematic review and meta-analysis of randomized, controlled weight-loss trials found that about a quarter teaspoon of black cumin powder every day appears to reduce body mass index within a span of a couple of months. Note that black cumin is different from regular cumin, for which the dosing is different. (See below.)

Garlic Powder (¼ tsp)

Randomized, double-blind, placebo-controlled studies have found that as little as a daily quarter teaspoon of garlic powder can reduce body fat at a cost of perhaps two cents a day.

Ground Ginger (1 tsp) or Cayenne Pepper (½ tsp)

Randomized controlled trials have found that ¼ teaspoon to 1½ teaspoons a day of ground ginger significantly decreased body weight for just pennies a day. It can be as easy as stirring the ground spice into a cup of hot water. Note: Ginger may work better in the morning than evening. Chai tea is a tasty way to combine the green tea and ginger tweaks into a single beverage. Alternately, for BAT activation, you can add one raw jalapeño pepper or a half teaspoon of red pepper powder (or, presumably, crushed red pepper flakes) into your daily diet. To help beat the heat, you can very thinly slice or finely chop the jalapeño to reduce its bite to little prickles, or mix the red pepper into soup or the whole-food vegetable smoothie I featured in one of my cooking videos on NutritionFacts.org.[4985]

Nutritional Yeast (2 tsp)

Two teaspoons of baker's, brewer's, or nutritional yeast contains roughly the amount of beta 1,3/1,6 glucans found in randomized, double-blind, placebo-controlled clinical trials to facilitate weight loss.

Cumin (Cuminum cyminum) (½ tsp with lunch and dinner)

Overweight women randomized to add a half teaspoon of cumin to their lunches and dinners beat out the control group by four more pounds and an extra inch off their waists. There is also evidence to support the use of the spice saffron, but a pinch a day would cost a dollar, whereas a teaspoon of cumin costs less than ten cents.

Green Tea (3 cups)

Drink three cups a day *between* meals (waiting at least an hour after a meal so as to not interfere with iron absorption). *During* meals, drink water, black coffee, or hibiscus tea mixed 6:1 with lemon verbena, but never exceed three cups of fluid an hour (important given my water preloading advice).

Take advantage of the reinforcing effect of caffeine by drinking your green tea along with something healthy you wish you liked more, but don't consume large amounts of caffeine within six hours of bedtime. Taking your tea without sweetener is best, but if you typically sweeten your tea with honey or sugar, try yacon syrup instead.

Stay Hydrated

Check this box if your urine never appeared darker than a pale yellow all day. Note that if you're eating riboflavin-fortified foods (such as nutritional yeast), then base this instead on getting nine cups of unsweetened beverages a day for women (which would be taken care of by the green tea and water preloading recommendations) or thirteen cups a day for men. If you have heart or kidney issues, don't increase fluid intake at all without first talking with your physician. Remember, diet soda may be calorie-free, but it's not consequence-free, as we learned in the Low in Added Sugar section.

Deflour Your Diet

Check this box every day your whole grain servings are in the form of intact grains. The powdering of even 100 percent whole grains robs our microbiomes of the starch that would otherwise be ferried down to our colons encapsulated in unbroken cell walls.

Front-Load Your Calories

There are metabolic benefits to distributing more calories to earlier in the day, so make breakfast (ideally) or lunch your largest meal of the day in true king/prince/pauper style.

Time-Restrict Your Eating

Confine eating to a daily window of time of your choosing under twelve hours in length that you can stick to consistently, seven days a week. Given the circadian benefits of reducing evening food intake, the window should end before 7:00 p.m.

Optimize Exercise Timing

The Daily Dozen's recommendation for optimum exercise duration for longevity is ninety minutes of moderately intense activity a day, which is also the optimum exercise duration for weight loss. Anytime is good, and the more the better, but there may be an advantage to exercising in a fasted state, at least six hours after your last meal. Typically, this would mean before breakfast, but if you timed it right, you could exercise midday before a late lunch or, if lunch is eaten early enough, before dinner. This is the timing for nondiabetics.

Diabetics and prediabetics should instead start exercising thirty minutes after the start of a meal and ideally go for at least an hour to completely straddle the blood sugar peak. If you had to choose a single meal to exercise after, it would be dinner, due to the circadian rhythm of blood sugar control that wanes throughout the day. Ideally, though, breakfast would be the largest meal of the day, and you'd exercise after that—or, even better, after every meal.

Weigh Yourself Twice a Day

Regular self-weighing is considered crucial for long-term weight control, but there is insufficient evidence to support a specific frequency of weighing. My recommendation is based on the one study that found that twice daily—upon waking and right before bed—appeared superior to once a day (about six versus two pounds of weight loss over twelve weeks).

Complete Your Implementation Intentions

Every two months, create three new implementation intentions—
"if *X*, then *Y*" plans to perform a particular behavior in a specific
context—and check each one off as you complete them every day.

Every Night

Fast After 7:00 p.m.

Because of our circadian rhythms, food eaten at night is more
fattening than the exact same food eaten earlier in the day, so fast
every night for at least twelve hours starting before 7:00 p.m. The
fewer calories after sundown, the better.

Get Sufficient Sleep

Check this box if you got at least seven hours of sleep at your regular
bedtime.

Experiment with Mild Trendelenburg

Try spending at least four hours a night lying with your body tilted
head-down six degrees by elevating the posts at the foot of your bed
by eight inches (or by nine inches if you have a California king). Be
extremely careful when you get out of bed, as this causes orthostatic
intolerance in most people, even if you're young and healthy—
meaning if you get up too fast, you can feel dizzy, faint, or light-
headed and could fall and hurt yourself. So get up *slowly*. Drinking
two cups of cold water thirty minutes before rising may also help
prevent this potentially hazardous side effect.

IMPORTANT: Do not try this at home *at all* if you have any
heart or lung issues, acid reflux, or problems with your brain (like
head trauma) or eyes (even a family history of glaucoma disqualifies
you). Also do not try this until you ask your physician if they think
it's safe for you to sleep in mild Trendelenburg.

Tick All the Right Boxes

Between the twenty-four checkboxes in the Daily Dozen and the thirty-seven new checkboxes in the Tweaks, you may feel a bit overwhelmed, but it's easy to knock off a bunch at a time. For example, starting a meal with a tomato salad sprinkled with some black cumin, garlic powder, and balsamic vinegar hits five boxes right there, including the "Preload with 'Negative Calorie' Foods" tweak and the Daily Dozen box for "Other Vegetables." And if that was one of your implementation intentions, make that six! Ten percent of your boxes nailed with a single appetizer.

Of course, you don't have to hit all the booster boxes every day. You don't even have to hit any. A healthy diet, as encapsulated by the Daily Dozen, should be all you need to lose as much weight as you want, but the more of these extra tweaks you can hit, the more successful you may be. I'm working on an entire *How Not to Diet Cookbook* to try to fit as many of these combinations together into delicious recipes and hearty meal plans—but in the meanwhile, please feel free to download the free, updated Dr. Greger's Daily Dozen app on your Android or iPhone. Start experimenting with a few of the Twenty-One Tweaks and see which ones work for you. My goal is to provide you with the broadest palette of tools to choose from.

Remember, it's not what you eat today that matters, or tomorrow, or next week, but rather what you eat over the next months, years, and decades, so you have to find lifestyle changes that fit into your lifestyle.

VI. Conclusion

Joining *U.S. News & World Report*'s expert panel to rank the "Best Diets" has been an eye-opening experience. Each year, we're asked to score dozens of trending diets on a scale from one to five based on seven criteria—most of which, to my surprise, are weighted equally. For example, in ranking which diet is best, a diet that is given top marks for ease of compliance—a score of five for being "extremely easy" to follow, based on factors such as "taste appeal"—could rank just as a high (all other things being equal) as a diet that was ranked as "extremely effective" in reducing the risk of heart disease, the number-one killer of men and women. That's like ranking bulletproof vest materials and concluding Kevlar does stop bullets better but, from a comfort standpoint, flannel wins the day.

After all, the Standard American Diet is easy to comply with—so much so it's the *Standard American Diet*—but it's killing us, more so than any other factor, including cigarettes.[4986]

For me, the best diet is the one that saves your life.

To *U.S. News*'s credit, the "health risks" category is counted twice because, in its words, "no diet should be dangerous."[4987] But even with double counting, a diet rated as "extremely unsafe" but "extremely effective" (for short-term weight loss) and "extremely easy" (like popping laxatives) would rank just as high (all else being equal) as a diet that was only moderately easy and effective but safe. How could "extremely unsafe" not disqualify a diet right off the bat? (Yes, cyanide is poisonous, but let's not discount its fragrant almondy aroma.)

Nearly every year since the rankings started in 2011, Dr. Ornish's plant-based diet has been ranked number one for heart health but has yet to be ranked number one overall. Isn't the goal of a diet to achieve a long, healthy life? Once he proved back in 1990 that his diet could reverse our leading killer, it seems to me that the competition should have been over.

We should eat real food that grows out of the ground, natural foods that come from fields, not factories, and gardens, not garbage. The same diet that has been shown to prevent, treat, and reverse some of our leading killer diseases just so happens to be the one with the greatest potential for permanent weight loss. Inspired by my grandmother's story, I went on this deep dive into the medical literature searching for an answer to the obesity epidemic and came full circle. Not only did I succeed in finding a plain solution to the crisis, I discovered the same solution: a diet centered around whole plant foods.

This may not be what people want to hear. This may not be what you want to hear. This certainly isn't what the food industry wants to hear—or wants you to hear. But I believe everyone deserves at least access to this knowledge.

At the end of the day, it's your body, your choice. As a physician and researcher, all I can do is share with you what I can discern from the best available balance of evidence at present, and the rest is up to you.

When I was in training, I remember witnessing a doctor grab a pack of cigarettes out of a patient's shirt pocket and crumple it into the trash. I'm not here to grab anyone's cheeseburger, but I'm also not one to soft-pedal the message. It's true that a healthy diet is like exercise: It's by no means an all-or-nothing proposition, and every little bit helps. But I'm not going to shy away from sharing what the science says for fear it would be considered "impractical" or "unrealistic" (as the Sugar Association calls advice to reduce sugar intake).[4988] When deciding how many daily servings of fruits and vegetables to recommend, dietary guidelines are advised to set "ambitious" goals but not recommend so many as to be "regarded as threatening."[4989] (It doesn't help that ten of the fourteen members of the current U.S. Dietary Guidelines Advisory Committee apparently have financial conflicts of interest with meat, dairy, or processed food companies.[4990]) Rather than patronizing the public, I think they should just tell everyone the truth.

The healthiest commodities are the least profitable. It's that simple. This isn't some grand conspiracy to make us all fat. It's just how the system works. So it's up to us to reclaim our health destinies from companies that may not have the best interests of our families' health at heart.

Thankfully, the solution is simple. You don't need to follow any expensive plans, swallow any questionable pills, or undergo any surgical procedures. There are no magic-bullet infomercial gadgets "As Seen on TV." No meal replacements or meetings to attend. We don't have to compromise our health to lose weight, or our life spans. In fact, quite the opposite. The best diet for weight loss may just so happen to be the safest, cheapest way to eat for the longest, healthiest life.

References

To access all of the cited sources, each hyperlinked so you can read the original studies themselves, go to www.nutritionfacts.org/books/how-not-to-diet/citations or point your phone camera at the QR code below:

Scan for cited sources:

Or visit:

www.bit.ly/citedsources

Acknowledgments

To all the amazing NutritionFacts.org research volunteers who made this book possible: Adriana, Alexandra, Aliena, Allen, Allie, Amy, Andrew, Ann Marie, Annette, Anthony, Becky, Ben, Brenna, Brian, Cara, Carina, Carly, Carmen, Carolina, Chavy, Chetan, Chris, Christine, Clarissa, Cody, Courtney, Cristina, Damon, Darlene, Deanna, Deborah, Devra, Dorothy, Elijah, Eliot, Ellen, Emelyn, Emma, Erin, Frank, Giang, Greg, Hala, Hannah, Isabel, Ivy, Jack, Jakub, James, Jane, Janelle, Jared, Jason, Jeff, Jenna, Jennifer, Jeremy, Jerold, Jo, Julie, Kacie, Karen, Katie, Katy, Kevin, Kimberley, Krissy, Laura, Lisa, Lora, Lori, Lucie, Luis, Luke, Lynda, Margaret, Maria, Maricela, Mary, Matthew, Michele, Michelle, Mike, Natalie, Nick, Nika, Olga, Patricia, Patrick, Peter, Preethi, Renatta, Rob, Robert, Roberto, Sabrina, Sashwat, Shannon, Sharon, Shevonn, Shireen, Shirley, Silvia, Suzie, Tammy, Theo, Thuy, Todd, Toni, Tracy, Travis, Valeria, Veronica, Yashaar, and Yhonatan.

Index

About the Author

A founding member and fellow of the American College of Lifestyle Medicine, **Dr. Michael Greger** is a physician, *New York Times* bestselling author, and internationally recognized speaker on nutrition, food safety, and public health issues. He runs the popular website NutritionFacts.org, a nonprofit science-based public service site providing free daily updates on the latest in nutrition research. All the proceeds he receives from his books and speaking are donated to charity.

NutritionFacts.org